CHAPTER 1

Anatomy
Questions

DIRECTIONS (Questions 1 through 25): Each of the numbered items or incomplete statements in this section is followed by answers or by completions of the statement. Select the ONE lettered answer or completion that is BEST in each case.

1. The horizontal fissure and the inferior part of the oblique fissure form the boundaries of which of the following?

    (A) apex of the left lung
    (B) lingula of the left lung
    (C) middle lobe of the right lung
    (D) superior lobe of the right lung
    (E) inferior lobe of the left lung

2. All of the following structures are included in the female pudendum EXCEPT the

    (A) ovaries
    (B) mons pubis
    (C) clitoris
    (D) bulb of the vestibule
    (E) greater vestibular glands

3. The broad ligament encloses all of the following structures EXCEPT the

    (A) uterine tubes
    (B) ovarian ligaments
    (C) part of the round ligament
    (D) the uterine artery
    (E) the greater vestibular glands

4. The bulbourethral glands of the male are embedded in the fibers of which of the following muscles?

    (A) sphincter urethrae
    (B) ischiocavernosus
    (C) superficial transverse perineus
    (D) bulbospongiosus
    (E) corpora cavanosus

5. Which of the following structures are lined by ciliated, pseudostratified epithelium containing goblet cells and have cartilage plates, mucous glands, and smooth muscle?

    (A) alveolar ducts
    (B) terminal bronchioles
    (C) respiratory bronchioles
    (D) alveolar sacs
    (E) secondary bronchi

6. Which of the following statements correctly applies to the left bronchus?

    (A) It is shorter than the right bronchus.
    (B) It passes under the aortic arch.
    (C) It is the more direct continuation of the trachea.
    (D) It is usually larger in diameter than the right bronchus.
    (E) Foreign bodies are more apt to lodge in it.

7. Which of the following types of joints permit movements of flexion and extension only?

    (A) plane
    (B) ginglymus
    (C) trochoidal
    (D) condyloid
    (E) saddle

8. The digastric muscle is a two-bellied muscle that attaches by an intermediate tendon to which of the following structures?

    (A) the 6th cervical vertebra
    (B) the mandible
    (C) the mastoid process
    (D) the cricoid cartilage
    (E) the hyoid bone

9. The omohyoid, the sternocleidomastoid, and the posterior belly of the digastric muscles form the boundaries for which of the following triangles?

(A) the submandibular
(B) the mental
(C) the carotid
(D) the omoclavicular
(E) the muscular

10. Which of the following nerves characteristically ascends in the neck along the posterior border of the sternocleidomastoid muscle?

(A) the greater occipital
(B) the great auricular
(C) the lesser occipital
(D) the transverse cervical
(E) the medial supraclavicular

11. All of the following nerves are formed from ventral primary rami EXCEPT the

(A) greater occipital nerve
(B) greater auricular
(C) lateral supraclavicular
(D) lesser occipital
(E) transverse cervical

12. Which of the following veins cross perpendicularly the superficial surface of the sternocleidomastoid surface directly beneath the platysma muscle?

(A) the retromandibular
(B) the anterior jugular
(C) the posterior auricular
(D) the external jugular
(E) the internal jugular

13. Which of the following structures is located within the prevertebral layer of cervical fascia?

(A) the vagus nerve
(B) the common carotid artery
(C) the internal jugular vein
(D) the esophagus
(E) the middle scalene muscle

14. The fascia on the deep aspect of the scalene muscles, which spread over the cervical pleura, reinforcing it and giving it a superior support, is known as which of the following fasciae?

(A) buccopharyngeal
(B) Sibson's
(C) axillary
(D) pretracheal
(E) alar

15. The lateral pharyngeal space is traversed by which of the following muscles?

(A) the stylopharyngeus
(B) the stylohyoid
(C) the salpingopharyngeus
(D) the omohyoid
(E) the cricothyroideus

16. All of the following muscles are innervated by the cervical plexus EXCEPT the

(A) sternohyoid
(B) sternothyroid
(C) omohyoid
(D) thyrohyoid
(E) mylohyoid

17. The superior thyroid artery is usually the first branch of which of the following arteries?

(A) the thyrocervical
(B) the internal carotid
(C) the external carotid
(D) the facial
(E) the costocervical

18. The isthmus of the thyroid gland is located at which of the following structures?

(A) the cricoid cartilage
(B) tracheal rings two, three, and four
(C) the jugular notch
(D) the thyroid cartilage
(E) the sixth cervical vertebra

19. The superior thyroid veins drain into which of the following veins?

(A) the internal jugular
(B) the facial
(C) the thyrocervical
(D) the subclavian
(E) the brachiocephalic

20. The superior parathyroid glands are located at the level of which of the following structures?

(A) the carotid bifurcation
(B) the thyroid cartilage
(C) the hyoid bone
(D) the cricoid cartilage
(E) the jugular notch

21. Beginning below at the sternoclavicular joint and terminating above midway between the angle of the mandible and the mastoid process describes the course of which of the following?

(A) the thyroglossal duct

(B) the common carotid artery

(C) the pyramidal lobe

(D) the recurrent laryngeal nerve

(E) the sternocleidomastoid muscle

22. Which of the following nerves is connected to the carotid sinus?

(A) the eleventh cranial

(B) the glossopharyngeal

(C) the ansa cervicalis

(D) the fifth cranial

(E) the fourth cervical

23. The posterior auricular artery arises from the external carotid artery at the level of which of the following structures?

(A) the hyoid

(B) the carotid bifurcation

(C) the sternoclavicular articulation

(D) the upper border of the posterior belly of the digastric muscle

(E) the common tendon of the omohyoid muscle

24. All of the following structures drain into the internal jugular vein EXCEPT the

(A) lingual veins

(B) facial veins

(C) superior thyroid veins

(D) inferior petrosal sinus

(E) azygos vein

25. All of the following functional components are associated with the vagus nerve EXCEPT the

(A) general somatic afferent

(B) general somatic efferent

(C) general visceral efferent

(D) general visceral afferent

(E) special visceral afferent

DIRECTIONS (Questions 26 through 50): Each set of matching questions in this section consists of a list of up to twenty-six lettered options followed by several numbered items. For each item, select the ONE best lettered option that is most closely associated with it. Each lettered heading may be selected once, more than once, or not at all.

Questions 26 through 30

(A) the vagus nerve

(B) the glossopharyngeal nerve

(C) the facial nerve

(D) the trigeminal nerve

(E) the hypoglossal nerve

26. It provides motor innervation of the voluntary muscles of the larynx and pharynx.

27. It provides parasympathetic preganglionic fibers to involuntary muscles and glands of the heart, esophagus, stomach, trachea, bronchi, intestines, and other abdominal viscera.

28. It provides taste fibers from the posterior one-third of the tongue.

29. It provides parasympathetic fibers for the parotid gland after synapse in the otic gland.

30. It provides special visceral efferent fibers to the tensor veli palatini and the tensor tympani muscles.

Questions 31 through 35

(A) the superior ganglion of the vagus nerve

(B) the inferior ganglion of the vagus nerve

(C) the superior cervical ganglion

(D) the middle cervical ganglion

(E) the cervicothoracic ganglion

31. The cell bodies of this ganglion are concerned with the visceral afferent components of the nerve.

32. The cell bodies of this ganglion are concerned primarily with the general somatic afferent component of the nerve.

33. It commonly lies at the level of the cricoid cartilage in the bend of the inferior thyroid artery.

34. It supplies gray rami communicans to the sixth, seventh, and eighth cervical and first thoracic spinal nerves.

35. This ganglion is located in the jugular foramen.

Questions 36 through 40

(A) the chorda tympani nerve

(B) the lingual nerve

(C) the ansa cervicalis

(D) the lesser petrosal nerve

(E) the deep petrosal nerve

36. This provides the innervation for the infrahyoid muscles and the geniohyoid muscle.

37. This nerve leaves the petrous portion of the temporal bone through the petrotympanic fissure.

38. This nerve provides general sensation to the anterior two-thirds of the tongue.

39. This nerve ends in the otic ganglion.

40. This nerve is a branch of the internal carotid plexus.

Questions 41 through 50

Match each of the numbered entries below with the following structures.

(A) foramen cecum
(B) optic canal
(C) superior orbital fissure
(D) foramen rotundum
(E) foramen ovale
(F) foramen lacerum
(G) foramen spinosum
(H) internal acoustic meatus
(I) jugular foramen
(J) hypoglossal canal
(K) foramen magnum
(L) condyloid canal
(M) mastoid foramen
(N) cribriform plates

41. the vertebral arteries

42. the anterior and posterior spinal arteries

43. filaments of the olfactory nerves

44. the ophthalmic artery

45. the maxillary division of the trigeminal nerve

46. the facial nerve

47. the mandibular division of the trigeminal nerve

48. the middle meningeal artery

49. the trochlear nerve

50. the abducens nerve

DIRECTIONS (Questions 51 through 127): Each of the numbered items or incomplete statements in this section is followed by answers or by completions of the statement. Select the ONE lettered answer or completion that is BEST in each case.

51. The spinal portion of the accessory nerve arises from motor cells in which of the following areas?

(A) the dorsal root of the first cervical nerve

(B) the medulla
(C) the ventral gray column of the first cervical segment of the spinal cord
(D) the first four cervical segments of the spinal cord
(E) the superior ganglion of the vagus nerve

52. Which of the following nerves provides the innervation to the infrahyoid muscles?

(A) the vagus
(B) the brachial plexus
(C) the hypoglossal nerve
(D) the ansa cervicalis
(E) the 11th cranial nerve

53. Which of the following nerves makes its appearance at the lateral border of the anterior scalene muscle, descends vertically over the ventral surface of this diverging muscle, and enters the chest along its medial border?

(A) the superior cervical cardiac
(B) the phrenic
(C) the spinal accessory
(D) the vagus
(E) the ansa subclavia

54. Which of the following arteries lies between the anterior and middle scalene muscles?

(A) the second part of the subclavian
(B) the first part of the axillary
(C) the vertebral
(D) the dorsal scapular
(E) the internal thoracic

55. Which of the following arteries arise from the costocervical trunk?

(A) the inferior thyroid
(B) the dorsal scapular
(C) the internal thoracic
(D) the suprascapular
(E) the deep cervical

56. Which of the following arteries frequently pass either above or below the middle trunk of the brachial plexus?

(A) the costocervical
(B) the dorsal scapular
(C) the suprascapular
(D) the transverse cervical
(E) the highest intercostal

57. All of the following muscles are considered to be muscles of inspiration EXCEPT the

(A) middle scalene

(B) anterior scalene

(C) diaphragm

(D) intercostals

(E) sternocleidomastoid

58. All of the following statements apply to the larynx EXCEPT that

(A) the larynx lies in front of the 4th, 5th, and 6th cervical vertebrae

(B) the larynx lies between the carotid sheaths laterally

(C) there are nine laryngeal cartilages

(D) the cartilages of the larynx are united by true joints

(E) the cricothyroid membrane suspends the larynx from the hyoid bone

59. Which of the following laryngeal muscles abduct the vocal folds?

(A) the cricothyroid

(B) the posterior cricoarytenoid

(C) the thyroarytenoid

(D) the transverse arytenoid

(E) the oblique arytenoid

60. The inferior laryngeal nerve innervates all of the following muscles EXCEPT the

(A) cricothyroid

(B) lateral cricoarytenoid

(C) posterior cricoarytenoid

(D) transverse arytenoid

(E) thyroarytenoid

61. All of the following statements concerning the trachea are correct EXCEPT that

(A) it begins at the lower border of the cricoid cartilage

(B) it terminates at the sternal angle

(C) it begins at the level of the sixth cervical vertebra

(D) it terminates at the upper border of the fifth thoracic vertebra

(E) it is about 24 cm in length

62. All of the following statements concerning the pharynx are correct EXCEPT that

(A) it begins at the level of the thyroid cartilage

(B) it terminates at the level of the lower border of the cricoid cartilage

(C) it is somewhat funnel-shaped in form

(D) it is approximately 12 cm in length

(E) the pharyngeal wall is almost entirely posterior and lateral to its cavity

63. All of the muscles of the pharynx are innervated by the vagus EXCEPT the

(A) palatopharyngeus

(B) salpingopharyngeus

(C) superior constrictor

(D) stylopharyngeus

(E) inferior constrictor

64. Taste from the posterior one-third of the tongue is provided by which of the following nerves?

(A) the trigeminal

(B) the facial

(C) the vagus

(D) the hypoglossal

(E) the glossopharyngeal

65. The vocalis muscles are composed of internal fibers of which of the following muscles?

(A) the posterior cricoarytenoid

(B) the lateral cricoarytenoid

(C) the aryepiglottic

(D) the thyroarytenoid

(E) the thyroepiglottic

66. A laterally directed, slitlike space behind the salpingopharyngeal fold is known as which of the following?

(A) the laryngeal vestibule

(B) the pharyngeal recess

(C) the piriform recess

(D) the glottis

(E) the rima glottidis

67. All of the following statements concerning the hypoglossal nerve are correct EXCEPT that

(A) it passes below the hyoid bone

(B) it passes between the external carotid and jugular vessels

(C) it divides into terminal branches between the mylohyoid and genioglossus muscles

(D) it enters the submandibular triangle deep to the posterior belly of the digastric muscle

(E) it crosses the occipital artery

68. All of the following nerves are cutaneous branches of the ophthalmic division of the trigeminal nerve EXCEPT the

(A) supratrochlear
(B) infraorbital
(C) external nasal branches
(D) lacrimal
(E) supraorbital

69. Which of the following nerves is the principal cutaneous nerve of the cheek?

(A) the auriculotemporal
(B) the mental
(C) the buccal branch of the trigeminal
(D) the zygomaticofacial
(E) the zygomaticotemporal

70. All of the following muscles are muscles of facial expression EXCEPT the

(A) zygomaticus major
(B) orbicularis oculi
(C) levator anguli oris
(D) procerus
(E) masseter

71. All of the following muscles are innervated by the mandibular division of the trigeminal nerve EXCEPT the

(A) lateral pterygoid
(B) masseter
(C) buccinator
(D) anterior belly of the digastric
(E) temporalis

72. All of the following statements concerning the parotid duct are correct EXCEPT that

(A) it extends forward about 2 cm above the zygoma
(B) it crosses the masseter muscle and the buccal fat pad
(C) it penetrates the buccinator muscle
(D) it opens in the interior of the mouth opposite the second upper molar tooth
(E) it has a length of 4 to 6 cm

73. The facial nerve provides the parasympathetic innervation for all of the following glands EXCEPT the

(A) lacrimal
(B) submandibular
(C) parotid

(D) nasal
(E) palatine

74. The designation of sphenomeniscus is sometimes given to the uppermost portion of which of the following muscles?

(A) the lateral pterygoid
(B) the buccinator
(C) the masseter
(D) the levator labii superioris
(E) the temporalis

75. The lingula of the mandible provides an attachment for which of the following structures?

(A) the stylomandibular ligament
(B) the mylohyoid muscle
(C) the articular disk
(D) the sphenomandibular ligament
(E) the sphenomeniscus

76. All of the following structures are associated with branches of the trigeminal nerve EXCEPT the

(A) foramen ovale
(B) foramen rotundum
(C) superior orbital fissure
(D) infraorbital foramen
(E) stylomastoid foramen

77. Which of the following arteries commonly pass between the two roots of the auriculotemporal nerve?

(A) the inferior alveolar
(B) the middle meningeal
(C) the anterior tympanic
(D) the masseteric
(E) the sphenopalatine

78. Which of the following structures passes inferiorly to the superior transverse ligament of the scapula?

(A) the transverse cervical artery
(B) the suprascapular nerve
(C) the axillary nerve
(D) the subscapular artery
(E) the scapular circumflex artery

79. Which of the following nerves innervates the serratus anterior muscle?

(A) the dorsal scapular
(B) the suprascapular
(C) the subscapular

(D) the axillary

(E) the long thoracic

80. The long head of the biceps arises from which of the following structures?

(A) the coracoid process

(B) the radial tuberosity

(C) the supraglenoid tubercle

(D) the bicipital aponeurosis

(E) the head of the humerus

81. Which of the following bones is located on the distal row of carpal bones, starting on the radial side?

(A) the trapezoid

(B) the capitate

(C) the hamate

(D) the trapezium

(E) the scaphoid

82. Approximately 70% of carpal fractures involve which of the following bones?

(A) the scaphoid

(B) the pisiform

(C) the hamate

(D) the capitate

(E) the lunate

83. Lesions of which of the following nerves may produce a "wristdrop"?

(A) the axillary

(B) the musculocutaneous

(C) the radial

(D) the median

(E) the ulnar

84. Which of the following structures passes anteriorly to the flexor retinaculum?

(A) the palmaris longus tendon

(B) the tendons of the long flexors of the fingers

(C) the median nerve

(D) the radial nerve

(E) the tendon of the extensor pollicis longus

85. Abductors of the fingers from the midline of the middle finger includes which of the following muscles?

(A) the palmaris brevis

(B) the opponens digiti minimi

(C) the lumbricals

(D) the pronator quadratus

(E) the dorsal interossei

86. A "claw hand" is usually associated with injury to which of the following nerves?

(A) the median

(B) the radial

(C) the ulnar

(D) the axillary

(E) the musculocutaneous

87. The transverse foramina of the upper five or six cervical vertebrae transmit which of the following structures?

(A) the cervical plexus

(B) the vertebral artery

(C) the internal carotid artery

(D) the internal jugular vein

(E) the vagus nerve

88. Costal foveae or facets are characteristically associated with which of the following vertebrae?

(A) the atlas

(B) the axis

(C) the third lumbar

(D) the fifth thoracic

(E) the sacrum

89. Intervertebral disks may protrude or rupture in any direction, but are most common in which of the following directions?

(A) anterior

(B) posterior

(C) anterolateral

(D) posterolateral

(E) lateral

90. Which of the following is commonly associated with a lateral curvature of the vertebral column?

(A) kyphosis

(B) a ruptured disk

(C) scoliosis

(D) lordosis

(E) a "Gorilla" rib

91. Which of the following muscles is included in the sacrospinalis?

(A) the spinalis

(B) the rotators

(C) the multifidi

(D) the semispinalis

(E) the intertransversari

92. The vertebral artery penetrates which of the following structures?

(A) the anterior longitudinal ligament
(B) the ligamenta flava
(C) the transverse ligament of the atlas
(D) the posterior longitudinal ligament
(E) the posterior atlantooccipital membrane

93. Which of the following structures is located within epidural space?

(A) the anterior external venous plexus
(B) the anterior internal venous plexus
(C) the anterior spinal artery
(D) the posterior spinal arteries
(E) the middle cerebral artery

94. The caudal end of the spinal cord is anchored to the coccyx by which of the following structures?

(A) the denticulate ligament
(B) the filum terminale
(C) the cauda equina
(D) the conus medullaris
(E) the anterior longitudinal ligament

95. Which of the following structures crosses the posterior surfaces of the obturator internus and gemelli and the quadratus femoris?

(A) the femoral artery
(B) the common iliac veins
(C) the obturator nerve
(D) the sciatic nerve
(E) the superior gluteal nerve and artery

96. The femoral canal contains which of the following structures?

(A) the femoral artery
(B) the femoral vein
(C) the femoral branch of the genitofemoral nerve
(D) connective tissue and lymph nodes
(E) the great saphenous vein

97. Which of the following *do not* pass under the flexor retinaculum of the foot?

(A) the tendon of the peroneus longus
(B) the tendon of the tibialis posterior
(C) the tendon of the flexor digitorum longus
(D) the tibial nerve
(E) the tendon of the flexor hallucis longus

98. The jugular notch lies on one level with which of the following vertebrae?

(A) the fourth cervical
(B) the third thoracic
(C) the first lumbar
(D) the second cervical
(E) the sixth thoracic

99. The costal notch for the seventh rib articulates with which of the following structures?

(A) the jugular notch
(B) the sternal angle
(C) the xiphiosternal junction
(D) the xiphoid process
(E) the manubrium

100. The limbus fossae ovalis forms a prominent margin for which of the following structures?

(A) the sinus venarum cavarum
(B) the right atrioventricular ostium
(C) the pulmonary trunk
(D) the interventricular foramen
(E) the fossa ovalis

101. The outflow tract leading into the pulmonary trunk through the pulmonary orifice is known as which of the following?

(A) the crista terminalis
(B) the infundibulum
(C) the crista supraventricularis
(D) the limbus fossa ovalis
(E) the ostium of the coronary sinus

102. the largest branch of the right coronary artery is which of the following?

(A) the posterior interventricular
(B) the marginal
(C) the sinuatrial
(D) the atrioventricular node
(E) the conus arteriosus

103. Which of the following structures is located in the posterior interventricular sulcus?

(A) the oblique vein of the left atrium
(B) the great cardiac vein
(C) the coronary sinus
(D) the middle cardiac vein
(E) the small cardiac vein

104. In quiet breathing, and in the supine position, where is the apex beat of the heart located?

(A) left of the sternal angle at the level of the second rib

(B) in the left fifth intercostal space in the midclavicular line

(C) in the midaxillary line

(D) at the xiphisternal junction

(E) in the second intercostal space left of the sternum

105. Sounds generated by the mitral valve are best heard at which of the following structures?

(A) over the apex, in the left fifth intercostal space

(B) over the wall of the right ventricle

(C) along the ascending aorta, second left intercostal space

(D) along the left sternal border, second intercostal space

(E) along the right sternal border, fifth intercostal space

106. The foramen secundum is formed by the breakdown of an area in which of the following structures?

(A) the septum primum

(B) the septum secundum

(C) the pars muscularis

(D) the pars membranacea of the interventricular septum

(E) the endocardial cushions

107. The superior mediastinum is situated chiefly behind which of the following structures?

(A) the heart

(B) the xiphoid process

(C) the manubrium

(D) the arch of the aorta

(E) the pulmonary trunk

108. Which of the following structures is located within the middle mediastinum?

(A) the esophagus

(B) the aorta

(C) the thoracic duct

(D) the heart

(E) the trachea

109. The superior thyroid artery is usually the first branch of which of the following arteries?

(A) the thyrocervical

(B) the internal carotid

(C) the external carotid

(D) the facial

(E) the costocervical

110. Which of the following structures is located between the aorta and the azygos vein?

(A) the left phrenic nerve

(B) the esophagus

(C) the thoracic sympathetic trunk

(D) the left vagus nerve

(E) the thoracic duct

111. The median umbilical ligament is the remnant of which of the following structures?

(A) the umbilical arteries

(B) the urachus

(C) the umbilical vein

(D) the ductus arterosus

(E) the septum primum

112. The deep perineal space contains which of the following structures?

(A) the prostate

(B) the bladder

(C) the uterus

(D) the urethra

(E) the superficial perineal muscles

113. The fossa navicularis is located within which of the following structures?

(A) the glans penis

(B) the corpus spongiosum

(C) the bulb of the penis

(D) the urogenital diaphragm

(E) the prostatic urethra

114. Which of the following structures is not located in the vulva?

(A) the mons pubis

(B) the labia majora

(C) the labia minora

(D) the clitoris

(E) the superficial traverse perineus

115. The urethra does not traverse which of the following structures?

(A) the prostate

(B) the clitoris

(C) the urogenital diaphragm

(D) the corpus spongiosum

(E) the glans penis

116. Which of the following muscles does not attach to the central tendon of the perineum?

    (A) the bulbospongiosus
    (B) the superficial traverse perineus
    (C) the ischiocavernosus
    (D) the pubovaginalis
    (E) the deep transversus perinei

117. Which of the following structures enters the deep inguinal ring?

    (A) the round ligament of the uterus
    (B) the uterine tubes
    (C) the suspensory ligament of the ovary
    (D) the mesosalpinx
    (E) the mesovarium

118. Which of the following statements regarding the common bile duct is correct?

    (A) It lies to the left of the hepatic artery.
    (B) It descends anteriorly to the first part of the duodenum.
    (C) It crosses the uncinate process of the pancreas.
    (D) It joins the main pancreatic duct and they together pass into the second part of the duodenum.
    (E) It lies in front of the superior vena cava.

119. Which of the following statements applies to the right kidney?

    (A) The second portion of the duodenum lies anteriorly to its medial border.
    (B) Its superior extremity reaches the upper border of the 5th thoracic vertebra.
    (C) Its inferior extremity is closer to the median plane than its superior pole.
    (D) It is usually somewhat longer than the left kidney.
    (E) It is in contact laterally with the spleen.

120. Which of the following structures is associated with the small intestine?

    (A) teniae coli
    (B) mesentery
    (C) sacculations
    (D) epiploic appendages
    (E) haustra coli

121. Which of the following structures passes through the scapular notch?

    (A) suprascapular nerve
    (B) subscapular artery
    (C) long thoracic nerve
    (D) suprascapular artery
    (E) subscapular nerve

122. The beginning of the thoracic duct is known as the

    (A) intestinal lymph trunk
    (B) bronchomediastinal lymph trunk
    (C) jugular lymph trunk
    (D) subclavian lymph trunk
    (E) cisterna chyli

123. The root of the left lung is ventral to which of the following structures?

    (A) inferior vena cava
    (B) thoracic aorta
    (C) left phrenic nerve
    (D) pericardiacophrenic vessels
    (E) anterior pulmonary plexuses of nerves

124. Which of the following nerves innervates the gluteus maximus muscle?

    (A) pudendal
    (B) sciatic
    (C) femoral
    (D) inferior gluteal
    (E) obturator

125. The saphenous nerve is the terminal branch of which of the following nerves?

    (A) peroneal
    (B) tibial
    (C) femoral
    (D) obturator
    (E) pudendal

126. The term sphenomeniscus is sometimes given to which of the following structures?

    (A) piriformis muscle
    (B) sphenomandibular ligament
    (C) terminal end of the maxillary artery
    (D) pterygopalatine fossa
    (E) superior belly of the lateral pterygoid muscle

127. Which of the following structures is located in the wall of the left atrium?

    (A) terminal crest
    (B) opening of the coronary sinus
    (C) limbus fossae ovalis
    (D) septomarginal trabecula
    (E) valvula foraminis ovalis

Answers and Explanations

1. **(C)** The oblique fissure separates the superior lobe from the inferior lobe. A further subdivision of the superior lobe of the right lung is made by the horizontal fissure. The horizontal fissure and the inferior part of the oblique fissure form the boundaries of the middle lobe of the right lobe. *(Woodburne, p 392)*

2. **(A)** Both the urethral and vaginal openings come to the surface in the vestibule. Also included in the female pudendum are the mons pubis, the clitoris, an erectile mass known as the bulb of the vestibule, and the greater vestibular glands. The internal female genital organs include the ovaries, the uterine tubes, the uterus, and the vagina. *(Woodburne, pp 511,537)*

3. **(E)** The broad ligament encloses the uterine tube, the ovarian ligament, part of the round ligament, the uterine artery and venous plexus, the uterovaginal plexus of nerves, and part of the ureter. The greater vestibular glands are located in the pudendum. *(Woodburne, pp 538,540)*

4. **(A)** The bulbospongiosus muscle in the male overlies the bulb of the penis. The ischiocavernosus muscles cover the crura of the penis. The superficial transverse perineus muscles arise on either side from the anterior and medial portions of the ischial tuberosity. The pea-size bulbourethral glands of the male are embedded in the fibers of the sphincter urethrae muscle. *(Woodburne, pp 513–514)*

5. **(E)** The secondary bronchi are lined with ciliated, pseudostratified epithelium containing goblet cells and have cartilage plates, mucous glands, and smooth muscle. Bronchioles have ciliated columnar epithelium and goblet cells and lack cartilage in their walls. Terminal bronchioles are lined by ciliated cuboidal epithelium and are completely invested by smooth muscle. The respiratory bronchioles exhibit scattered alveoli and functional units. *(Woodburne, pp 394–396)*

6. **(B)** The right bronchus is shorter, straighter, and larger, and, since it is the more direct continuation of the trachea, foreign bodies are more apt to lodge in it. The bronchus is smaller in diameter but almost twice as long as the right bronchus. The left bronchus passes under the aortic arch. *(Woodburne, p 389)*

7. **(B)** The ginglymus or hinge joint permits movements of flexion and extension only. The plane joints provide simple gliding of sliding movements. The pivot joint or trochoidal permits movement around a single axis, but around a longitudinal axis through the bone. A condyloid articulation allows movement in the directions at right angles to one another. The saddle joint is a biaxial type. *(Woodburne, pp 47–48)*

8. **(E)** The digastric muscle is a two-bellied muscle that attaches by an intermediate tendon to the hyoid bone. With the border of the mandible for a base, the digastric muscle completes the definition of the submandibular triangle, the apex of which is directed inferiorly. *(Woodburne, p 179)*

9. **(C)** The omohyoid muscle passes downward and laterally from the hyoid bone to disappear behind the sternocleidomastoid muscle and thus subdivides this area of the anterior triangle into the carotid and muscular triangles. The carotid is bordered by the omohyoid, sternocleidomastoid, and the posterior belly of the digastric muscles. *(Woodburne, p 179)*

10. **(C)** The lesser occipital nerve ascends in the neck along the posterior border of the sternocleidomastoid muscle. The great auricular nerve crosses the sternocleidomastoid obliquely in a course toward the auricle. The transverse cervical nerve crosses the sternocleidomastoid muscle horizontally to reach the anterior triangle of the neck. The medial supraclavicular nerves cross the clavicular head of the sternocleidomastoid. The greater occipital nerve turns upward over the obliquus capitis inferior muscle. *(Woodburne, pp 181,183)*

11. (A) The greater occipital nerve is a dorsal rami of the second cervical nerve. The ventral rami of the first four cervical nerves form the cervical plexus. The cutaneous branches of the plexus are the lesser occipital, great auricular, transverse cervical, and supraclavicular nerves. *(Woodburne, pp 181,211)*

12. (D) The external jugular vein crosses perpendicularly the superficial surface of the sternocleidomastoid muscle directly under the platysma muscle. The anterior jugular descends near the median line. The posterior auricular joins the retromandibular to form the external jugular. The internal jugular runs in the carotid sheath deep to the sternocleidomastoid muscle. *(Woodburne, p 181)*

13. (E) The prevertebral fascia crosses the midline anterior to the prevertebral muscles continuing laterally to cover the scalene muscles. The esophagus is surrounded by the visceral fascia. The vagus nerve, internal jugular vein, and common carotid artery are surrounded by the carotid sheath. *(Woodburne, pp 185–187)*

14. (B) Scalene fascia spread over the cervical pleura, reinforcing it and giving it a superior support. The buccopharyngeal and pretracheal form the cervical visceral fasciae. The alar fascia forms a subdivision of the retropharyngeal space and extends from the skull to the level of the seventh cervical vertebra. The axillary sheath is an extension of the prevertebral fascia over the subclavian artery. *(Woodburne, pp 186–187)*

15. (A) The lateral pharyngeal space is a fat-filled area between the lateral aspect of the pharynx and pterygoid muscles. The space is traversed by the stylopharyngeus and styloglossus muscle. This area can be invaded by infections from the base of the tongue, the teeth, the tonsils, and the pharynx, and by its continuities with the retropharyngeal space, pass such material on as far as the posterior mediastinum. *(Woodburne, pp 187–188)*

16. (E) All of the infrahyoid muscles, sternohyoid, omohyoid, sternothyroid and thyrohyoid muscles are innervated by branches of the cervical plexus. The mylohyoid is innervated by the mandibular division of the trigeminal nerve. *(Woodburne, pp 189,258)*

17. (C) The superior thyroid artery is usually the first branch of the external carotid. The internal carotid gives off no major branches in the neck. The inferior thyroid is the largest branch of the thyrocervical trunk. The facial is a branch of the external carotid. The costocervical is a branch of the subclavian. *(Woodburne, pp 191,213)*

18. (B) The isthmus of the thyroid gland unites the two lateral lobes across trachea rings two, three, and four. Both the cricoid and thyroid cartilages are superior to the isthmus. The cricoid cartilage is located at the level of the 6th cervical vertebra. *(Woodburne, pp 190–191)*

19. (A) The superior thyroid veins cross the common carotid artery and empty into the internal jugular veins above the thyroid cartilage. The inferior thyroid veins drain into the brachiocephalic veins. Occasionally, they make a common entry into the jugular with the lingual and facial veins. The two inferior thyroid veins empty into the left and right brachiocephalic veins. The middle thyroid veins empty into the lower end of the internal jugular vein. *(Woodburne, p 192)*

20. (D) The superior parathyroid glands lie, normally, at the level of the lower border of the cricoid cartilage. The inferior parathyroid glands are located near the inferior pole of the thyroid gland. The carotids bifurcate at the level of the superior margin of the thyroid cartilage and thus lie superior to the superior parathyroid glands. *(Woodburne, pp 192–193)*

21. (B) The course of the carotid artery may be defined by a line beginning below at the sternoclavicular joint and terminating above midway between the angle of the mandible and the mastoid process of the temporal bone. This is the "carotid line." It represents the common carotid artery as high as the upper border of the thyroid cartilage. *(Woodburne, pp 193–194)*

22. (B) The carotid sinus region is important in blood pressure regulation. Its walls are especially elastic and contain modified end organs that respond to changes in blood pressure. The peripheral nerve connected with these end organs is the carotid branch of the glossopharyngeal nerve. *(Woodburne, p 194)*

23. (D) The posterior auricular artery rises from the posterior aspect of the external carotid at the level of the upper border of the posterior belly of the digastric muscle. It ascends through the carotid fossa to the notch between the external acoustic meatus and the mastoid process. Aside from muscular branches and a supply to the parotid gland, the posterior auricular artery provides stylomastoid, auricular, and occipital branches, which distribute largely in the scalp. *(Woodburne, p 195)*

24. (E) The azygos vein empties into the superior vena cava. The inferior petrosal sinus, lingual, facial, superior, and middle thyroid veins drain into the internal jugular veins. The azygos vein receives the drainage of the esophageal veins, the

mediastinal and pericardial veins, and the right bronchial vein. It frequently has some imperfect valves. (*Woodburne, pp 196,401*)

25. **(B)** The functions of the vagus nerve include special visceral efferent, general visceral efferent, general visceral afferent, special visceral afferent, and general somatic afferent but not general somatic efferent. (*Woodburne, pp 196–197*)

26. **(A)** The vagus nerve provides motor innervation to the voluntary muscles of the larynx, pharynx, and palate (except the tensor veli palatini), and of the upper two-thirds of the esophagus. The vagus nerve arises intracranially by the convergence of eight or ten rootlets, which emerge from the medulla oblongata in the groove dorsal to the infection olive. The vagus nerve leaves the skull through the jugular foramen. (*Woodburne, p 196*)

27. **(A)** The vagus nerve provides parasympathetic preganglionic fibers to involuntary muscles and glands of the heart, esophagus, stomach, trachea, bronchi, intestines, and other abdominal viscera. The vagus nerve descends through the neck in the carotid sheath, lying in a separate compartment formed in the sheath behind and between the artery and vein. The vagus nerve gives rise to meningeal and auricular branches while in the jugular fossa. (*Woodburne, p 196*)

28. **(B)** The glossopharyngeal nerve provides taste fibers to the posterior one-third of the tongue. As its name implies, the ninth cranial nerve is primarily related to the tongue and pharynx. It carries the same type of nerve fibers as does the vagus. The nerve passes through the jugular foramen to supply the tongue and pharynx. (*Woodburne, p 230*)

29. **(B)** The glossopharyngeal nerve provides parasympathetic innervation for the parotid gland after synapse in the otic ganglion. The postganglionic neurons arising in the ganglion distribute by way of the auriculotemporal branch of the trigeminal nerve to the parotid gland. The carotid sinus nerve arises from the glossopharyngeal nerve just beyond its emergence from the jugular foramen. (*Woodburne, pp 230–231*)

30. **(D)** The trigeminal nerve (mandibular division) provides motor fibers to the mylohyoid, anterior belly of the digastric, the tensor veli palatini, tensor tympani lateral and medial pterygoid, masseter, and temporalis. (*Woodburne, p 255*)

31. **(B)** The cell bodies of the inferior ganglion of the vagus are concerned with the visceral afferent components of the vagus. After the vagus exits from the jugular foramen, the nerve exhibits a fusiform swelling of approximately 1 inch length, which is the inferior ganglion (nodose ganglion); the ganglion communicates with the hypoglossal, the superior cervical sympathetic ganglion, and the loop between the first and second cervical nerves. (*Woodburne, p 197*)

32. **(A)** The cell bodies of the superior ganglion of the vagus are concerned primarily with the general somatic afferent (cutaneous) component of the nerve. The superior ganglion (jugular ganglion) forms a spherical swelling of about 4 mm diameter on the vagus nerve in the jugular foramen. In the region of the superior ganglion, a number of communications are made with other nerves; the cranial portion of the accessory nerve, the inferior ganglion of the glossopharyngeal, and the superior cervical sympathetic ganglion. (*Woodburne, p 197*)

33. **(D)** The middle cervical ganglion commonly lies at the level of the cricoid cartilage in the bend of the inferior thyroid artery or superior to the arch of the artery. The middle cervical ganglion is the smallest of the cervical ganglia and the most variable in form and position. It has an average length of 13.5 mm, but it may be double or absent. (*Woodburne, pp 203–204*)

34. **(E)** The cervicothoracic ganglion supplies gray rami communicans to the sixth, seventh, and eighth cervical and first thoracic spinal nerves. The cervicothoracic ganglion represents a combination of the inferior cervical and the first or the second thoracic ganglia. The inferior cervical portion of the cervicothoracic ganglion lies anteriorly to the base of the transverse process of the seventh cervical vertebra and is usually posteromedial to the origin of the vertebral artery. (*Woodburne, p 204*)

35. **(A)** The superior ganglion of the vagus is located in the jugular foramen. At the root of the neck, the right vagus passes anteriorly to the first part of the subclavian artery and behind the brachiocephalic vein and so enters the thorax. The left vagus descends between the left common carotid and the left subclavian arteries and, in the chest, passes to the left of the arch of the aorta. (*Woodburne, p 197*)

36. **(C)** The ansa cervicalis complex provides the innervation of the infrahyoid muscles and the geniohyoid muscle. From the loop between the first and second cervical nerves, a short nerve trunk joins the hypoglossal nerve just distal to its exit from the skull. Most of these fibers run in the hypoglossal nerve for only two or three centimeters and then leave it to descend in front of the internal

and common carotid arteries as the superior root of the ansa cervicalis. *(Woodburne, p 211)*

37. **(A)** The chorda tympani nerve leaves the petrous portion of the temporal bone through the petrotympanic fissure, crosses the medial surface of the spine of the sphenoid, and, high in the infratemporal fossa, joins the posterior aspect of the lingual nerve. *(Woodburne, p 207)*

38. **(B)** The lingual nerve is a branch of the mandibular division of the trigeminal and provides general sensation to the anterior two-thirds of the tongue. In its course to the tongue, it descends into the submandibular triangle, passes across the duct, and then, curving forward and upward into the tongue, spirals the underside of the duct and passes it again medially. *(Woodburne, p 207)*

39. **(D)** The lesser petrosal nerve ends in the otic ganglion. The continuation of the tympanic nerve beyond the tympanic plexus is the lesser petrosal nerve. The tympanic nerve supplies parasympathetic fibers, through the otic ganglion, to the parotid gland and sensory fibers to the mucous membrane of the middle ear. *(Woodburne, p 230)*

40. **(E)** The deep petrosal nerve is a branch of the internal carotid plexus, the continuation of the cervical sympathetic trunk in the cranium. The deep petrosal nerve consists of postganglionic sympathetic fibers that have their cells of origin in the superior cervical sympathetic ganglion and separate from the internal carotid plexus in the foramen lacerum. *(Woodburne, p 278)*

41. **(K)** The spinal cord, vertebral arteries, spinal roots of the cranial nerve XI, dural veins, and anterior and posterior spinal arteries pass through the foramen magnum. The foramen magnum, at the center of the base of the skull, is bordered anteriorly by the oval occipital condyles, which articulate with the superior facets on the lateral masses of the first cervical vertebra. *(Woodburne, pp 308,312)*

42. **(K)** The anterior and posterior spinal arteries traverse the foramen magnum. Through the foramen magnum pass the spinal cord and its meningeal coverings, the ascending rootlets of the accessory nerve, the vertebral arteries, the anterior and posterior spinal arteries, and the ligaments passing between the occipital bone and the axis. *(Woodburne, pp 308,312)*

43. **(N)** The filaments of the olfactory nerves pass through the cribriform plates. Behind the foramen cecum, the crista galli (Cock's Comb) of the ethmoid bone gives attachment to the falx cerebri. On either side of the crista galli, the perforated cribriform plate of the ethmoid provides passage for the olfactory nerve fibers to the olfactory bulb, which lies on the cribriform plate. *(Woodburne, pp 310,312)*

44. **(B)** Cranial nerve II and the ophthalmic artery pass through the optic canals. The central part of the middle cranial fossa contains anteriorly the chiasmatic groove, which leads at either side into the optic canal for the optic nerve and ophthalmic artery. Behind the chiasmatic groove the deep concavity of the sella turcica provides the hypophyseal fossa for the hypophysis. *(Woodburne, pp 311–312)*

45. **(D)** The maxillary division of cranial nerve V passes through the foramen rotundum. Behind the superior orbital fissure is the foramen rotundum, which leads to the pterygopalatine fossa and transmits the maxillary division of the trigeminal nerve. The foramen rotundum is located in the sphenoid bone. *(Woodburne, pp 311–312)*

46. **(H)** The facial nerve and cranial nerve VIII enter the internal acoustic meatus. Above the jugular foramen is the internal acoustic meatus for the facial and vestibulocochlear nerves and the labyrinthine artery. Behind and lateral to this is the aqueductus vestibuli transmitting the endolymphatic duct from the membranous labyrinth of the ear. *(Woodburne, p 312)*

47. **(E)** The mandibular division of the trigeminal nerve and accessory meningeal artery passes through the foramen ovale. The large, oval foramen ovale lies behind and lateral to the foramen rotundum. Through it pass the mandibular division of the trigeminal nerve and the accessory meningeal artery. *(Woodburne, pp 311–312)*

48. **(G)** The middle meningeal artery and vein and meningeal branch of the mandibular nerve pass through the foramen spinosum. The small foramen spinosum, behind and lateral to foramen ovale, transmits the middle meningeal artery and the meningeal branch of the mandibular nerve. *(Woodburne, pp 311–312)*

49. **(C)** The ophthalmic vein, ophthalmic division of the trigeminal nerve, cranial nerves III, IV, and VI, and sympathetic fibers pass through the superior orbital fissure. The lateral portions of the middle cranial fossa are deep and receive the temporal lobes of the brain, the bone being modeled in accordance with its gyri and sulci. Anteriorly, the superior orbital fissure provides communication with the orbit in the interval between the lesser and greater wings and the body of the sphenoid bone. *(Woodburne, pp 311–312)*

50. **(C)** The abducens, oculomotor, and trochlear nerves pass through the superior orbital fissure. The superior orbital fissure transmits many of the nerves entering the orbit together with the ophthalmic vein. *(Woodburne, pp 311–312)*

51. **(C)** The spinal portion of the accessory nerve arises from motor cells in the lateral part of the ventral gray column of the first segments of the cervical spinal cord. The rootlets of the nerve emerge on the side of the cord between the ventral and dorsal denticulate ligament and the dorsal rootlets of the cervical nerves. *(Woodburne, p 209)*

52. **(D)** The ansa cervicalis complex provides the innervation of the infrahyoid muscles and the geniohyoid muscle. The vagus supplies muscles of the larynx and pharynx. The hypoglossal nerve innervates the muscles of the tongue and the eleventh cranial nerve innervates the trapezius and sternocleidomastoid muscles. *(Woodburne, pp 196,209,211, 231)*

53. **(B)** The phrenic nerve is the sole motor nerve to the diaphragm. The nerve arises by a large root from the third, fourth, and fifth cervical nerves. It appears at the lateral border of the anterior scalene muscle, descends vertically over the ventral surface of the diverging muscles, and enters the chest along its medial border. The spinal accessory does not enter the chest. The superior cervical cardiac and vagus nerves descend in the carotid sheath. *(Woodburne, pp 147,204,209,302)*

54. **(A)** The second part of the subclavian artery represents the highest part of the arch of the vessel. It is short and lies between the anterior scalene muscle in front and the middle scalene muscle behind. The first part of the axillary begins at the outer margin of the first rib. The vertebral and internal thoracic arteries arise from the first part of the subclavian. The dorsal scapular arises from the third part of the subclavian artery. *(Woodburne, pp 213–214)*

55. **(E)** The costocervical trunk arises from the posterior aspect of the subclavian artery behind the anterior scalene muscle. It divides into the highest intercostal and the deep cervical arteries. The inferior thyroid, and suprascapular internal thoracic arteries arise from the first part of the subclavian artery. The dorsal scapular artery rises from the third part of the subclavian artery. *(Woodburne, pp 214–215)*

56. **(B)** The dorsal scapular artery is usually a branch of the second or third part of the subclavian artery. The dorsal scapular artery has an intimate relation to the brachial plexus, passing posteriorly through it, most frequently either above or below the middle trunk. The highest intercostal is a branch of the costocervical, which arises from the second part of the subclavian artery. Both the transverse cervical and suprascapular arise from the thyrocervical trunk. *(Woodburne, pp 214–215)*

57. **(E)** The diaphragm is the principal muscle of inspiration. When the scalene muscles act together from above, they elevate the first and second ribs; they are muscles of inspiration. The sternocleidomastoid muscles, acting together, project the head forward and the chin upward. *(Woodburne, pp 209,218,489)*

58. **(E)** The thyrohyoid membrane suspends the larynx from the hyoid bone. The cartilages of the larynx are united by true joints. The larynx lies in front of the fourth, fifth, and sixth cervical vertebrae. The larynx lies between the carotid sheaths laterally and there are nine laryngeal cartilages. *(Woodburne, pp 218–219)*

59. **(B)** The vocal folds are abducted and the rima glottidis is widened by the posterior cricoarytenoid muscle. Adduction of the fold is followed by contraction of the lateral cricoarytenoid and the transverse arytenoid muscles. The thyroarytenoid muscles may contract for complete glottic closure. Tension of the vocal ligaments is increased by the action of the cricothyroid muscles. *(Woodburne, p 223)*

60. **(A)** The long slender external branch of the superior laryngeal nerve descends along the oblique line of the thyroid cartilage to the cricothyroid muscle, which it supplies. All of the other intrinsic muscles of the larynx are innervated by the inferior laryngeal nerve. *(Woodburne, p 224)*

61. **(E)** The trachea is about 12 cm long, of which 6 cm is above the upper border of the manubrium sterni and about 6 cm is in the chest. The corrugated cylindrical trachea has a maximum diameter of about 2 cm. The trachea begins at the lower border of the cricoid cartilage at the level of the sixth cervical vertebra and terminates at the sternal angle at the upper border of the fifth thoracic vertebra. *(Woodburne, p 225)*

62. **(A)** The pharynx is approximately 12 cm long. It begins at the base of the skull and terminates below at the level of the lower border of the cricoid cartilage. The pharyngeal wall is almost entirely posterior and lateral to its cavity. The pharynx is somewhat funnel-shaped in form. Its greatest breadth is about 5 cm at its attachment to the base of the skull, and it tapers below to the 1.5 cm width of the upper esophagus. *(Woodburne, pp 225–226)*

63. **(D)** The nerve to the stylopharyngeus muscle arises from the glossopharyngeal nerve. The pharyngeal plexus innervates the muscles of the pharynx with the exception of the stylopharyngeus. The inferior pharyngeal constrictor muscle receives an additional supply from the external branch of the superior laryngeal nerve. *(Woodburne, p 229)*

64. **(E)** The glossopharyngeal nerves carries taste from the posterior one-third of the tongue. The lingual nerve proper, a branch of the mandibular division of the trigeminal nerve, is concerned with general sensation from the anterior two-thirds of the tongue and the mucous membrane of the floor of the mouth. The chorda tympani branch of the facial nerve conveys the special sense of taste from the anterior two-thirds of the tongue. The vagus carries tastes from the epiglottic region. The hypoglossal nerve is motor to the tongue. *(Woodburne, p 267)*

65. **(D)** The vocalis muscles are composed of those internal fibers of the thyroarytenoid muscles most closely related to the vocal ligament. Two muscular cones are described for each vocalis muscle. The broad bases of these muscular cones are represented in the attachments of their fibers into the vocal ligament, especially into its elastic tissue. *(Woodburne, p 223)*

66. **(B)** A laterally directed, slitlike recess behind the salpingopharyngeal fold is the pharyngeal recess. Lateral to the laryngeal opening and internal to the thyroid cartilage and thyrohyoid membrane is the deep depression of the piriform recess. The vocal folds and the space between them are designated as the glottis and are the part of the larynx most directly concerned in the production of sound. The rima glottis is the space between opposed vocal folds and arytenoid cartilages. *(Woodburne, p 221)*

67. **(A)** The hypoglossal nerve turns forward near the angle of the mandible, loops around the occipital artery, and passes between the external carotid and jugular vessels. It enters the submandibular triangle deep to the posterior belly of the digastric muscle. The nerve passes above the hyoid bone. It divides into terminal branches between the mylohyoid and genioglossus muscles. *(Woodburne, p 231)*

68. **(B)** The cutaneous branches of the ophthalmic division of the trigeminal nerve include the supraorbital, supratrochlear, lacrimal, infratrochlear, and external nasal branches. The cutaneous branches of the maxillary division of the trigeminal nerve includes the infraorbital, inferior palpebral, external nasal, zygomatiofacial, and the zygomaticotemporal. *(Woodburne, pp 233–234)*

69. **(C)** The buccal branch of the mandibular nerve is the principal cutaneous nerve of the cheek. The auriculotemporal nerve reaches the subcutaneous tissues from the infratemporal fossa at a point between the condyle of the mandible and the external acoustic meatus. The mental nerve supplies the skin of the chin and mucous membrane of the lower lip. The zygomaticofacial supplies the skin over the prominence of the cheek. The zygomaticotemporal nerve is cutaneous to the anterior temporal region. *(Woodburne, p 234)*

70. **(E)** The masseter is a muscle of mastication. The zygomaticus major, orbicularis oculi, levator anguli oris, and procerus are muscles of facial expression. The muscles of facial expression are subcutaneous voluntary muscles. In general, they arise from bones or fascia of the head and insert into the skin. *(Woodburne, pp 235–236,250)*

71. **(C)** The buccinator is a muscle of facial expression and is therefore innervated by the facial nerve. The lateral pterygoid, masseter, anterior belly of the digastric, and temporalis are all muscles of mastication and are therefore innervated by the mandibular division of the trigeminal nerve. *(Woodburne, pp 234,250–251)*

72. **(A)** The parotid duct has a length of 4 to 6 cm and extends forward about 1 cm below the zygoma. Crossing the masseter muscle and the buccal fat pad, the duct turns deeply at the anterior border of the buccal pad of fat and penetrates the buccinator muscle, opening in the interior of the mouth opposite the second upper molar tooth. *(Woodburne, p 251)*

73. **(C)** The facial nerve provides the parasympathetic innervation of the submandibular, sublingual, lacrimal, nasal, and palatine glands. The glossopharyngeal nerve provides parasympathetic innervation for the parotid gland. *(Woodburne, pp 230,243)*

74. **(A)** The designation of sphenomeniscus is sometimes given to the uppermost portion of the lateral pterygoid, reflecting its separate origin and special insertion. A smaller upper head arises from the infratemporal surface of the greater wing of the sphenoid. The two heads merge posteriorly but show a regional distinction at their insertion, the lower part ending in the pterygoid fovea of the neck of the mandible. The upper head of the muscle inserts into the articular disk of the temporomandibular joint and into the upper part of the neck of the condyle. *(Woodburne, p 252)*

75. **(D)** The sphenomandibular ligament descends from the spine of the sphenoid bone (or the petrotympanic fissure) to the lingula of the

mandible. The stylomandibular ligament extends from the styloid process to the posterior border of the ramus of the mandible. The mylohyoid muscle extends from the mylohyoid groove to the hyoid bone. The articular disk is located within the temporomandibular capsule. The sphenomeniscus are the uppermost fiber of the lateral pterygoid muscle. *(Woodburne, pp 205,252)*

76. **(E)** The ophthalmic division of the trigeminal nerve enters the orbit through the superior orbital fissure. The maxillary division of the trigeminal nerve leaves the cranial cavity through the foramen rotundum, travels through the infraorbital groove, canal, and foramen. The mandibular division leaves the skull via the foramen ovale and enters the mandibular foramen to exit the mandible at the mental foramen. The facial nerve exits the cranial cavity via the stylomastoid foramen. *(Woodburne, pp 243,257)*

77. **(B)** The middle meningeal artery is the principal artery of the cranial dura mater. It passes upward, superficial to the sphenomandibular ligament and between the two roots of the auriculotemporal nerve, and enters the middle cranial fossa via the foramen spinosum. *(Woodburne, p 259)*

78. **(B)** The suprascapular artery is joined by the suprascapular nerve in its course backward toward the scapular notch. It runs above the superior transverse scapular ligament, which separates it from the suprascapular nerve located below or inferior to the ligament. The transverse cervical artery passes more medially to reach the levator scapulae muscle. The subscapular artery arises from the lower part of the axillary artery and divides into the thoracodorsal and scapular circumflex arteries; the axillary nerve arises from the posterior cord and passes below the teres minor to supply the deltoid muscle. *(Hollinshead, pp 202–204)*

79. **(E)** The long thoracic nerve innervates the serratus anterior. The subscapular nerve innervates the subscapularis muscle. The dorsal scapular nerve innervates the rhomboids. The axillary nerve innervates the deltoid muscle. The suprascapular nerve innervates the supraspinatus and infraspinatus muscles. *(Hollinshead, p 202)*

80. **(C)** The long head of the biceps brachii arises from the supraglenoid tubercle of the scapula. It inserts into the radial tuberosity and the bicipital aponeurosis. The short head of the biceps brachii arises from the tip of the coracoid process. *(Hollinshead, p 209)*

81. **(D)** The distal row, starting on the radial side, is made up of the trapezium, trapezoid, capitate,

and hamate bones. The proximal row, beginning on the radial side, is made up of the scaphoid, lunate, triquetral, and pisiform bones. The proximal row of carpal bones articulate proximally with the radius and the articulate disk of the ulna to form the radiocarpal or wrist joint proper. The pisiform, the fourth bone in the proximal row, lies on the anterior surface of the triquetral and articulates with that bone only. *(Hollinshead, p 225)*

82. **(A)** Approximately 70% of carpal fractures involves the scaphoid only. A fracture through its narrow middle part may deprive the scaphoid of its blood supply, causing the proximal part of the scaphoid to undergo avascular necrosis. *(Hollinshead, p 228)*

83. **(E)** Lesions of the radial nerve in the lower part of the arm may paralyze all of the extensor muscles of the forearm, producing a "wristdrop" (flexion of the hand by gravity when the forearm is horizontal), as well as inability to extend the metacarpophalangeal joints at the digits. *(Hollinshead, p 245)*

84. **(A)** The palmaris longus tendon passes in front of the flexor retinaculum as do the ulnar nerve and vessels. The median nerve and tendons of the long flexors of the fingers and of the thumb pass behind it, in the carpal canal. *(Hollinshead, p 248)*

85. **(E)** The dorsal interossei are abductors of the fingers from the midline of the middle finger. The palmaris brevis tightens the skin of the hypothenar eminence. The opponens digiti minimi carries out the small amount of flexion and lateral rotation allowed by the fifth metacarpal. The pronator quadratus takes part in all movements of pronation. The lumbricals are primarily extensors of the interphalangeal joints; secondarily, they flex the metacarpophalangeal joints. *(Hollinshead, pp 263,267,271)*

86. **(A)** A "claw hand" is usually associated with injury to the ulnar nerve. Injuries to the radial nerve produce a "wristdrop." The median nerve injury interferes with pronation of the forearm and with flexion of the phalanges of digits two and three. The axillary injury involves the deltoid muscle and abduction of the upper limb. The musculocutaneous nerve injury involves the flexors of the forearm and abductors of the arm. *(Hollinshead, pp 210,245,280)*

87. **(B)** The transverse foramina of about the upper five or six cervical vertebrae transmit the vertebral arteries and veins, the cervical plexus. The major structures in the carotid sheath are the internal jugular vein, the carotid vessels, and the

vagus nerve. The cervical spinal nerves leave the vertebral canal through the intervertebral foramina. (Hollinshead, pp 278,286,830)

88. (D) A distinguishing feature of the thoracic vertebrae is that they articulate with ribs and therefore bear costal foveae or facets. Both the atlas and axis are cervical vertebrae that are distinguished by transverse processes with transverse foramina. The sacral vertebrae are fused to form the sacrum, and lumbar vertebrae do not articulate with ribs and hence no costal foveae. (Hollinshead, pp 287–292)

89. (D) Intervertebral disks may protrude or rupture in any direction, but most common is a posterolateral direction, just lateral to the strong central portion of the posterior longitudinal ligament. This is usually the weakest part of the disk, since the annulus is thinner here and is not supported by other ligaments. (Hollinshead, p 297)

90. (C) Abnormal curvatures of the vertebral column are designated as kyphosis (hunchback), lordosis (swayback), and scoliosis (a lateral curvature). Since spinal nerves pass over the posterolateral part of the intervertebral disk, a protruded or ruptured disk frequently causes irritation of one or more nerves. When there is a rib on the first lumbar vertebra, that rib is called a lumbar or "Gorilla" rib. (Hollinshead, pp 286,297,301)

91. (A) The sacrospinalis is the largest muscular mass of the back. It includes the iliocostalis, the longissimus, and the spinalis. The transversospinalis muscles lie deep to the sacrospinalis and include the semispinalis, multifidi, and rotators. The segmental muscles include the interspinales and intertransversarii. (Hollinshead, pp 313,314,316)

92. (E) The vertebral artery ascends through the transverse foramina of the upper cervical vertebrae and, after passing through that of the atlas, turns medially and posteriorly in the vertebral sulcus and turns forward to penetrate the posterior atlantooccipital membrane. (Hollinshead, p 317)

93. (B) The spinal cord and its meninges do not fill the vertebral canal. The space between the walls of this canal and the outer menix of the cord, the dura mater, is the epidural space, which is filled with fat, connective tissue, and a plexus of veins. The venous plexuses in the epidural space are divided into anterior and posterior internal vertebral venous plexuses. The external venous plexuses, anterior to the vertebral bodies and posterior to the vertebral arches, are connected to the internal venous plexus. (Hollinshead, p 320)

94. (B) The terminal tapered part of the cord is the conus medullaris, and the tough thread continued from the conus is the filum terminale. The conus and filum terminale are surrounded by longitudinally directed roots of the more caudal spinal nerves called the cauda equina. The anterior longitudinal ligament is located on the anterior surface of the vertebral bodies. (Hollinshead, p 323)

95. (D) The sciatic nerve is the largest nerve in the body and emerges below the piriformis. It runs across the posterior surfaces of the obturatus internus and gemelli and the quadratus femoris. The femoral artery is formed below the inguinal ligament and the common iliac veins from within the pelvis. (Hollinshead, pp 368,386)

96. (D) Within the femoral sheath are three compartments. The lateral compartment contains the femoral artery and the femoral branch of the genitofemoral nerve. The intermediate compartment contains the femoral vein and the medial compartment. The femoral canal contains only a slight amount of loose connective tissue and one or two lymphatic vessels and nodes. (Hollinshead, p 386)

97. (A) The flexor retinaculum of the foot runs between the medial malleolus and the calcaneus. It sends three septa to the tibia and thus contains four compartments that contain tendons of the tibialis posterior, flexor digitorum longus, flexor hallucis longus and the tibial nerve, and posterior tibial vessels. The peroneus longus and brevis pass beneath the superior and inferior peroneal retinacula. (Hollinshead, pp 416–417)

98. (B) The jugular notch lies on the level with the third thoracic vertebra. The manubriosternal joint is palpable as the sternal angle, a smooth ridge produced by the angulation of the bones and their slightly everted articular edges. The sternal angle is level with the second costal cartilage and with the lower border of the fourth thoracic vertebra. (Hollinshead, p 469)

99. (C) The costal notches for the third, fourth, fifth, and sixth ribs lie on the sides of the body of the sternum. The costal notches for the seventh rib, the lowest to articulate with the sternum, lies at the junction of the body and xiphoid process. On either side of the jugular notch, the manubrium receives the sternal end of the clavicles in a shallow concave facet, thus forming the sternoclavicular joints. (Hollinshead, p 469)

100. (E) The interatrial septum has a depression which is the fossa ovalis, and its prominent margin is the limbus fossae ovalis. The cavity posterior to the crista terminalis is the sinus venarum

cavarum, into which the two venae cavae open. The right atrioventricular ostium is guarded by the tricuspid valve. *(Hollinshead, p 527)*

101. **(B)** The funnel-shaped infundibulum, or conus arteriosus, leads into the pulmonary trunk through the pulmonary orifice. The crista supraventricularis divides the interior of the right ventricle into two portions, inflow and outflow tracts. The interior of the right atrium is partially divided into two main parts by the crista terminalis. The limbus fossae ovalis forms a prominent margin for the fossa ovalis. Medial to the opening of the inferior vena cava is the ostium of the coronary sinus. *(Hollinshead, pp 527–528)*

102. **(A)** The largest branch of the right coronary artery is the posterior interventricular branch, which runs forward in the posterior interventricular sulcus toward the apex and supplies the diaphragmatic surface of both ventricles and approximately the posterior one-third of the interventricular septum. Smaller named branches include the marginal, sinuatrial, atrioventricular nodes, and the conus arteriosus. *(Hollinshead, p 535)*

103. **(D)** The middle cardiac vein runs in the posterior interventricular sulcus, and the small cardiac vein runs in the coronary sulcus along the right coronary artery. The great cardiac vein lies in the anterior interventricular sulcus. The coronary sinus continues to the right in the coronary sulcus. The oblique vein is usually very small and empties into the coronary sinus. *(Hollinshead, pp 526–537)*

104. **(D)** The middle cardiac vein runs in the posterior interventricular sulcus, and the small cardiac vein runs in the coronary sulcus along the right coronary artery. The great cardiac vein lies in the anterior interventricular sulcus. The coronary sinus continues to the right, is usually very small, and empties into the coronary sinus. *(Hollinshead, pp 536–537)*

105. **(A)** Sounds generated by the mitral valve are best heard over the apex, and those of the tricuspid valve are best heard over the anterior wall of the right ventricle. Sounds of the aortic valve radiate along the ascending aorta to the 2nd costal cartilage at the sternal border on the right where the aorta is closest to the chest wall; the pulmonary artery is along the left sternal border in the second space, where the pulmonary trunk divides. *(Hollinshead, p 544)*

106. **(A)** The foramen secundum is formed by the breakdown of an area in the septum primum. The septum secondary gives rise to the limbus fossa

ovalis. The interventricular septum is derived from the endocardial cushions, a muscular portion, the pars muscularis, and a membranous portion, the pars membranacea. *(Hollinshead, pp 546–547)*

107. **(C)** The superior mediastinum is situated chiefly behind the manubrium sterni. The mediastinum is arbitrarily subdivided by a transverse plane that passes through the sternal angle and the lower border of the fourth thoracic vertebra. The superior mediastinum is above this plane and the inferior mediastinum is below this plane. *(Hollinshead, p 555)*

108. **(D)** The pericardial sac and its contents comprise the middle mediastinum. The posterior mediastinum is between the vertebral bodies and the pericardial sac. The heart is found in the middle mediastinum. The esophagus, vagi, descending aorta, azygos veins, and thoracic duct are located in the posterior mediastinum. *(Hollinshead, pp 522,566)*

109. **(C)** The superior thyroid artery is usually the first branch of the external carotid. The internal carotid gives off no major branches in the neck. The inferior thyroid is the largest branch of the thyrocervical trunk. The facial is a branch of the external carotid. The costocervical is a branch of the subclavian. *(Woodburne, pp 191,213)*

110. **(E)** In the posterior mediastinum, the thoracic duct ascends on the front of the vertebral bodies, running between the aorta and the azygos vein. In most of its course, the thoracic duct lies behind the esophagus and is anterior to the right intercostal arteries and to the transverse, terminal portions of the hemiazygos and accessory hemiazygos veins as these vessels cross the vertebrae. *(Hollinshead, p 572)*

111. **(B)** The median umbilical ligament, attached to the apex of the bladder, is the remnant of the embryonic urachus. The umbilical arteries, ductus arterosus, septum primum, and umbilical veins are all embryonic structures associated with fetal circulation. *(Hollinshead, pp 548,767)*

112. **(D)** The deep perineal space contains, in addition to the deep perineal muscles and the urethra and vagina, the bulbourethral glands in the male. The prostate, bladder, and uterus are superior to the deep perineal space. The superficial perineal muscles are inferior to the deep perineal space. *(Hollinshead, pp 797–798)*

113. **(A)** Within the glans, the urethra dilates to form the fossa navicularis. The posterior expanded end of the corpus spongiosum, the bulb of the penis, is tightly attached to the inferior fascia of the uro-genital diaphragm. The prostatic urethra is superior to the urogenital diaphragm. *(Hollinshead, p 801)*

114. (E) The female external genitalia are collectively referred to as the vulva. The vulva consists of the mons pubis, the labia majora and minora, the clitoris, and the bulb of the vestibule and the vestibule of the vagina, into which open the orifices of the vagina, the urethra, and the ducts of the paraurethral and vestibular glands. *(Hollinshead, p 803)*

115. (B) The clitoris is the homologue of the penis, but it consists of only two erectile bodies, the corpora cavernosa clitoridis, and it is not traversed by the urethra. The male urethra has a prostatic part, membranous portion, and a spongy part. It passes through the prostate, urogenital diaphragm, and the corpus spongiosum of the penis. *(Hollinshead, pp 769,804)*

116. (E) The muscles whose fibers are interlaced in the central tendon of the perineum include the pubovaginalis, pubococcygeus, both deep perineal muscles, the sphincter ani externus, the superficial perineal muscles, the bulbospongiosus, and the superficial traverse perinei. The ischiocavernosus muscles are attached to the ischiopubic ramus and insert into the corpus cavernosum. *(Hollinshead, pp 796,803)*

117. (A) The round ligament of the uterus runs retroperitoneally from the uterotubal junction to enter the deep inguinal ring. The mesovarium attaches to the ovary and is a reduplication of the posterior lamina of the broad ligament. The ligament of the ovary attaches to the uterus in the inferior angle of the uterotubal junction. The mesosalpinx is located between the uterine tube and the base of the mesovarium. *(Hollinshead, pp 777,783)*

118. (D) The common bile duct lies to the right of the hepatic artery and anteriorly to the portal vein. It descends behind the first portion of the duodenum and then crosses the posterior surface of the head of the pancreas. It lies in front of the inferior vena cava. The common bile duct and the main pancreatic duct meet one another and, together, pass obliquely through the posteromedial wall of the second part of the duodenum. *(Woodburne, p 462)*

119. (A) The second portion of the duodenum lies anteriorly to the medial border of the right kidney. The superior extremities reach the upper border of the body of the twelfth thoracic vertebra; their inferior extremities lie at the level of the third lumbar vertebra and farther from the median

plane than are the superior poles. The left kidney is somewhat longer than the right kidney. *(Woodburne, p 448)*

120. (B) Three surface features serve to distinguish isolated loops of the small or large intestine. The large intestine has teniae coli, sacculations or haustra coli, and epiploic appendages. The mesentery is the peritoneal reflection from the body wall to the small intestine. *(Woodburne, pp 472–473)*

121. (A) The suprascapular nerve passes through the scapular notch and is separated from the suprascapular artery by the superior traverse scapular ligament. The suprascapular nerve (C5, 6) from the superior trunk of the brachial plexus enters the supraspinatus fossa through the scapular notch. Passing under the superior transverse scapular ligament, it is deep to the muscle and supplies it from its underside. The suprascapular artery from the thyrocervical trunk of the subclavian artery passes over the ligament and distributes with the suprascapular nerve. *(Woodburne, pp 88–89)*

122. (E) The cisterna chyli, or the beginning of the thoracic duct, receives the right and left lumbar trunks. The cisterna lies on the bodies of the upper two lumbar vertebrae between the right crus of the diaphragm and the abdominal aorta and represents a dilated receptacle for the lymph gathered from the lower part of the body. *(Woodburne, p 493)*

123. (B) The root of the left lung is ventral to the thoracic aorta and inferior to its arch. Ventral to both roots are the phrenic nerves, the pericardiacophrenic vessels, and the anterior pulmonary plexuses of nerves. Dorsal to the roots lie the vagus nerves and the posterior pulmonary plexuses. The superior pulmonary veins are ventral, the bronchi are dorsal, and the pulmonary arteries are between them. *(Woodburne, p 346)*

124. (D) The inferior gluteal nerve, a postaxial branch of the sacral plexus with fibers from L5, S1, and S2, is the sole supply of the gluteus maximus. The pudendal nerve innervates muscles of the perineum. The femoral, sciatic, and obturator nerves innervate muscles of the lower limb. *(Woodburne, p 577)*

125. (C) The saphenous nerve is the terminal branch of the femoral nerve. Arising from the femoral nerve in the femoral triangle, it enters the abductor canal, where it crosses the femoral vessels anteriorly from their lateral to their medial side. Opposite the knee joint, the nerve becomes cutaneous, emerging between the tendons of the sartorius and gracilis muscles. It descends in the leg in company with the greater saphenous vein. *(Woodburne, p 570)*

126. **(E)** The designation of sphenomeniscus is sometimes given to the uppermost portion of the lateral pterygoid muscle, reflecting its separate origin and special insertion. The lateral pterygoid muscle lies deeply in the infratemporal fossa almost completely under cover of the temporalis. It is supplied by a branch of the mandibular division of the trigeminal nerve, which enters at the upper medial border of the upper head of the muscle. *(Woodburne, p 252)*

127. **(E)** The right atrium has a posteriorly situated, thin-walled sinus venarum and an anterior, more muscular portion. The terminal crest separates the two parts. The posterior, or interatrial, septal wall contains an oval, depressed, thinned-out area, the fossa ovalis. Its prominent oval margin is known as the limbus fossae ovalis. The coronary sinus opens into the right atrium. The valvula formainis ovalis is located on the interseptal wall of the left atrium. *(Woodburne, p 380)*

BIBLIOGRAPHY

Hollinshead, W. *Textbook of Anatomy*. 4th ed. Philadelphia: Harper & Row; 1985

Moore, KL. *Clinically Oriented Anatomy*. 3rd ed. Baltimore: Williams & Wilkins; 1992

NoBack CR, Strominger NL, Demarest RJ. *The Human Nervous System*. 4th ed. Philadelphia: Lea & Febiger; 1991

Sadler TW. *Langman's Medical Embryology*. 6th ed. Baltimore: Williams & Wilkins; 1990

Woodburne RT, Burckel WE. *Essentials of Human Anatomy*. 8th ed. New York: Oxford University Press; 1988

Subspecialty List: Anatomy

Question Number and Subspecialty

1. Respiratory system
2. Female genital system
3. Female genital system
4. Male genital system
5. Respiratory system
6. Respiratory system
7. Musculoskeletal system
8. Musculoskeletal system
9. Musculoskeletal system
10. Peripheral nervous system
11. Peripheral nervous system
12. Cardiovascular system
13. Musculoskeletal system
14. Musculoskeletal system
15. Musculoskeletal system
16. Peripheral nervous system
17. Cardiovascular system
18. Endocrine system
19. Cardiovascular system
20. Endocrine system
21. Cardiovascular system
22. Peripheral nervous system
23. Cardiovascular system
24. Cardiovascular system
25. Peripheral nervous system
26. Peripheral nervous system
27. Peripheral nervous system
28. Peripheral nervous system
29. Peripheral nervous system
30. Nervous system
31. Nervous system
32. Nervous system
33. Peripheral nervous system
34. Peripheral nervous system
35. Peripheral nervous system
36. Peripheral nervous system
37. Peripheral nervous system
38. Peripheral nervous system
39. Peripheral nervous system
40. Peripheral nervous system
41. Skeletal system
42. Skeletal system
43. Skeletal system
44. Skeletal system
45. Skeletal system
46. Skeletal system
47. Skeletal system
48. Skeletal system
49. Skeletal system
50. Skeletal system
51. Peripheral nervous system
52. Peripheral nervous system
53. Peripheral nervous system
54. Cardiovascular system
55. Cardiovascular system
56. Cardiovascular system
57. Muscular system
58. Respiratory system
59. Muscular system
60. Peripheral nervous system
61. Respiratory system
62. Digestive system
63. Peripheral nervous system
64. Peripheral nervous system
65. Muscular system
66. Digestive system
67. Peripheral nervous system
68. Peripheral nervous system
69. Peripheral nervous system
70. Muscular system
71. Peripheral nervous system
72. Digestive system
73. Peripheral nervous system
74. Muscular system
75. Skeletal system
76. Skeletal system
77. Cardiovascular system
78. Skeletal system
79. Peripheral nervous system
80. Muscular system
81. Skeletal system
82. Skeletal system
83. Peripheral nervous system
84. Skeletal system
85. Muscular system
86. Peripheral nervous system
87. Skeletal system
88. Skeletal system

89. Skeletal system
90. Skeletal system
91. Muscular system
92. Cardiovascular system
93. Skeletal system
94. Central nervous system
95. Peripheral nervous system
96. Peripheral nervous system
97. Muscular system
98. Skeletal system
99. Skeletal system
100. Cardiovascular system
101. Cardiovascular system
102. Cardiovascular system
103. Cardiovascular system
104. Cardiovascular system
105. Cardiovascular system
106. Cardiovascular system
107. Cardiovascular system
108. Cardiovascular system
109. Cardiovascular system
110. Lymphatic system
111. Embryology
112. Urogenital system
113. Male reproductive system
114. Female reproductive system
115. Urogenital system
116. Male reproductive system
117. Male reproductive system
118. Digestive system
119. Urogenital system
120. Digestive system
121. Skeletal system
122. Lymphatic system
123. Respiratory system
124. Peripheral nervous system
125. Peripheral nervous system
126. Musculoskeletal system
127. Cardiovascular system

CHAPTER 2

Physiology
Questions

DIRECTIONS (Questions 128 through 193): Each of the numbered items or incomplete statements in this section is followed by answers or by completions of the statement. Select the ONE lettered answer or completion that is BEST in each case.

128. The sodium concentration of cerebrospinal fluid (CSF) is approximately equal to that of plasma, whereas the potassium concentration of CSF is approximately 40 percent less than that found in plasma. The reason for this discrepancy is that

    (A) CSF is a serum filtrate that is modified by the resorptive activity of the choroid plexus
    (B) CSF is a serum filtrate, and potassium is not filtered as well as sodium
    (C) CSF is a serum filtrate that is modified by the secretory activity of the choroid plexus
    (D) CSF is a serum filtrate whose potassium concentration is depleted by the glial potassium sequestration
    (E) none of the above

129. Tremor that is caused by a cerebellar lesion is most readily differentiated from that caused by loss of the dopaminergic nigrostriatal tracts in that

    (A) it is present at rest
    (B) it is decreased during activity
    (C) it only occurs during voluntary movements
    (D) its frequency is very regular
    (E) its amplitude remains constant during voluntary movements

130. Although both vasopressin (ADH) and aldosterone significantly contribute to fluid and electrolyte balance, they do not appear to closely regulate blood volume in the long run. Blood volume is maintained at near normal levels in diabetes insipidus (absence of ADH) or Addison's disease (absence of aldosterone) because

    (A) the peripheral renin–angiotensin system is stimulated

    (B) salt and water intake are appropriately adjusted
    (C) plasma oncotic pressure increases
    (D) sympathetic reflexes decrease glomerular filtration
    (E) renal blood flow decreases

131. Under normal conditions, the major mechanism of body heat loss is

    (A) radiation
    (B) evaporation
    (C) perspiration
    (D) insensible perspiration
    (E) conduction

132. Choreiform movements in humans are most likely to be associated with degeneration of the

    (A) subthalamic nuclei
    (B) nigrostriatal tracts
    (C) cerebellum
    (D) lateral spinothalamic tracts
    (E) caudate nucleus

133. The stimulation of electrodes implanted in the medial forebrain bundle of experimental animals is most likely to lead to

    (A) repeated self-stimulation
    (B) rage reactions
    (C) avoidance reactions
    (D) temporary paralysis
    (E) repeated turning movements

134. Many neurons in the basal ganglia are observed to begin to discharge

(A) in association with somatosensory stimulation

(B) at the onset of acoustic stimulation

(C) before the onset of slow movements

(D) at a low rate that is independent of motor activity

(E) during visual accommodation

135. The introduction of cold water into one ear may cause giddiness and nausea. The primary cause of this effect of temperature is

(A) temporary immobilization of otoliths

(B) decreased movement of ampullar cristae

(C) increased discharge rate in vestibular afferents

(D) decreased discharge rate in vestibular afferents

(E) convection currents in endolymph

136. Reflex sneezing is most likely to be initiated by

(A) inhibition of olfactory receptor neurons

(B) stimulation of olfactory receptor neurons

(C) stimulation of nasal trigeminal nerve endings

(D) stimulation of gustatory receptors

(E) stimulation of efferent fibers from olfactory striae

137. Which of the following physiologic responses occurs as the pitch of a sound is increased?

(A) the frequency of action potentials in auditory nerve fibers increases

(B) units in the auditory nerve become responsive to a wider range of sound frequencies

(C) a greater number of hair cells become activated

(D) the location of maximal basilar membrane displacement moves toward the base of the cochlea

(E) the latency with which units in the auditory cortex are activated is decreased

138. Stimulation of retinal rod cells with light results in

(A) increased influx of Na^+ and hyperpolarization

(B) increased influx of Na^+ and depolarization

(C) decreased influx of Na^+ and hyperpolarization

(D) decreased influx of Na^+ and depolarization

(E) none of the above

139. The peptide substance P may play an important role in primary afferent fibers that conduct responses to noxious stimuli. Sectioning the dorsal roots close to the spinal cord leads to

(A) increased substance P levels in the substantia gelatinosa

(B) an increase in substance P in the dorsal root distal to the section

(C) an increase in substance P in the dorsal root proximal to the section

(D) a decrease in substance P in dorsal root ganglion cell somata

(E) an increase in substance P levels in ventral roots

140. The stimulation of nerve endings in the Golgi tendon organs leads directly to

(A) contraction of intrafusal muscle fibers

(B) contraction of extrafusal muscle fibers

(C) reflex inhibition of motor neurons

(D) increased γ-efferent discharge

(E) increased activity in group II afferent fibers

141. Which of the following types of receptors would normally show the greatest degree of adaptation?

(A) muscle spindles

(B) nociceptors

(C) touch receptors

(D) visceral chemoreceptors

(E) stretch receptors in the lungs

142. A motor neuron receives an excitatory stimulus at its dendritic terminus. In order for that stimulus to result in an action potential, there must be

(A) electrotonic spread of the resultant hyperpolarization to the axon hillock, where it induces the opening of voltage-gated sodium channels

(B) electrotonic spread of the resultant depolarization to the soma, where it induces the opening of voltage-gated sodium channels

(C) electrotonic spread of the resultant hyperpolarization to the soma, where it induces closing of voltage-gated sodium channels

(D) electrotonic spread of the resultant depolarization to the axon hillock, where it induces opening of voltage-gated sodium channels

(E) electrotonic spread of the resultant depolarization to the axon hillock, where it induces closing of voltage-gated sodium channels

143. Vagal nerve endings release acetylcholine. The expected effect of stimulating the vagus nerve would be to

(A) decrease the rate of rhythmicity of the sinoatrial (SA) node by inducing hyperpolarization

(B) increase conductivity at the atrioventricular (AV) junction by inducing depolarization

(C) depolarize cells of the SA node by opening potassium channels under the control of the muscarinic acetylcholine receptor

(D) increase the force of myocardial contractions

(E) decrease the rate of rhythmicity of the SA node by increasing the upward drift in membrane potential caused by sodium leakage

144. Which of the following types of movements occurs in the colon and not in the small intestine?

(A) segmental contractions

(B) mass action contractions

(C) 5 cm/sec peristaltic waves

(D) 20 cm/sec peristaltic waves

(E) peristaltic rushes

145. When the bile duct is blocked, jaundice develops. This jaundice is most likely to be associated with a rise in the plasma concentrations of

(A) glucuronic acid

(B) glucuronyl transferase

(C) free bilirubin

(D) bilirubin glucuronide

(E) urobilinogens

146. Glucagon is secreted by the alpha cells of the pancreatic islets. Which of the following is most likely to induce glucagon secretion?

(A) low serum concentrations of amino acids

(B) low serum concentrations of glucose

(C) high serum concentrations of glucose

(D) secretion of somatostatin by the delta cells

(E) sympathetic stimulation

147. Vitamin B_{12} is required for a number of metabolic processes. Which of the following lesions would not lead to a deficiency of this vitamin?

(A) chronic gastritis resulting in achlorhydria

(B) autoimmune destruction of gastric parietal cells

(C) surgical resection of the jejunum

(D) surgical resection of the ileum

(E) total gastrectomy

148. The major fate of triglycerides within cells of the intestinal mucosa is

(A) hydrolysis to 2-monoglycerides and free fatty acids

(B) incorporation into chylomicrons, followed by exocytosis

(C) incorporation into micelles in conjunction with bile salts

(D) passive diffusion into portal blood

(E) hydrolysis to glycerol and free fatty acids

149. When measuring skeletal muscle tension that develops during isometric contractions, it is observed that

(A) total tension is inversely proportional to the length of the fiber

(B) total tension increases monotonically with the length of the fiber

(C) active tension increases monotonically with the length of the fiber

(D) active tension first increases then decreases with the length of the fiber

(E) passive tension first increases then decreases with the length of the fiber

150. A neuronal soma has a resting membrane potential of –65 mV. Opening potassium channels in the neuronal membrane will most likely cause

(A) depolarization to about –30 mV

(B) hyperpolarization to about –86 mV

(C) initiation of an action potential

(D) no change in membrane potential

(E) depolarization to about +61 mV

151. Electrical synapses conduct electricity directly from one cell to the next. The subcellular structure that mediates this process is the

(A) tight junction

(B) desmosome

(C) zonula adherens

(D) adhesion plaque

(E) gap junction

152. Which of the following statements most accurately describes the response of a cell to a decrease in the conductance of the cell membrane to chloride ions?

   (A) the cell will hyperpolarize if its membrane potential is positive with respect to the equilibrium potential for chloride ions
   (B) the cell will depolarize if its membrane potential is positive with respect to the equilibrium potential for chloride ions
   (C) the cell will hyperpolarize if the external chloride concentration is greater than the internal chloride concentration
   (D) the cell will hyperpolarize if the external chloride concentration is less than the internal chloride concentration
   (E) no change in membrane potential will occur if the external and internal chloride ion concentrations are equal

153. The drug captopril prevents the action of angiotensin-converting enzyme (ACE). Its clinical usefulness, therefore, is

   (A) as an antihypertensive because it prevents renin secretion
   (B) as an antihypertensive because it prevents the action of renin on angiotensinogen
   (C) as an antihypertensive, since ACE converts the inactive angiotensin I to the active angiotensin II
   (D) as a pressor, since ACE converts the active angiotensin I to the inactive angiotensin II
   (E) as a pressor, since the action of ACE prevents angiotensin's stimulation of aldosterone secretion

154. Miniature end-plate potentials that can be recorded from a muscle fiber are believed to represent

   (A) the postsynaptic action of a single neurotransmitter molecule released from the presynaptic terminal
   (B) the opening of a single receptor-ion channel in the muscle membrane
   (C) the opening of multiple ion channels in the muscle membrane because of the spontaneous release of a small amount of transmitter
   (D) the spontaneous opening of ion channels in the muscle membrane in the absence of presynaptically released transmitter
   (E) the opening of multiple ion channels in the postsynaptic membrane in response to a single presynaptic action potential

155. A lesion that produces partial or total blindness but that spares the pupillary light response is most likely to be located in the

   (A) optic nerve
   (B) optic chiasm
   (C) optic tract
   (D) pretectal area
   (E) geniculocalcarine tract

156. All of the following might be expected to occur in an animal whose bile duct has been ligated EXCEPT

   (A) total inhibition of cholesterol absorption
   (B) total inhibition of monoglyceride absorption
   (C) decreased triglyceride hydrolysis
   (D) decreased free fatty acid absorption
   (E) none of the above

157. If an electrode that records the activity of neuronal units were placed in the spiral ganglion, it would be most likely to detect

   (A) afferent impulses from inner hair cells of the cochlea
   (B) afferent impulses from outer hair cells of the cochlea
   (C) afferent impulses from the utricle
   (D) afferent impulses from the semicircular canals
   (E) efferent impulses to inner hair cells of the cochlea

158. If a person suffered a stab injury and air entered the intrapleural space (pneumothorax), the most likely response would be for the

   (A) lung to expand outward and the chest wall to spring inward
   (B) lung to expand outward and the chest wall to spring outward
   (C) lung to collapse inward and the chest wall to collapse inward
   (D) lung to collapse inward and the chest wall to spring outward
   (E) lung volume to be unaffected and chest wall to spring outward

159. Normally, O_2 transfer is perfusion limited—that is, the amount of O_2 taken up is a function of pulmonary blood flow. All of the following may, however, favor diffusion limitation of transfer of O_2 from alveolus to pulmonary capillary blood EXCEPT

   (A) increased extravascular lung water
   (B) breathing hypoxic gas mixture
   (C) interstitial fibrosis

(D) increased ventilatory rate

(E) strenuous exercise

160. All of the following statements accurately describe the interaction of respiratory centers in the CNS and their effect on respiration EXCEPT that

(A) sectioning the brain stem above the pons, near the inferior colliculus of the midbrain, does not alter respiration in animals

(B) the apneustic and pneumotaxic centers of the pons are not necessary for maintenance of the basic rhythm of respiration

(C) transection above the apneustic center results in prolonged inspiration and very short expiration

(D) prolonged inspiration and very short expiration may be exacerbated by transection of the afferent fibers of the vagus and glossopharyngeal nerves

(E) the medullary rhythmicity center is a discrete group of neurons whose rhythmicity is abolished when the brain is transected above and below this area

161. There is very little protein in the glomerular filtrate. This is because

(A) all serum proteins are too large to fit throug the glomerular pores

(B) of the positive charges lining the pores, which repel serum proteins

(C) of the combination of pore size and negative charges lining the pores

(D) of active reabsorption of filtered protein by glomerular epithelial cells

(E) none of the above

162. The extra energy required for a burst of vigorous physical activity lasting between 10 and 20 sec comes from

(A) the breakdown of glycogen to lactic acid

(B) the breakdown of adenosine triphosphate (ATP) in muscle cells

(C) the breakdown of creatine phosphate

(D) oxidative reactions

(E) gluconeogenesis

163. All of the following are true statements regarding mechanisms of sweating EXCEPT that

(A) acclimatization to hot weather includes increased sweating with increased concentration of sodium chloride (NaCl)

(B) stimulation of the preoptic area of the anterior hypothalamus excites sweating

(C) atropine will decrease the rate of sweating by inhibition of postganglionic cholinergic fibers to sweat glands

(D) aldosterone decreases concentration of Na^+ in sweat by increasing reabsorption of Na+ in the sweat gland

(E) profuse sweating can seriously affect electrolyte balance

Questions 164 and 165

The figure below represents a pressure–volume loop of the left ventricle for a single cardiac cycle.

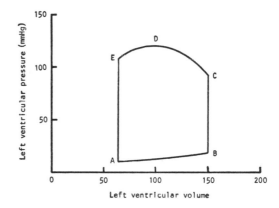

164. The point in the figure at which the aortic valve opens is

(A) point A

(B) point B

(C) point C

(D) point D

(E) point E

165. According to the figure above, if aortic pressure is maintained at constant level, a sudden transfusion of blood will result in

(A) a shift in B to the left

(B) a shift in B to the right

(C) a shift in C to the left

(D) a decrease in the area inscribed by $\overline{ABCDE}$

(E) a decrease in segment $\overline{CDE}$

166. A major difference between the heart muscle and skeletal muscle is that

    (A) only cardiac cells are made up of sarcomeres
    (B) the sliding filament hypothesis explains only skeletal muscle contraction
    (C) length–tension relationship in the heart does not depict an optimum length
    (D) graded contraction occurs only in the skeletal muscles
    (E) only skeletal muscle has both thick and thin filaments

167. The figure below represents the effect of drug A on mean systemic blood pressure (BP), both before and after the administration of drug B. These drugs are most likely

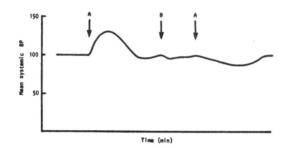

Time (min)

DRUG A	DRUG B
(A) acetylcholine	atropine
(B) histamine	diphenhydramine (H_1 blocker)
(C) epinephrine	propranolol (beta blocker)
(D) norepinephrine	propranolol (beta blocker)
(E) epinephrine	phenoxybenzamine (alpha blocker)

168. The pituitary hormone follicle-stimulating hormone (FSH) differs from ACTH in that FSH

    (A) is sensitive to proteolysis
    (B) is secreted by the intermediate lobe
    (C) is a single-peptide chain
    (D) is a glycoprotein
    (E) regulates the function of another endocrine gland

169. Insulin stimulates facilitated diffusion of glucose into cells of all of the following tissues EXCEPT

    (A) fat
    (B) lymphatic
    (C) muscle
    (D) brain
    (E) none of the above

170. Which of the following is a strong stimulus to the secretion of growth hormone?

    (A) insulin-like growth factor I
    (B) rapid-eye-movement (REM) sleep
    (C) nerve growth factor
    (D) glucagon
    (E) free fatty acids

171. All of the following statements concerning CO_2 transport are true EXCEPT that

    (A) compared to O_2, dissolved CO_2 plays a significant role in its transport
    (B) the bulk of CO_2 transport involves reversible combination of CO_2 with water in red blood cells (RBCs)
    (C) CO_2 is rapidly converted to bicarbonate ions in plasma
    (D) chloride ions diffuse into RBCs
    (E) CO_2 combines with terminal amine groups, and these carbamino compounds are important in CO_2 unloading

172. The cellular volume of human erythrocytes will decrease when

    (A) they are suspended in a medium whose osmotic strength is 300 mOsm and that has a sodium concentration of 140 mmol/L
    (B) the cells' sodium pump is inhibited with ouabain
    (C) they are suspended in a medium whose osmotic strength is 200 mOsm
    (D) they are suspended in a medium whose osmotic strength is 450 mOsm
    (E) they are suspended in a medium whose osmotic strength is 300 mOsm and that has a sodium concentration of 100 mmol/L

173. In chronic renal insufficiency (glomerulonephritis, pyelonephritis, renal vascular disease), there is a net functional loss of nephrons. If we assume that production of urea and creatinine is constant and that the patient is in a steady state, a 50 percent decrease in the normal glomerular filtration rate (GFR) will

    (A) not affect plasma creatinine
    (B) decrease plasma urea concentration
    (C) greatly increase plasma Na^+
    (D) increase the percent of filtered Na^+ excreted
    (E) significantly decrease plasma K^+

174. Before inspiration, alveolar pressure (PA) is atmospheric and intrapleural pressure (Ppl) is –5 cm H_2O. At the end of an inspiration in a healthy person, with the glottis open, these readings would be

(A) PA of +2, Ppl of −8 cm H_2O

(B) PA of −2, Ppl of −8 cm H_2O

(C) PA of 0, Ppl of +5 cm H_2O

(D) PA of 0, Ppl of −5 cm H_2O

(E) PA of 0, Ppl of −8 cm H_2O

175. If alveolar ventilation is halved (while breathing room air and if CO_2 production remains unchanged), then

(A) alveolar CO_2 pressure ($P_{A}CO_2$) will be halved

(B) arterial O_2 pressure (PaO_2) will double

(C) arterial CO_2 pressure ($PaCO_2$) will double

(D) alveolar O_2 pressure ($P_{A}O_2$) will double

(E) PaO_2 will not change

176. Bronchoalveolar segments of the lung with low ventilation/perfusion ratios may collapse when 100 percent O_2 is inhaled for 1 hr because

(A) pulmonary surfactant is inactivated

(B) O_2 toxicity causes alveolar edema

(C) CO_2 elimination is greater than normal

(D) interstitial edema around small airways causes airway closure

(E) gas is removed by blood faster than it enters the unit by ventilation

177. A patient has a plasma volume of 4 L, extracellular fluid (ECF) volume of 20 L, and intracellular volume of 30 L. If the patient is hyponatremic, to raise plasma Na^+ by 10 mmol/kg water would require administration of

(A) 40 mmol of NaCl

(B) 200 mmol of NaCl

(C) 300 mmol of NaCl

(D) 500 mmol of NaCl

(E) 1000 mmol of NaCl

178. A patient is admitted to the hospital with a respiratory acidosis. The patient's renal excretion of potassium would be expected to

(A) rise, since acid and potassium excretion are coupled

(B) rise, since acidosis is a stimulus to renin secretion by the juxtaglomerular apparatus

(C) rise, since acidosis increases the affinity of the aldosterone receptor for aldosterone

(D) fall, since the filtered load of potassium to the tubules falls in acidosis

(E) fall, since tubular secretion of potassium is inversely coupled to acid secretion

179. If the cabin of an airplane is pressurized to an equivalent altitude of 10,000 ft (barometric pressure of 523 mm Hg), the $P_{A}O_2$ in a healthy person compared with his or her predicted $P_{A}O_2$ at sea level will

(A) decrease to < 100 mm Hg because the fraction of inspired air that is O_2 (F_{IO_2}) will be < 0.21

(B) not change because $P_{A}CO_2$ will decrease because of hyperventilation

(C) not change because the cabin is pressurized

(D) decrease to < 100 mm Hg even though the F_{IO_2} is still around 0.2

(E) remain approximately the same because water vapor pressure is low at high altitude

180. In a normal person, PaO_2 is slightly less than $P_{A}O_2$ primarily because of

(A) shunted blood

(B) significant diffusion gradients

(C) reaction time of O_2 with hemoglobin

(D) unloading of CO_2

(E) none of the above

181. The slowest conduction rate is found in which of the following cardiac pathways?

(A) from the sinoatrial (SA) node to the atrioventricular (AV) node

(B) in the AV node

(C) in the bundle of His

(D) in the Purkinje fibers

(E) in the ventricular muscle

182. Radiolabeled inulin is most useful for the determination of which of the following body fluid volumes?

(A) plasma volume

(B) total blood volume

(C) interstitial fluid volume

(D) extracellular fluid (ECF) volume

(E) intracellular fluid volume

183. The anatomic dead space in an individual with a tidal volume of 500 ml is 125 ml when determined by plotting nitrogen concentration vs. expired volume after a single inspiration of 100 percent O_2 (Fowler's method). If the patient's lungs are healthy and the $PaCO_2$ is 40 mm Hg, the mixed expired CO_2 tension ($P_{E}CO_2$) should be about

(A) 0 mm Hg

(B) 10 mm Hg

(C) 20 mm Hg

(D) 30 mm Hg

(E) 40 mm Hg

184. A patient is given 100 percent O_2 to breathe, and arterial blood gases are determined. A Pao_2 of 125 mm Hg is associated with

(A) diffusion abnormality
(B) ventilation/perfusion inequality
(C) anatomic right-to-left shunting
(D) the normal response
(E) profound hypoventilation

185. All of the following statements concerning the regulation of respiration are true EXCEPT that

(A) the increase in pulmonary ventilation is linearly related to end-tidal $Paco_2$
(B) the main stimulus to increase ventilation comes from central chemoreceptors
(C) arterial hypoxemia potentiates the ventilatory drive to elevations in $Paco_2$
(D) central chemoreceptors respond to increases in local H^+ ion concentration or decreases in local Pao_2
(E) an increase in the work of breathing may be associated with a decreased ventilatory response to CO_2

186. In a normal kidney, with a low filtration coefficient, a large increase in glomerular filtration rate (GFR) may be expected to occur

(A) on afferent arteriolar constriction
(B) with strong sympathetic stimulation of the kidney
(C) after modest increases in renal blood flow
(D) with an increase in systemic arterial pressure
(E) on constriction of efferent arterioles

Questions 187 and 188

The figure below is a schematic diagram of renal clearance. In this diagram, Px is plasma concentration, Cx is plasma clearance, Ux is urine concentration, and $\dot{V}$ is urine flow.

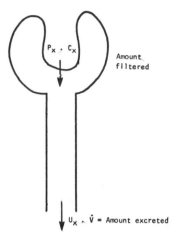

187. If Px = 20 mg/100 ml, $\dot{V}$ = 1 ml/min, Ux = 25 mg/ml, renal blood flow is 500 ml/min, and glomerular filtration fraction is 0.25, then substance x is

(A) glucose
(B) inulin
(C) p-aminohippurate (PAH)
(D) actively reabsorbed
(E) actively secreted

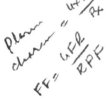

188. In the figure above, Px = 1 mg/100 ml, $\dot{V}$ = 1 ml/min, and Ux = 6 mg/ml. If these data were obtained from a healthy adult male under normal physiologic conditions, with a glomerular filtration rate (GFR) of 125 ml/min, then x is most likely to be

(A) inulin
(B) Na^+
(C) glucose
(D) p-aminohippurate (PAH)
(E) none of the above

189. Head injuries can lead to a syndrome in which the hormone vasopressin (ADH) is secreted at abnormally high levels. Patients manifesting the symptoms of the syndrome of inappropriate ADH secretion (SIADH) would be expected to have

(A) low serum sodium due to the dilutional effect of ADH-induced water retention in the collecting tubules
(B) low serum sodium due to a direct inhibitory effect of ADH on distal tubular sodium resorption
(C) no change in serum sodium, since the dilutional effect of ADH-induced water retention is balanced by a direct stimulatory effect of ADH on distal tubular sodium resorption

(D) high serum sodium due to the direct stimulatory effect of ADH on distal tubular sodium resorption

(E) high serum sodium due to the concentrating effect of ADH-induced water excretion in the collecting tubules

190. All of the following statements regarding physiologic adjustments to exercise are true EXCEPT that

(A) alveolar ventilation increases because of an increase in tidal volume and respiratory rate

(B) cardiac output increases with an increase in heart rate and stroke volume

(C) body temperature falls because of increased evaporative heat loss

(D) arteriolar vasodilation occurs in working muscle, with an accompanying vasoconstriction in skin and viscera

(E) the oxyhemoglobin dissociation curve shifts to the right, enhancing O_2 use

191. If O_2 consumption (measured by analysis of mixed expired gas) is 300 ml/min, arterial O_2 content is 20 ml/100 ml blood, pulmonary arterial O_2 content is 15 ml/100 ml blood, and heart rate is 60/min, what is the stroke volume?

(A) 1 ml

(B) 10 ml

(C) 60 ml

(D) 100 ml

(E) 200 ml

192. All of the following statements about the fetal circulation are true EXCEPT that

(A) a significant portion of inferior vena cava flow is shunted through the foramen ovale to the left

(B) the major portion of right ventricular output passes through the ductus arteriosus to the aorta

(C) Po_2 of fetal blood leaving the placenta is slightly greater than maternal mixed venous Po_2

(D) the presence of fetal hemoglobin shifts the oxyhemoglobin dissociation to the left

(E) the liver, heart, and head of the fetus receive the most highly O_2-saturated blood

193. The resistance to blood flow in the cerebral circulation of humans will increase when

(A) Pao_2 decreases to < 50 mm Hg

(B) an individual inhales a gas mixture enriched with CO_2

(C) an individual's hematocrit is decreased to < 0.30 by isovolemic exchange transfusion

(D) systemic arterial pressure increases from 100 to 130 mm Hg

(E) an individual suffers an epileptic seizure

DIRECTIONS (Questions 194 through 247): Each set of matching questions contains lettered options, followed by several items. For each item, select the ONE lettered option that is most closely associated with it. Each lettered heading may be selected once, more than once, or not at all.

Questions 194 through 196

For each condition listed, choose the set of arterial blood gas values with which it is most likely associated.

(A) $Paco_2$ decreased, pH decreased

(B) $Paco_2$ increased, pH increased

(C) $Paco_2$ increased, pH decreased

(D) $Paco_2$ decreased, pH increased

(E) $Paco_2$ normal, pH decreased

194. Partly compensated metabolic acidosis

195. Hyperventilation

196. Uncompensated hypoventilation

Questions 197 through 199

For each cell type in the visual system, choose the visual stimulus that is likely to bring about the largest change in the firing rate of the cell.

(A) a small stationary spot or annulus

(B) a small moving spot or annulus

(C) a stationary bar in a specific orientation

(D) a moving bar in a specific orientation

(E) a moving bar in any orientation

197. Retinal ganglion cells

198. Lateral geniculate neurons

199. Simple cells of the visual cortex

Questions 200 through 204

For each of the electroencephalographic (EEG) patterns named below, select the phase of sleep most likely to be associated with it.

(A) alpha waves

(B) beta waves

(C) theta waves

(D) delta waves

(E) low voltage punctuated by occasional sleep spindles

200. Rapid eye movement (REM) sleep

201. Light sleep (first stage of slow wave sleep)

202. Deep sleep (stage 4 of slow wave sleep)

203. Alert wakefulness

204. Quiet wakefulness

Questions 205 through 207

For each process listed below, choose the hormone that is most likely to directly stimulate it.

    (A) estradiol

    (B) estriol

    (C) luteinizing hormone (LH)

    (D) follicle-stimulating hormone (FSH)

    (E) inhibin

205. Induction of LH surge

206. Ovulation

207. Stimulate Sertoli cells to convert spermatids to sperm

Questions 208 and 209

A middle-aged male with smaller than normal-sized kidneys (by X-ray) and a history of chronic glomerulonephritis has the following laboratory analyses:

ARTERIAL BLOOD	URINE
pH = 7.33	pH = 6.0
Pao_2 = 95 mm Hg	protein = positive
$Paco_2$ = 35 mm Hg	glucose = negative
HCO_3^- = 18 mEq/L	

208. This patient most likely has

    (A) metabolic acidosis with no respiratory compensation

    (B) metabolic acidosis with some respiratory compensation

    (C) respiratory acidosis with no renal compensation

    (D) respiratory acidosis with some renal compensation

    (E) condition of diabetic ketoacidosis

209. The most likely cause of his acid/base imbalance is

    (A) hypoventilation

    (B) hyperventilation

    (C) decreased ability to produce adequate urinary NH_4^+ excretion

    (D) excess beta-hydroxybutyric and acetoacetic acids in his blood

    (E) decreased catabolism of sulfur-containing amino acids (e.g., methionine, cysteine)

Questions 210 and 211

The illustration below represents a pair of action potentials.

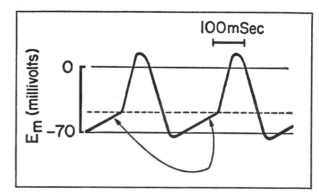

210. The action potentials shown represent those of

    (A) myelinated motor axons

    (B) skeletal muscle fibers

    (C) pharmacomechanically coupled smooth muscle fibers

    (D) cardiac nodal cells

    (E) ventricular Purkinje cells

211. The gradual depolarization between action potentials (see arrows) is mainly the result of

    (A) a gradual increase in inward Na^+ current through fast Na^+ channels (I_{Na})

    (B) an increase in the "delayed rectifier" current due to outward movement of K^+ (I_K)

    (C) a combination of gradual inactivation of outward I_K along with the presence of an inward "funny" current (I_f) due to the opening of channels permeable to both Na^+ and K^+ ions

    (D) changes in permeability of cells to the principal extracellular anions, Cl^- and HCO_3^-

    (E) a gradual change in the ratio of extracellular to intracellular ion concentrations across the cell membrane

Questions 212 through 216

Below is a Davenport diagram plotting arterial plasma bicarbonate against arterial blood pH. Dashed lines are different levels of arterial Pco_2 (isobars). On the diagram are nine different points (letters A through I). Match each numbered description below with one of these lettered points. For this set of questions, letters may be used once, more than once, or not at all.

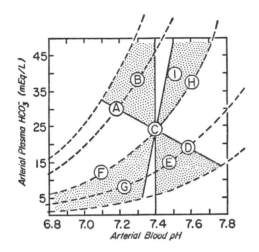

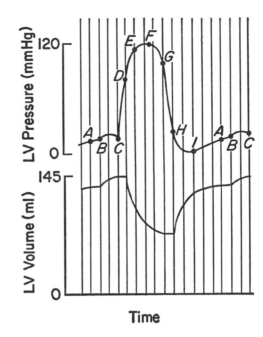

212. Simple respiratory acidosis without any renal compensation

213. Respiratory acidosis with some renal compensation

214. Simple respiratory alkalosis without any renal compensation

215. Metabolic alkalosis with some respiratory compensation

216. Metabolic acidosis with some respiratory compensation

Questions 217 through 223

Below are illustrated simultaneous changes in left ventricular pressure (LV pressure) and volume (LV volume) over time. There are nine lettered points on the LV pressure curve (points A through I). Match each numbered event named below with one of the lettered points. For this set of questions, letter choices may be used once, more than once, or not at all.

217. Beginning of second heart sound (S_2)

218. LV pressure essentially equal to diastolic aortic blood pressure

219. Aortic valve closes

220. Peak of left atrial v wave

221. End of left ventricular systole

222. Beginning of first heart sound (S_1)

223. Peak of T wave of electrocardiogram (ECG)

Questions 224 through 226

The graph below represents a patient who has a febrile episode. Temperatures measured are rectal and in degrees C. Match each numbered statement with the appropriate letter choice from the graph (letters A through G). For this set of questions, letter choices may be used once, more than once, or not at all.

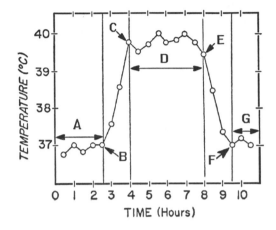

224. Period during which patient claims to be fairly comfortable (although the patient's set point is above normal)

225. Point at which patient begins to behave as if in a hot environment (sweats and complains of "burning up")

226. Point at which patient begins to behave as if in a cold environment (complains of chills and has shivering)

Questions 227 through 229

Illustrated below are four different patterns of forced expiratory volume in one second (FEV_1) and forced vital capacity (FVC). Match each of the numbered conditions below with one of the lettered patterns (A through D). For this set of questions, letter choices may be used once, more than once, or not at all.

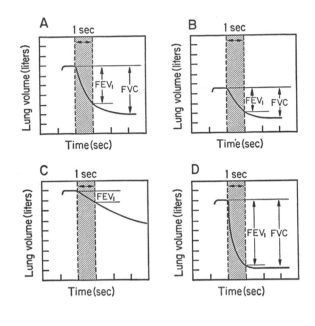

227. Patient with emphysema

228. Patient with pulmonary fibrosis

229. Patient with asthma

Questions 230 through 232

Below is illustrated an electrocardiogram, such as might be recorded from standard limb lead II. There are several lettered points (A through H) indicating different parts of the electrocardiogram. Below the illustration are several numbered descriptions. Match each number with the appropriate letter choice nearest the event described. For this set of questions, letter choices may be used once, more than once, or not at all.

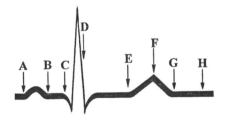

230. Ventricular repolarization has just ended

231. Ventricular depolarization has just begun

232. Beginning of atrial depolarization

Questions 233 through 235

Illustrated below is a left ventricular pressure–volume loop from a normal healthy adult. Four different points are indicated by letters W through Z. Below the illustration are three multiple choice questions based on this illustration. For each question choose the one most nearly correct answer.

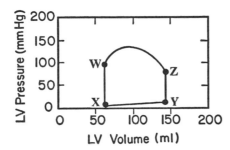

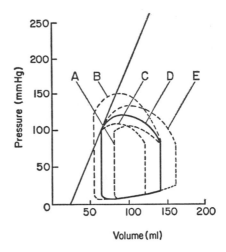

233. The part of the cardiac cycle described as 150-volumetric relaxation is between points

   (A) W and X
   (B) X and Y
   (C) Y and Z
   (D) Z and W

234. The part of the cardiac cycle that has the highest rate of energy consumption (highest rate of ATP hydrolysis) is between points

   (A) W and X
   (B) X and Y
   (C) Y and Z
   (D) Z and W

235. The part of the cardiac cycle that does the most physical work (external work as force acting through distance) is between points

   (A) W and X
   (B) X and Y
   (C) Y and Z
   (D) Z and W

Questions 236 and 237

Below is an illustration representing five left ventricular pressure–volume loops, each labeled by a letter (letters A through E). Loop D represents the normal pressure–volume loop of a healthy adult at rest. Match each numbered description below the illustration with the appropriate letter choice. For this series of questions, letter choices may be used once, more than once, or not at all.

236. The pressure–volume loop that represents an increase in stroke volume (above normal) by an increase in contractility (positive inotropic effect)

237. The pressure–volume loop that represents a decrease in preload (below normal)

Questions 238 through 240

Below is an illustration of changes in body oxygen consumption (LVM$\dot{V}_{O_2}$) and energy requirements (dashed lines) with moderate dynamic exercise. Several different periods are indicated by letters A through E. Below the illustration are several numbered descriptions. Match each number with the appropriate letter choice from the illustration. For this series of questions, choices may be used once, more than once, or not at all.

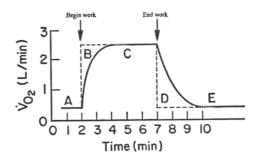

238. Period during which $\dot{V}_{O_2}$ exceeds metabolic needs

239. Period during which O_2 delivery to exercising muscles is less than that required for aerobic metabolism

240. Period during which cardiac output and pulmonary ventilation are at their highest

Questions 241 and 242

Below are five different areas of the nephron (letter choices A through E). Below these letter choices are two numbered descriptions. Match each number with the appropriate letter choice. For this series of questions, letter choices may be used once, more than once, or not at all.

(A) glomerulus

(B) proximal tubule

(C) juxtaglomerular apparatus

(D) thick ascending limb of Henle's loop

(E) collecting duct

241. Primary site for majority of salt and water reabsorption

242. Low water permeability under all circumstances

Questions 243 through 245

Below are four hormones (letter choices A through D). Below these choices are three numbered descriptions. Match each number with the appropriate letter choice. For this series of questions, letter choices may be used once, more than once, or not at all.

(A) aldosterone

(B) antidiuretic hormone

(C) atrial natriuretic peptide

(D) angiotensin II

243. Increases urea permeability in the collecting duct

244. Is produced by the adrenal glands

245. Increases urinary excretion of sodium

Questions 246 and 247

Below are eight letter choices (A through H). Below these choices are two numbered descriptions. Match each number with the appropriate letter choice. For this series of questions, letter choices may be used once, more than once, or not at all.

(A) skeletal muscle only

(B) cardiac muscle only

(C) smooth muscle only

(D) both skeletal and cardiac muscle

(E) both cardiac and smooth muscle

(F) both skeletal and smooth muscle

(G) all three muscle types (skeletal, cardiac, and smooth muscle)

(H) none of the above

246. The one(s) in which electrical signals pass from muscle cell to muscle cell through connexons

247. All of the calcium required for contractile activation comes from inside the cells.

DIRECTIONS (Questions 248 through 254): Each of the numbered items or incomplete statements in this section is followed by answers or by completions of the statement. Select the ONE lettered answer or completion that is BEST in each case.

248. Which of the following describes the compliance of the lungs measured under static conditions?

(A) change in lung volume divided by the corresponding change in distending pressure $(P_{alv} - P_{pl})$

(B) change in distending pressure $(P_{alv} - P_{pl})$ multiplied by the change in lung volume

(C) lung volume divided by recoil pressure $(P_{alv} - P_{pl})$

(D) change in elastic recoil pressure $(P_{alv} - P_{pl})$

(E) change in distending pressure $(P_{alv} - P_{pl})$ divided by change in lung volume

249. During normal isotonic skeletal muscle contraction

(A) thick filaments decrease in length

(B) thin filaments decrease in length

(C) thick filaments increase in length

(D) overlap between thick and thin filaments increases

(E) thick and thin filaments slide away from one another

250. Skeletal muscle resembles heart muscle in that

(A) both are activated to contract by acetylcholine

(B) calcium currents across the sarcolemma are responsible for excitation-contraction coupling

(C) both have similar contractile filaments and banding patterns

(D) both can be tetanized

(E) both have action potentials of similar duration

251. Residual volume

(A) is part of the expiratory reserve volume

(B) is part of vital capacity

(C) cannot be measured directly with a spirometer

(D) represents the resting volume of the lungs

(E) is the volume at which the lungs tend to recoil outward

252. When the diaphragm contracts

    (A) intrapleural pressure becomes more negative
    (B) alveolar pressure increases
    (C) the recoil tendency of the lung decreases
    (D) intraabdominal pressure decreases
    (E) functional residual capacity decreases

253. An individual has an alveolar ventilation of 6000 ml/minute, a tidal volume of 600 ml, and a breathing rate of 12 breaths/minute. What is this individual's anatomic dead space?

    (A) 100 ml
    (B) 120 ml
    (C) 150 ml
    (D) 200 ml
    (E) 250 ml

254. A patient's laboratory analysis of arterial plasma showed a pH of 7.56, bicarbonate 21 mEq/L (slightly below normal), abnormally low P_{O_2}, and abnormally low P_{CO_2} (25 mm Hg). This patient probably

    (A) has severe chronic lung disease
    (B) is a lowlander who has been vacationing at high altitude for two weeks
    (C) is a subject in a clinical research experiment who has been breathing a gas mixture of 10% oxygen and 90% nitrogen for a few minutes
    (D) is an emergency room patient with severely depressed respiration as a result of a heroin overdose
    (E) is an adult psychiatric patient who swallowed an overdose of aspirin

Answers and Explanations

128. **(E)** The CSF is not a serum filtrate. The ionic and proteinaceous composition of the CSF is caused by active transport (secretion and resorption) by the epithelial cells of the choroid plexus. These cells actively pump sodium into the CSF. Water and chloride passively follow the active sodium transport. Potassium is not actively transported into the CSF and, in fact, is resorbed to some extent by the choroid plexus. *(Guyton, pp 681–682)*

129. **(C)** The cerebellum is generally considered to play an important role in the coordination and smoothing out of voluntary movements. Intention tremor, which may be observed in cerebellar disease, is absent at rest but appears at the onset of voluntary movements. This aspect of the tremors readily differentiates them from those observed with the degeneration of the nigrostriatal dopaminergic tracts in Parkinson's disease, which produces tremors that are present at rest. The amplitude of oscillations caused by cerebellar deficits is not generally constant throughout a voluntary movement. *(Ganong, pp 181–184)*

130. **(B)** In both diabetes insipidus and Addison's disease, appropriate water and salt intake will adequately compensate for the potential excess volume loss. If access to appropriate intake is prevented, however, tremendous volume loss will occur. All of the other changes listed in the question would tend to maintain blood volume, but all are either short-term effects or the result of extreme stimuli, such as hemorrhage or intense sympathetic activity. *(Guyton, pp 315–318)*

131. **(A)** A wide variety of environmental conditions provoke several mechanisms to come into play to maintain body temperature by balancing heat production and heat loss. The loss of heat via infrared rays (radiation) accounts for more than 60 percent of the normal heat loss. Conduction of heat to objects or to air (i.e., convection) accounts for 15 percent, and evaporation accounts for about 25 percent. Sweating is an important form of heat loss and is regulated by various body mechanisms. Insensible perspiration through the skin and lungs, although important, remains relatively constant despite environmental changes and thus does not provide a major mechanism to regulate body temperature. *(Guyton, pp 799–800)*

132. **(E)** Huntington's disease in humans is characterized by the degeneration of the caudate nuclei. This is associated with the appearance of disorganized, choreiform movements. Damage to other regions of the nervous system involved in the control of movements may produce other forms of movement disorders. For example, damage to the subthalamic nuclei may result in sudden, intense, and involuntary movements, termed ballistic movements. Degeneration of the nigrostriatal dopaminergic system characterizes Parkinson's disease, which is associated with akinesia and tremor. Lesions of the cerebellum may result in the incoordination of voluntary movements, termed ataxia. The spinothalamic tracts convey sensory information to the thalamus, and their loss does not produce choreiform movements. *(Ganong, pp 178–179)*

133. **(A)** Experiments have been performed in which stimulating electrodes were implanted in certain regions of the nervous system of rats and the animals were allowed to control the stimulus by pressing a bar that triggered the application of the stimulating current. Electrodes implanted in the medial forebrain bundle, as well as in areas of the frontal cortex, caudate nucleus, ventral tegmentum, and the septal nuclei, frequently led to repeated self-stimulation by the animals. The neural circuits that subserve this self-stimulation behavior have been considered to constitute an endogenous reward system within the brain. Rage reactions and avoidance reactions may be induced by stimulation of other parts of the CNS, such as regions of the hypothalamus. Temporary paralysis or repeated turning movements are not normally observed on stimulation of the medial forebrain bundle. *(Ganong, pp 196–198)*

134. **(C)** The basal ganglia constitute part of the extrapyramidal system concerned with the control of movement. Many neurobiologists believe that the basal ganglia play an important role in the initiation of voluntary movement. Consistent with such a notion is the experimental observation that unit activity in the basal ganglia is associated with movements and that many units start to fire before the onset of slow, sustained movements. Basal ganglia units are less likely to discharge during rapid movements. The discharge of units in basal ganglia has not been linked to somatosensory stimulation, acoustic stimulation, or visual accommodation. *(Ganong, pp 168–169)*

135. **(E)** Water that is either higher or lower than body temperature and that is introduced into the external auditory meatus may set up convection currents within the endolymph of the inner ear. These currents may result in the stimulation of the semicircular canals by causing movements of the ampullar cristae. Conflicting, different information from the right and left sides, in turn, may result in vertigo and nausea. Decreased movement or immobilization of the otoliths or of the ampullar cristae is not caused by such changes in temperature. Furthermore, changes in the discharge rate of vestibular afferents, which must occur with caloric stimulation, are most likely to be caused by the changes in the activity of the receptors rather than being a direct response of the afferents to changes in temperature. *(Ganong, p 139)*

136. **(C)** The olfactory mucous membranes are rich in trigeminal nerve endings, which may respond to nasal irritants and initiate a variety of reflex reactions that include sneezing and lacrimation. Neither olfactory nor gustatory receptors nor the efferent pathways to the olfactory bulb are believed to be involved in the initiation of such reflex responses. The activation of trigeminal nerve endings by certain olfactory stimuli may, however, contribute to the characteristics of certain odors. *(Ganong, p 152)*

137. **(D)** The primary change in the cochlea that registers an increase in the frequency of a sound wave is a change in the position of maximal displacement of the basilar membrane. A sound of low pitch produces the greatest displacement toward the apex of the cochlea and produces the greatest activation of hair cells at that location. As the pitch is increased, the position of greatest displacement moves closer to the base of the cochlea. Increases in the number of hair cells that are activated and in the frequency of discharge of units in the auditory nerve fibers, together with an increase in range of frequencies to which such units respond, are all more likely to be observed in response to increases in the intensity of a sound

stimulus rather than to increases in pitch. In the auditory cortex, sound frequencies are organized topographically so that a change in pitch may be represented by a change in the location of activated cortical units. A change in the latency with which cortical units are activated would not be expected, however. *(Ganong, pp 140–145)*

138. **(C)** Light-induced decomposition of rhodopsin results in closure of sodium channels. This results in decreased Na+ influx and a consequent hyperpolarization of the membrane potential. *(Guyton, p 549)*

139. **(B)** Much evidence has accumulated that certain dorsal root ganglion cells synthesize substance P. This peptide is carried, by axoplasmic transport, to both the central and peripheral branches of these sensory neurons. Centrally, most of these substance P-containing processes end in the substantia gelatinosa, and a variety of experimental approaches have led to the hypothesis that substance P is the transmitter used by the sensory cells that mediate responses to pain. Sectioning the dorsal roots results in a fall in substance P levels in the substantia gelatinosa and in the dorsal roots proximal to the section. The peptide, however, continues to be manufactured in the dorsal root ganglion cells and to be transported along the branches of the cells, leading to a buildup of substance P distal to the section. Sectioning the dorsal roots does not produce an increase in substance P concentration in the ventral roots. *(Takahashi and Otsuka)*

140. **(C)** The stimulation of receptors in the Golgi tendon organs leads to the inverse stretch reflex. This reflex is responsible for the relaxation that is observed when a muscle is subjected to a strong stretch. Impulses from the organs travel in type Ib fibers to the spinal cord, where they activate inhibitory interneurons. These in turn suppress the activity of motor neurons and therefore lead to the relaxation of the extrafusal muscle fibers attached to the tendons. The activity in group II afferent fibers, the γ-efferent discharge rate, and the state of contraction of intrafusal fibers control the stretch reflex, which is distinct from the inverse stretch reflex mediated by the Golgi tendon organs. *(Ganong, pp 103–104)*

141. **(C)** When a constantly maintained stimulus is applied to a receptor cell, the firing rate in the sensory nerve fibers may remain approximately constant during the time that the stimulus is present. Such a response may be termed a tonic receptor response. Alternatively, a stimulus may produce a bout of action potentials whose frequency declines markedly as the stimulus is maintained. This is known as a phasic response, and the decline or cessation of firing is called adaptation. Muscle spindles, pain receptors (nociceptors), visceral chemoreceptors, and stretch receptors in the lungs generally show little adaptation. Cutaneous touch receptors, on the other hand, are characterized by strong adaptation to a maintained stimulus. *(Ganong, pp 76–79)*

142. **(D)** The excitatory stimulation at the dendritic terminus results in a depolarization, which spreads electronically toward the soma. The concentration of voltage-gated sodium channels is highest at the axon hillock. If it is of sufficient magnitude, the depolarization results in the opening of these sodium channels and the initiation of an action potential. *(Guyton, p 488)*

143. **(A)** Acetylcholine released by the vagal nerve stimulates muscarinic receptors in the cells of the SA node, resulting in the opening of potassium channels and, consequently, in hyperpolarization. It, therefore, takes longer for sodium leakage to cause the membrane potentials of these cells to reach the threshold required for an action potential. The rate of rhythmicity is thus decreased. A similar hyperpolarization of the fibers at the AV junction decreases conduction of atrial impulses to the ventrical. *(Guyton, p 116)*

144. **(B)** Segmental contractions appear as alternating regions of contraction and relaxation within both the small intestine and the colon. Peristaltic waves also may occur at a variety of rates in both regions and are responsible for the movement of the contents of the small intestine toward the colon and those of the colon toward the rectum. Peristaltic rushes are intense intestinal peristaltic waves that are not normally observed unless a blockage occurs within the intestine. Mass action contractions, which are only observed in the colon, are due to the simultaneous contraction of colon smooth muscle over a large area. *(Ganong, pp 431–432)*

145. **(D)** Within the liver, bilirubin is conjugated to glucuronic acid through the action of the enzyme glucuronyl transferase. Although some bilirubin glucuronide that is formed in the liver may enter the blood, most of it is transported to the bile canaliculi, from where it may enter the bile ducts and then the duodenum. When bile ducts are blocked, bilirubin glucuronide levels in the blood increase and produce symptoms of jaundice. Jaundice may, however, also develop under a variety of conditions in which the blood concentrations of free, unconjugated bilirubin are elevated. *(Ganong, p 426)*

146. **(B)** Hypoglycemia is the most potent stimulus for glucagon secretion. High serum levels of amino acids (especially alanine and arginine) also will induce glucagon release. Somatostatin inhibits glucagon secretion. *(Guyton, p 863)*

147. **(C)** Absorption of vitamin B_{12} requires that it form a complex with intrinsic factor, which is secreted by the parietal cells of the stomach. Destruction of these cells thus results in a vitamin B_{12} deficiency. The vitamin B_{12}-intrinsic factor complex is absorbed in the ileum. Thus, surgical resection of the ileum will also produce a deficiency but not surgical resection of the jejunum. *(Guyton, pp 360,737,784)*

148. **(B)** Within mucosal cells, the major source of triglycerides is the acylation of 2-monoglycerides, which enter the cells by diffusion across their luminal membranes. The triglycerides, together with cholesterol, cholesteryl esters, phospholipids, and proteins, then form chylomicrons. These are released to the extracellular space by exocytosis, after which they enter the lymphatic system. *(Ganong, pp 401–404)*

149. **(D)** The total tension that is developed on stimulating a muscle isometrically is the sum of the passive tension of the unstimulated muscle and the active tension exerted by stimulation. The passive tension increases monotonically with the length of the fiber. Active tension, however, increases up to the resting length of the fiber and then declines as the length is increased further. The total tension therefore also shows first an increase and then a decrease as a fiber is lengthened. *(Ganong, p 56)*

150. **(B)** Increasing the membrane's conductance to potassium will result in the membrane potential approaching the value dictated by the potassium Nernst potential, which is about –86 mV. *(Guyton, p 488)*

151. **(E)** Gap junctions form channels that join the cytoplasmic compartments of two adjoining cells, thus allowing electrical current to flow between them. *(Guyton, p 482)*

152. **(B)** Although electrogenic pumps may contribute to the membrane potential of certain cells, the major determinants of membrane potential are the external and internal concentrations of permeant ions and their relative permeabilities in the membrane. Increasing the conductance for an ion causes the membrane potential to approach the equilibrium potential for that ion. Conversely, decreasing the conductance causes the membrane potential to move away from the equilibrium potential for that ion. Thus a decrease in the conductance of a membrane to chloride ions causes the cells to depolarize—that is, become more positive—if the membrane potential is positive with respect to the chloride equilibrium potential. *(Kandel and Schwartz, pp 82–84,88)*

153. **(C)** ACE cleaves the inactive angiotensin I (which is produced by the action of renin on angiotensinogen) to the active angiotensin II. Angiotensin II is a powerful vasoconstrictor and also induces decreased renal excretion of salt and water through its stimulation of aldosterone secretion. These actions of angiotensin II tend to raise blood pressure. Therefore, inhibition of the action of ACE has an antihypertensive effect. *(Guyton, pp 211–214)*

154. **(C)** The transmitter at the muscle end-plate, acetylcholine, may be released spontaneously in small packets or quanta, without the presynaptic terminal's being invaded by an action potential. These quanta are believed to represent the contents of single transmitter vesicles. Release of acetylcholine activates multiple ion channels in the muscle to produce a miniature end-plate potential. *(Ganong, pp 81–82)*

155. **(E)** The constriction of the pupil of the eye in response to light is mediated by a pathway that travels from the retina through the optic nerves, the optic chiasm, and the optic tracts. Lesions in these areas are, therefore, likely to impair this reflex. The pathway leaves the optic tracts anterior to the lateral geniculate to enter the pretectal area. Lesions in this area would, therefore, also prevent normal functioning of the reflex. A lesion of the geniculocalcarine tracts, which convey visual information from the lateral geniculate bodies to the occipital cortex, would cause partial or total blindness in humans but would not, however, affect the pupillary reflex. *(Ganong, pp 121–122)*

156. **(B)** Bile acid micelles serve a ferrying function in the intestine, carrying free fatty acids, monoglycerides, and cholesterol to the epithelial cells, where they are absorbed. The bile acid micelles also accelerate triglyceride digestion by sequestering the products of the reversible digestion reactions. Bile acid ferrying is absolutely necessary for cholesterol absorption. In contrast, the absence of bile acids that would follow bile duct ligation would reduce monoglyceride and free fatty acid absorption by only approximately 50 percent. *(Guyton, pp 728–729,734)*

157. **(A)** The spiral ganglion contains neurons whose processes project from both the inner and outer hair cells of the cochlea to the cochlear nuclei. Although there are more than five times as many outer hair cells in the cochlea as there are inner hair cells, more than 90 percent of the neurons within the spiral ganglion receive inputs from the less numerous inner hair cells. Efferent activity to hair cells is primarily generated by neurons in the olivary nucleus. Vestibular information from the semicircular canals and the utricle is relayed via the vestibular ganglion. *(Ganong, pp 139–140)*

158. **(D)** The response to a stab wound that punctures the lung demonstrates the elasticity of the lung and chest wall. The tendency of the lung to collapse is normally balanced by the tendency of the chest wall to spring out. Thus intrapleural pressures are subatmospheric. Introduction of air in this space allows the lung to collapse and the chest wall to spring out. *(West, 1991, p 566)*

159. **(D)** Normally, O_2 is transferred from air spaces to blood via a perfusion-limited process. Thus, O_2 moves across the alveolar–capillary membrane by a process of simple diffusion, and the amount of gas taken up depends entirely on the amount of blood flow. Processes that impair diffusion of O_2 transform the normal relationship to a diffusion-limited process. Thus if the O_2 must move a greater distance because of a thickened barrier, as would occur with increased extravascular lung water or cell components (interstitial fibrosis), the diffusion process is limited. Furthermore, decreasing the driving passage (by lowering inspired O_2 concentrations or decreasing the residence time of blood in the lungs), as occurs with strenuous exercise, may also alter the normal relationship. Increasing the ventilatory rate will not have this effect and will only serve to maintain a high gradient of O_2 from air to blood. *(West, 1991, pp 548–551)*

160. **(E)** The respiratory center of the CNS consists of a diffuse group of neurons whose inherent activity persists even after all known afferent stimuli have been eliminated. Although sectioning the brain and observing respiratory changes are a useful approach to locating important central areas of respiratory regulation, this approach interferes with many complex pathways that may interact. Nonetheless, transectioning of the brain above the pons has little effect. An apneustic center may be located in the pons. Transection above the center results in prolonged inspiration and short expiration. Apparently, a pneumotaxic center in the upper pons modulates this effect along with vagal impulses. The medullary center is capable of initiating and maintaining sequences of respiration. *(Guyton, pp 444–445)*

161. **(C)** Glomerular pores have a diameter of approximately 8 nm. Albumin, the smallest serum protein (with a molecular weight of 69,000) has a diameter of approximately 6 nm. However, albumin is prevented from passing through the pores by

electrostatic repulsion, since the pores are lined by negative charges, and albumin, like most serum proteins, is itself negatively charged. *(Guyton, p 290)*

162. **(A)** Energy can be derived from either aerobic or anaerobic sources. Although aerobic oxidative processes can provide a significant amount of energy, these processes are too slow to provide all of the energy required. Although stores of ATP and creatinine phosphate are present in muscle, they provide sufficient energy for only very brief periods of exercise (a few seconds). Deaminated proteins may undergo gluconeogenesis, in which they are converted to glucose or glycogen. This pathway is not normally used for strenuous exercise. The breakdown of glycogen to lactic acid provides sufficient energy rapidly enough to support brief periods of strenuous exercise (many seconds to a few minutes). The depletion of glycogen and production of lactic acid contribute to an energy debt, which is repaid via oxidative metabolism in the period after exercise. *(Guyton, pp 790–791)*

163. **(A)** Sweating is a function of eccrine glands that are innervated with sympathetic postganglionic cholinergic fibers, and thus atropine will depress the rate of sweating. Stimulation of the preoptic area of the anterior hypothalamus will stimulate sweating. Normal sweat is low in Na+ and Cl– because reabsorptive mechanisms are in part regulated by circulating aldosterone. Serious fluid electrolyte imbalance may occur if sodium chloride (NaCl) is not properly reabsorbed. Acclimatization to hot weather involves increased sweat production with decreased concentration of NaCl, thus allowing appropriate heat balance with electrolyte conservation. *(Guyton, pp 800–802)*

164. **(C)** In the figure that accompanies the question, diastolic filling of the left ventricle starts at A and terminates at B (mitral valve closes). Depolarization of the ventricles causes contraction of the ventricle. This contraction causes an abrupt increase in ventricular pressure with no change in ventricular volumes (BC), since the aortic valve remains closed. Opening of the aortic valve at point C marks onset of the ejection phase, and thereafter ventricular volume falls rapidly (CD) and then somewhat more slowly (DE). Closure of the aortic valve (E) occurs at the end of systole. At this point, pressure in the aorta is greater than that in the ventricles, blood flow is reversed in the aorta, and the aortic valve closes. In an aortic pressure curve, this is depicted by the isovolumetric relaxation curve, where ventricular pressure decreases rapidly with no change in ventricular volumes. *(Berne and Levy, p 411)*

165. **(B)** An increase in filling by transfusion of blood will, at constant aortic pressure, increase the end-diastolic pressure (point B in the figure that accompanies the question). By the Frank-Starling law of the heart, an increase in filling will be accompanied by an increase in stroke volume. Thus C will be shifted to the right and CDE will increase. The area inside the curve represents stroke work and would be expected to be increased with an increase in cardiac output. *(Berne and Levy, p 412)*

166. **(D)** The heart is a functional syncyctium, since a wave of depolarization causes the entire myocardium to contract when a suprathreshold stimulus is applied. In skeletal muscle, graded contraction can occur and is a function of the number of muscle fibers that are stimulated. Although there are other differences, both cell types consist of sarcomeres with thick (myosin) and thin (actin) filaments. Similar length–tension curves for both cell types have been demonstrated, with optimal sarcomere length characteristic of both. Although still a hypothesis, the sliding filament theory appears to adequately describe muscle mechanics of both the heart and skeletal muscles. At rest, the thin actin filaments are separated but overlap the thick myosin filaments. During stimulation, the actin filaments are pulled inward among myosin filaments, resulting in muscle contraction. *(Guyton, pp 69–70,76,100–101)*

167. **(E)** Epinephrine has both α- and β-receptor effects. The α effect causes a rise in systemic BP. By blocking this α effect with phenoxybenzamine, the β effect is unmasked, which is usually a moderate decrease in systemic BP. Histamine usually depresses systemic BP, as might acetylcholine. Occasionally, high doses of acetylcholine increase BP because of stimulation of the adrenal gland and release of epinephrine. However, atropine would not antagonize this effect. β blockade will enhance the effect of both epinephrine and norepinephrine. *(Guyton, pp 671,677–678)*

168. **(D)** Both FSH and ACTH have a primary peptide structure and are therefore subject to degradation by proteolytic enzymes. FSH, however, belongs to that group of pituitary hormones that contain carbohydrates in their structure and are made up of two different protein subunits. Other glycoproteins in this group are thyroid-stimulating hormone (TSH) and luteinizing hormone (LH). ACTH, on the other hand, is a single-polypeptide chain. Both FSH and ACTH regulate the functions of other endocrine glands. *(Ganong, pp 204–206)*

169. **(D)** Insulin action stimulates the activation or membrane insertion of glucose carriers in most of

its target tissues. These glucose carriers greatly enhance the permeability of the cell membrane to glucose, thus allowing glucose to flow passively down its concentration gradient into the cytoplasm. Glucose uptake is not stimulated by insulin in liver and brain. *(Guyton, p 858)*

170. **(D)** A variety of stimuli are able to elicit an increase in the release of growth hormone, including elevations in the plasma concentration of glucagon. Growth hormone acts by increasing the circulating levels of certain growth factors. Among growth factors that have been described are insulinlike growth factor I and nerve growth factor, although the identity and actions of the growth factors controlled by growth hormone have not been fully elucidated. Although an increase in the rate of growth hormone secretion occurs at the onset of sleep, episodes of REM sleep are associated with a decrease in the secretion of this hormone. The release of growth hormone is also enhanced by fasting and by exercise and may be inhibited by glucose and free fatty acids. *(Ganong, pp 204–206)*

171. **(C)** The solubility of CO_2 in blood is 20 times that of O_2, and thus a small (5 percent) but considerable portion of CO_2 is dissolved in blood. More importantly, almost 10 percent of the total CO_2 transported is in the dissolved form. The bulk of CO_2 transport involves its reversible combination with water. This occurs rapidly enough because of the action of carbonic anhydrase, an enzyme located inside RBCs. As bicarbonate ion diffuses out of RBCs, chloride ions diffuse in according to Gibbs–Donnan equilibrium. Combination of CO_2 with amine groups, especially those of hemoglobin, also accounts for a considerable portion of CO_2 transport (30 percent). *(West, 1991, pp 540–542)*

172. **(D)** The normal osmolality of plasma is approximately 286 mOsm. In order to maintain a stable intracellular volume, therefore, cells such as erythrocytes work to maintain an intracellular osmolarity of about 286 mOsm. Placing red blood cells in a medium with an osmotic strength of 450 mOsm will result in net water loss and consequent cell shrinkage, since the cell membrane is permeable to water, and the osmotic driving force will cause water to flow from the more dilute to the more concentrated compartment. The cell volume will not be affected by the ionic composition of the extracellular medium as long as its ionic strength is 286 mOsm. Inhibiting the sodium pump will result in an increase in intracellular sodium, with a resultant increase in the osmotic strength of the intracellular fluid and will thus cause the cells to swell. *(Berne and Levy, pp 12–13)*

173. **(D)** Such substances as creatinine (almost exclusively excreted by glomerular filtration) and urea (some reabsorption) have no adaptive mechanisms to regulate plasma levels. Thus a significant decrease in GFR results in significant increases in plasma creatinine and urea (if production of both substances is constant). This is because the amount excreted ($U_x \cdot \dot{V}$) equals the amount produced. Furthermore, $U_x \cdot \dot{V}$ equals $GFR \cdot P_x$. If GFR decreases, P_x increases. However, both Na^+ and K^+ need to be closely regulated. Thus as GFR decreases in disease, the percentage of either Na^+ or K^+ excreted increases in order to maintain a normal amount of Na^+ or K^+ excretion. In kidney disease, some unknown natriuretic and kaliuretic substance may be responsible for this adaptive mechanism. *(Mountcastle, pp 1211–1215)*

174. **(E)** At any time in the respiratory cycle, when the glottis is open and no air is moving, P_A is equal to atmospheric pressure, or 0 cm H_2O. Inspiration is accomplished by a decrease in P_{pl} such that it is most subatmospheric at end-inspiration. The increase in thoracic volume lowers P_{pl}, and the elastic recoil of the lung (surface tension, tissue forces) determines the magnitude of the decrease. During expiration, P_A is > 0 and P_{pl} returns toward -5 cm H_2O in this case. With a forced expiratory maneuver, P_{pl} can be > 0 cm H_2O. *(West, 1991, pp 569–570)*

175. **(C)** The relationship between alveolar ventilation ($\dot{V}_A$) and alveolar CO_2 pressure (P_{ACO_2}) is represented as

$$\dot{V}_A = \frac{\dot{V}_{CO_2}}{P_{ACO_2}} \times K$$

where K is a constant such that $P_{ACO_2} = F_{ECO_2} = K$. ($F_{ECO_2}$ is the fraction of expired CO_2.) Since $\dot{V}_{CO_2}$ is constant, P_{ACO_2} will double if $\dot{V}_A$ is halved. In normal persons, P_{ACO_2} is virtually identical to arterial CO_2 pressure (P_{aCO_2}). Unless inspired air is enriched with O_2, arterial O_2 pressure (P_{aO_2}) and alveolar O_2 pressure (P_{AO_2}) will decrease. *(West, 1991, pp 546–547)*

176. **(E)** When ventilation/perfusion ($\dot{V}_A/\dot{Q}$) inspired ratios become very low, an unstable situation occurs. At the point beyond which all the gas is removed by blood, very little gas is available for expiration from this bronchoalveolar segment. A critical point then arises, and the unit tends to collapse. Neither O_2 toxicity nor surfactant inactivation would be expected to occur in this brief period of time. Although interstitial edema may occur, this would more likely produce trapped air segments than collapsed alveoli. CO_2 elimination will eventually decrease to zero as the unit collapses. *(West, 1992, pp 184–186)*

177. (D) A NaCl increase of 10 mmol/kg of body water is equivalent to an increase of 20 mOsm/kg body water, since NaCl rapidly ionizes. In the patient described in the question, whole body water is 20 L + 30 L, or 50 L. Thus, 50 L × 20 mOsm/L = 1,000 mOsm of solute. Since 500 mmol of NaCl is equal to 1,000 mOsm of NaCl, 500 mmol of NaCl is necessary for therapy. *(Mountcastle, p 1156)*

178. (E) Secretion of acid and of potassium by the renal tubule are inversely related. Thus, increased excretion of protons will result in decreased secretion (or increased retention) of potassium ions, with the result that the body's potassium store rises. *(Davenport, 1974, p 81)*

179. (D) Even though the cabin of the airplane described in the question is pressurized, the barometric pressure decreased to 523 mm Hg. Thus, the F_{IO_2} remains the same (0.21) but inspired P_{O_2} decreases, since it is the product of F_{IO_2} and barometric pressure. Water vapor pressure remains at 47 mm Hg as long as body temperature is normal, and thus P_{O_2} of humidified alveolar air must be less than that at sea level. Although a decrease in P_{ACO_2} (due to some hyperventilation) may slightly enhance P_{AO_2} and the rate of P_{AO_2} loss to body metabolism may decrease, neither is sufficient to prevent the decrease in P_{AO_2} due to the drop in barometric pressure. *(West, 1991, pp 588–590)*

180. (A) Shunted blood is blood that bypasses ventilated parts of the lung and directly enters the arterial circulation. In normal persons, this is largely due to mixing of arterial blood with bronchial venous and some myocardial venous blood, which drains into the left heart. Diffusion, although finite, is usually immeasurably small, as is reaction velocity with hemoglobin. *(West, 1991, pp 553–554)*

181. (B) Under normal circumstances, depolarization is initiated in the SA node and then propagates to the AV node. From there, action potentials are propagated through the bundle of His and through the Purkinje system to the ventricular muscle. Conduction in the AV node is slower than conduction either from the SA node to the AV node or from the AV node to ventricular muscle. The AV nodal delay is typically of the order of 100 msec. *(Ganong, p 459)*

182. (D) Inulin is an inert carbohydrate that fails to enter cells but readily enters extracellular space. It is therefore most useful in the determination of the ECF volume. If the plasma volume has been determined by some other method, the interstitial fluid volume may be calculated as the difference between the extracellular and plasma volumes. *(Ganong, pp 1–2)*

183. (D) Bohr's equation states that

$$\dot{V}_D/\dot{V}_T = (P_{ACO_2} - P_{ECO_2})/P_{ACO_2}$$

where P_{ECO_2} is mixed expired CO_2. In a normal person, P_{aCO_2} is virtually identical to P_{ACO_2}. Thus

$$\dot{V}_D/\dot{V}_T = (P_{aCO_2} - P_{ECO_2})/P_{aCO_2}$$

Since by Fowler's method, $\dot{V}_D/\dot{V}_T = 0.25$ in the patient described in the question, the $(P_{aCO_2} - P_{ECO_2})/P_{aCO_2} = 0.25$ $(40 - P_{ECO_2})/40 = 0.25$. Therefore $P_{ECO_2} = 30$ mm Hg. If considerable inequality of blood flow and ventilation were present, P_{ECO_2} could be much less than 30 mm Hg, and the patient's physiologic dead space would exceed the anatomic dead space. *(West, 1991, pp 526–527)*

184. (C) The choices given, except for normal, are patients with hypoxemia. Breathing 100% O_2 will greatly relieve the hypoxemia of all except the patient with an anatomical right to left shunt. The P_{aO_2} will greatly increase in the normal individual as well. Breathing 100% O_2 increases the P_{aO_2} to about 670 mm Hg. In the normal person the P_{aO_2} will be only slightly less than this. In abnormalities of diffusion (eg, alveolar wall thickening) the P_{aO_2} will be farther below 670 mm Hg, but not so low as 125 mm Hg. In V/Q abnormalities, P_{aO_2} will be quite high in all communicating air spaces after 100% O_2, and both alveolar and arterial P_{O_2} will be quite high. In true right to left shunt, breathing 100% O_2 will not substantially elevate the P_{aO_2} which could be 125 mm Hg. The small rise over normal P_{aO_2} comes mainly from a small amount of additional dissolved O_2 in blood passing through ventilated areas. 100% O_2 greatly increases the P_{aO_2} in profound hypoventilation. *(West, 1992, p 166)*

185. (D) Hypoxemia is an important stimulus to ventilatory drive but derives all its effects via stimulation of peripheral, *not* central, chemoreceptors. In humans, the most important regulating factor with respect to ventilation is the P_{aCO_2}. Ventilation increases linearly with a rise in P_{aO_2}. Although some of the response to CO_2 may be attributed to peripheral chemoreceptors, the largest percentage is the result of stimulation of central chemoreceptors. The effect of CO_2 presumably is via increase in H^+ in the cerebrospinal fluid (CSF) and cerebral extracellular fluid (ECF). Arterial hypoxemia will potentiate this effect, both by increasing the response to CO_2 and by reducing the level at which this response occurs. Increased work of breathing will reduce this ventilatory drive by depressing the effector organs involved. *(West, 1992, pp 584–585)*

186. **(E)** GFR is equal to the product of filtration pressure and a filtration coefficient. The glomerular capillary pressure is approximately 60 mm Hg and will *decrease* with afferent arteriolar vasoconstriction or *increase* with efferent arteriolar vasoconstriction. The hydraulic pressure in Bowman's capsule is approximately 18 mm Hg. The colloid osmotic pressure entering the capsule is 28 mm Hg and rises 20 to 25 percent as protein-free plasma is filtered. Alterations in these forces will produce expected changes in filtration. An increase in renal blood flow in a glomerulus with low filtration coefficient will produce only modest increases in GFR. This is because a low filtration coefficient causes fluid to be reabsorbed at the efferent artery, and colloid osmotic pressure promptly rises. Sympathetic stimulation will cause afferent vasoconstriction and thus lower plasma hydraulic pressure. A rise in blood pressure may be expected to increase GFR, but the kidney autoregulates and afferent vasoconstriction maintains GFR. *(Guyton, pp 291–293)*

Calculat- Plasma clearance, GFR if equal ✱

187. **(B)** Plasma clearance, or Cx, (ml/min) = (x · V̇)/Px. In the example that accompanies the question, Cx = (25 mg/ml) × 1 ml/min)/(20 mg/100 ml) = 125 ml/min. If renal blood flow is 500 ml/min and glomerular filtration fraction is 0.25, then the glomerular filtration rate (GFR) is 125 ml/min. If Cx = GFR, then substance x is neither reabsorbed nor secreted and may be inulin or perhaps creatinine. Glucose is normally totally reabsorbed, and PAH is actively secreted. *(Mountcastle, p 1175)*

✱ *His ruling if clearance more PAH or creatinine*

188. **(D)** Plasma clearance of substance x in the question is represented as

$$\frac{(6 \text{ mg/ml}) \times (1 \text{ ml/min})}{1 \text{ mg/100 ml}} = \frac{600 \text{ ml}}{\text{min}}$$

clearance more so

If the GFR = 125 ml/min, then 600 ml/min is a *PAH* reasonable value for effective renal plasma flow (ERPF). PAH is a substance that freely crosses the glomerular membrane, but unlike inulin, it is secreted into the tubules by tubular epithelium. A value of 600 mL/min is a reasonable normal value for ERPF. Actual flow is somewhat higher since extraction of PAH is not complete (< 85 percent). Plasma clearance of Na^+ in a normal subject is orders of magnitude less than the GFR, and in normal individuals there is no clearance of glucose. *(Mountcastle, p 1175)*

189. **(A)** ADH acts on the collecting tubules of the kidney to induce water retention. Inappropriately high levels of ADH, as are achieved in SIADH, result in the renal retention of free water, which consequently exerts a dilutional effect on serum ion concentrations. Thus, serum sodium can fall dramatically in SIADH. ADH does not exert any direct effect on the renal handling of sodium. *(Guyton, pp 314–315,828–829)*

190. **(C)** Strenuous exercise provides a good example of how various physiologic adjustments operate and are integrated. Although the underlying mechanisms are in large part unknown, it is clear that alveolar ventilation and cardiac output both increase. Regional blood flow is altered so that active muscles have increased blood flow and less active, nonessential areas, such as the skin and viscera, have temporally decreased blood flow. O_2 use is enhanced by decreases in tissue P_{O_2} in exercising muscle, as well as a shift to the right of the oxyhemoglobin dissociation curve due to increases in H^+, temperature, and CO_2. The body temperature rises, although sweating mechanisms are significantly increased. *(Mountcastle, pp 1401–1411)*

191. **(D)** The Fick principle is derived by applying the law of conservation of mass and states that

$$\dot{V}o_2 = \dot{Q}(Cao_2 - C\bar{v}o_2)$$

where $\dot{V}o_2$ is O_2 consumption, $\dot{Q}$ is cardiac output, and Cao_2 and $C\bar{v}o_2$ are arterial and mixed venous O_2 content, respectively.

Thus,

$$\dot{Q} = \frac{Vo_2}{(Cao_2 - C\bar{v}o_2)}; \ \dot{Q} = \frac{300 \text{ ml/min}}{(20 - 15)\text{ml}/100 \text{ ml}} = \frac{6000 \text{ ml}}{\text{min}}$$

Stroke volume × heart rate = cardiac output.

$$\text{Stroke volume} = \frac{\text{Cardiac output}}{\text{Heart rate}} = \frac{6000 \text{ ml/min}}{60/\text{min}} = 100 \text{ ml}.$$

(Berne and Levy, pp 412–413)

192. **(C)** The high rate of blood flow at the placenta and the significant resistance of the placenta to diffusion of O_2 result in blood in the umbilical vein that has a lower P_{O_2} (30 mm Hg) than maternal mixed venous blood. However, the shift in fetal oxyhemoglobin concentration and the Bohr effect all increase the transport of O_2 to fetal tissues. A number of significant differences in circulating patterns are present in the fetus, including shunting of blood across a patent foramen ovale and ductus arteriosus. The net effect of these shunts in the presence of high fetal pulmonary vascular resistance is very low fetal pulmonary blood flow. At birth, these patterns normally are quickly changed to ex utero patterns with high pulmonary perfusion. Since the liver is supplied by umbilical venous blood and the heart and head receive blood before it has mixed with significant amounts of desaturated blood, these important organs receive blood that is relatively high in saturated oxyhemoglobin. *(Berne and Levy, pp 527–529)*

Plasma clearance = Urine conc × Urine Flow / Plasma conc.

193. (D) Cerebral blood flow will increase when Pa_{O_2} is decreased to < 50 mm Hg or when Pa_{CO_2} increases above normal. A decrease in viscosity will also increase cerebral blood flow. Cerebral blood flow is closely linked to brain parenchymal metabolism, and intense activity during a seizure will result in large, widespread increases in blood flow. The brain autoregulates, and consequently an increase in blood pressure is offset by an *increase* in local vascular resistance to maintain constant cerebral blood flow. *(Berne and Levy, pp 523–524)*

194–196. (194-A, 195-D, 196-C) Metabolic acidosis as a result of diabetes mellitus, hypoxemia, or other factors causes HCO_3^- to fall and lower the pH. The increased H^+ ions increase the ventilatory rate by their actions on peripheral chemoreceptors, thus lowering the Pa_{CO_2} and returning the pH toward but not all the way back to normal values.

Hyperventilation will decrease Pa_{O_2} ($\dot{V}_A = [\dot{V}_{CO_2} \times K]/Pa_{CO_2}$) and thus increase $(HCO_3^-)/Pa_{CO_2}$, thereby elevating pH.

Hypoventilation due to overdosage of drugs or CNS pathology results in an increase in Pa_{CO_2}. When there is no renal compensation, the pH will decrease. Normal Pa_{CO_2} and decreased pH are most likely to occur during metabolic acidosis without respiratory compensation. *(West, 1991, pp 498–502)*

197–199. (197-A, 198-A, 199-C) Retinal ganglion cells relay visual information from the retina to other regions of the brain after it has been processed by the retinal network containing the photoreceptors and the horizontal, bipolar, and amacrine cells. The optimal stimulus for a retinal ganglion cell is typically a stationary spot or annulus of light in its circular receptive field. Two types of cell responses may be observed. A ganglion cell may be excited by a spot of light at the center of its receptive field and inhibited by an annulus of light that surrounds the center (an on-center cell). Conversely, inhibition by a central spot of light and excitation by the surrounding annulus may be observed (an off-center cell). Moving stimuli are not optimal for retinal ganglion cells. A stationary bar in any orientation within its receptive field also will generally evoke a brisk response in a retinal ganglion cell. Such a stimulus is not considered optimal, however, because it simultaneously activates both the center and, to a lesser extent, the surrounding area of the receptive field.

The response properties of neurons in the lateral geniculate are for the most part similar to those of retinal ganglion cells, the optimal stimulus also being a small stationary spot or annulus. For this reason, the lateral geniculate is widely considered to be a relay station that faithfully transmits information from the retina to the cortex, with little internal processing of visual information.

In contrast to cells in the retina and the lateral geniculate, the optimal stimulus for the simple cells that are found in layer III of the visual cortex is a stationary bar. To obtain a maximal response, the bar must be held at a specific orientation in the receptive field of the cell. Changes in the orientation of the bar away from this position cause the response to decline. The optimal orientation varies from cell to cell, but neurons within a cortical column tend to respond to the same orientation. The ability to provide a maximal response to moving visual stimuli, such as a bar that is moving across the visual field, is characteristic of complex cells of the visual cortex. *(Ganong, pp 130–134)*

200–204. (200-B, 201-E, 202-D, 203-B, 204-A) In the first stage of slow wave sleep, which is associated with very light sleep, the EEG pattern shows very low voltage waves punctuated by occasional bursts of alpha activity, called sleep spindles. As sleep progresses, frequency of the EEG waveform decreases until it is approximately 2 to 3 cycles per second. This pattern, called delta waves, is characteristic of the deep sleep of slow wave stage 4. Alert wakefulness and REM sleep are both characterized by beta waves, which indicate a high degree of brain activity. Quiet wakefulness is associated with alpha waves. *(Guyton, pp 661–663)*

205–207. (205-A, 206-C, 207-D) Although the early maturation of an ovarian follicle is dependent on the presence of FSH, ovulation is induced by a surge of LH. Although estrogen usually has a negative feedback effect on LH and FSH secretion, the LH surge seems to be a response to elevated estrogen levels. In concert with FSH, LH induces rapid follicular swelling. LH also acts directly on the granulosa cells to cause them to decrease estrogen production as well as to initiate production of small amounts of progesterone. These changes lead to ovulation. FSH is required for Sertoli cells to mediate the development of spermatids into mature sperm. *(Guyton, pp 877, 900–902, 908–910)*

208. (B) With arterial blood pH of 7.33, the patient clearly has an acidosis. The first question you should ask yourself is, "Is it respiratory or nonrespiratory (metabolic)?" If it were respiratory, the Pa_{CO_2} would have been above normal. Since it is lower than normal, this indicates the acidosis is metabolic with some respiratory compensation in response to the acidemia. The low arterial bicarbonate confirms the diagnosis of metabolic acidosis. It is unlikely that the metabolic acidosis is due to diabetic ketoacidosis; if this were the case, you would expect much glucose in the blood and urine. *(Guyton, pp 340–343)*

209. **(C)** In healthy subjects on a normal diet, about 70 mEq of hydrogen ion is produced each day (largely from oxidation of sulfur-containing amino acids). This would produce a progressive metabolic acidosis if the H^+ were not excreted in the urine as NH_4^+ and $H_2PO_4^-$. Both are decreased in the later stages of renal failure (e.g., from chronic glomerulonephritis). Since NH_4^+ excretion plays the major role in disposing of daily H^+, a deficiency in ammonium excretion explains the metabolic acidosis (probably simply a reflection of the diminished number of functioning nephrons). *(Rose, 1981, pp 427–428)*

210. **(D)** The action potentials illustrated must be those of cardiac nodal cells (SA node or AV node). The durations of the action potentials shown are too long for either motor axons (2 mSec) or skeletal muscle fibers (5 mSec). Also the configuration is different. They cannot represent pharmacomechanical coupling in smooth muscle, which has no appreciable action potential at all. They cannot be ventricular Purkinje action potentials as these have: 1) a more negative diastolic component that does not gradually depolarize, 2) a longer duration (200 mSec), and 3) a plateau region. *(Berne and Levy, pp 36,379)*

211. **(C)** One of the principal distinguishing features of nodal cell action potentials is the gradual diastolic depolarization, the so-called pacemaker potential. When the pacemaker potential reaches threshold (dashed line in illustration), an action potential is generated and propagated along conducting pathways to other cardiac fibers (the basis of autorhythmicity of cardiac pacemaker cells). During the diastolic period the outward I_K (or delayed rectifier current mainly responsible for repolarization) is slowly deactivated. At the same time there is activation of poorly selective channels (permeable to both Na^+ and K^+) which gives rise to a slow "funny" inward current due mainly to Na^+. *(Patton et al, pp 792–793)*

212. **(A)** A normal, healthy individual in acid–base balance is represented by point C (pH 7.4, bicarbonate 24 mEq/L, and $Paco_2$, 40 mm Hg). Changes in $Paco_2$, cause changes in pH along the line A-C-D, which is a CO_2 titration curve. Moving either upward or downward along this titration curve represents these changes in pH with changes in $Paco_2$ (to higher or lower CO_2 isobars). There are small secondary changes in bicarbonate due to buffer reactions with nonbicarbonate buffers. These are not *compensatory* changes in bicarbonate concentration. At point A no compensa-

tion in the form of increased renal production of bicarbonate has occurred yet.

213. **(B)** This is respiratory acidosis (as was the previous question) but with some renal compensation in the form of increased production of bicarbonate. Bicarbonate concentration increases upward along the same higher CO_2 isobar of the previous question (going from point A to B). This returns the pH partly back toward normal.

214. **(D)** Just as hypoventilation produces respiratory acidosis, hyperventilation produces respiratory alkalosis, another example of changes along the A-C-D line. In respiratory alkalosis there is a lower $Paco_2$ so that the point on the graph is at a lower CO_2 isobar. As no compensation has yet occurred, there is no reduction in bicarbonate due to renal action. Had there been some renal compensation, the new point would have been E.

215. **(I)** Noncompensated "metabolic" changes in pH occur along the normal CO_2 isobar (for 40 mm Hg), or dashed line F-C-H. If this were metabolic alkalosis with NO respiratory compensation (an unlikely situation), the answer would be point H. However, the alkaline pH causes some inhibition of alveolar ventilation with an increase in $Paco_2$. Thus, point I represents the correct answer for metabolic alkalosis with some respiratory compensation.

216. **(G)** Point F represents a simple uncompensated metabolic acidosis (a rare circumstance). But as the pH falls, alveolar ventilation is stimulated (e.g., Kussmaul breathing in ketoacidosis of diabetes) producing a lower $Paco_2$. Lowering the $Paco_2$ moves the pH back toward normal along a lower CO_2 isobar. *(Guyton, pp 340–343)*

217. **(G)** The second heart sound (S_2) begins with the abrupt closure of the semilunar valves (aortic and pulmonic valves) at the end of ventricular systole and the beginning of isovolumic relaxation.

218. **(D)** The aortic blood pressure oscillates between a peak (called the systolic blood pressure) and a nadir (called the diastolic blood pressure). This nadir is reached just after the beginning of systole when the rising left ventricular pressure equals, or just exceeds, the aortic blood pressure and forces the left ventricular blood to be ejected through the aortic valve. At this time (the end of the isovolumic contraction and the beginning of ejection) the left ventricular pressure essentially equals aortic diastolic blood pressure at point D.

219. **(G)** As the left ventricular pressure falls from its peak, it soon becomes less than that of the aorta. This causes an abrupt closure of the aortic valve,

as blood attempts to flow back into the left ventricle. This sudden closure produces a sharp onset of S_2 which has a snapping quality and is of shorter duration than S_1.

220. **(H)** During ventricular systole the blood returning to the heart from the pulmonary circulation causes a gradual rise in left atrial volume and pressure. When ventricular isovolumic relaxation ends, blood suddenly exits from the left atrium into the left ventricle (beginning of ventricular rapid filling). It is the opening of the mitral valve that brings an end to the rising left atrial pressure. Thus, the peak of the left atrial v wave and the opening of the mitral valve must be simultaneous at point H in the illustration.

221. **(G)** By definition, ventricular systole begins with the beginning of the first heart sound (S_1) and ends with the beginning of the second (S_2). That is, ventricular systole ends at the point at which the aortic valve snaps shut (point G in the illustration).

222. **(C)** At the beginning of isovolumic contraction (which is also the beginning of ventricular systole), the abrupt rise of ventricular pressure, acceleration of some blood back toward the atria, and tension and recoil of atrioventricular valve leaflets as they close, all give rise to the first heart sound (S_1).

223. **(F)** The T wave of the electrocardiogram represents ventricular repolarization (which leads to relaxation). By the peak of the T wave, enough ventricular muscle had begun to relax so that the ventricular pressure starts to fall. Thus, the peak of the T wave and the peak of the ventricular pressure (point F in the illustration) are simultaneous. *(Berne and Levy, pp 407–408)*

224. **(D)** Endogenous and exogenous pyrogens resulting from the presence of infecting pathogenic microorganisms raise the hypothalamic set point and thereby cause a rise in body temperature (fever). Once the patient's temperature has risen to match the newer higher set point, the patient is comfortable, and his new higher temperature is well-regulated around the new set point.

225. **(E)** If the factors originally responsible for the fever are gone (successfully eliminated by the body's immune system), the hypothalamic set point returns to normal. For a while the body's core temperature is above the now normal set point. This has the same effect as if the individual were too hot. The patient begins sweating and complains of "burning up" because of his hot skin (due to vasodilation).

226. **(B)** When the set point is first raised, due to pyrogens, the body temperature is temporarily below the new, higher set point, just as if the body were too cool. The hypothalamus causes the usual responses to produce additional heat (shivering) and to conserve the heat present (skin vasoconstriction, lack of sweating). The patient subjectively feels chilled and seeks to raise his body temperature until he is more comfortable (piles on blankets, sits by the fire, gets a heating pad, etc.). *(Guyton, pp 806–807)*

227. **(C)** What is recorded in all of the examples is the forced expiratory volume in one second (FEV_1). The patient is connected to a spirometer and after taking in as much air as possible (maximal inhalation) is asked to expire as forcefully as he/she can to exhale as much air as possible as rapidly as possible. The volume exhaled in the first second (shaded area of examples) is the FEV_1. The difference between the beginning total lung capacity (TLC) and the residual volume (RV) is the vital capacity. The forced vital capacity (FVC), shown in all but example C, is not always the same as in a less forced measurement. Pattern A represents a normal, healthy adult. The flow rate is high at first (steep downward slope) near the beginning TLC, but then becomes less and less steep as the lung volume decreases until it plateaus (becomes flat) at residual volume and zero flow. Record C represents a patient with an obstructive disease that makes it difficult to force large volumes of air out at a high rate of flow. Thus the slope is less steep than normal, and it takes a long time to reach the residual volume (may take 20 or 30 seconds; this is why pattern C doesn't include FVC). Emphysema, chronic bronchitis, and asthma are common obstructive diseases. Both the TLC and the RV are higher than normal in such patients.

228. **(B)** Record B represents the FEV_1 of a patient with restrictive lung disease (lungs are restricted in volume). Pulmonary fibrosis is a chronic condition that can follow pulmonary inflammation (pneumonitis) brought about by a number of conditions. Other examples of restrictive disease include problems with chest wall movement (Pickwickian syndrome, scoliosis, myasthenia gravis, etc.) and loss of lung compliance (e.g., lack of surfactant, pulmonary edema, fibrosis, etc.). Although flow rates are quite good at any given volume (comparable to that of a normal subject at that same lung volume), the TLC, VC, and RV are all below normal.

229. **(C)** Like the patient in question number 227, this patient (with asthma) has an obstructive disease that slows the rate of forced expiration and takes a long time to reach the reserve volume. At the bedside the same kind of information can be ob-

tained by asking the patient to blow out a lighted match. Patients with obstructive disease have difficulty doing so. *(West, 1992, pp 3–7)*

230. **(G)** Ventricular repolarization is not a propagated phenomenon and does not follow the same path and direction as the preceding depolarization. Rather, it is the result of individual muscle fibers independently undergoing repolarization. Not all ventricular myocardial fibers begin and end repolarization at the same time. Nevertheless, repolarization appears to spread throughout the ventricles over a prolonged period of time (about 0.15 seconds). The T wave is the electrocardiographic manifestation of ventricular repolarization and therefore the point nearest the end of the T wave (point G) marks the end of ventricular repolarization.

231. **(C)** The spread of depolarization through the ventricular conducting system (Bundle of His) has little or no contribution to the electrocardiogram because of its small mass. However, as soon as depolarization is propagated to the myocardial muscle fibers of the interventricular septum and they become depolarized, the Q wave of the QRS complex begins. Thus, point C is nearest the onset of ventricular depolarization.

232. **(A)** A wave of depolarization propagates from the sinoatrial node throughout the atrial myocardial fibers. The effect of this atrial depolarization on the electrocardiogram is to produce the P wave. Thus the point nearest the onset of atrial depolarization is A. *(Guyton, pp 118–128)*

233. **(A)** Isovolumetric relaxation involves a drop in left ventricular pressure with no change in left ventricular volume (hence the term "isovolumetric"). This occurs between points W (point at which the aortic valve closes) and X (point at which the mitral valve opens and ends the isovolumetric period).

234. **(C)** The production of pressure is not very energy efficient (compared with movement of blood). Since the period of isovolumetric contraction produces the majority of the pressure increase of ventricular systole, and over a rather short period of time, it has the highest rate of energy consumption (either measured by ml O_2 consumed per unit time or by mols ATP hydrolized per unit time).

235. **(D)** The left ventricle does positive external work (force acting through distance) only when it ejects blood under pressure. Stroke work is approximated by stroke volume times mean pressure (cm^3 × dynes/cm^2 = dynes–cm, or ergs). The most accurate measure of positive external work can be obtained from the area contained within the pres-

sure–volume loop. Until something is moved, no external work can be performed by definition. Movement of blood as ejection of stroke volume begins at point Z (point at which the aortic valve opens) and ends at point W (point at which the aortic valve shuts). *(Guyton, pp 104–106; West, 1991, pp 250–256)*

236. **(B)** Of the five pressure–volume loops illustrated, only two have stroke volumes greater than normal (loops B and E). Which one of the two that has increased contractility can be determined from the location of the end–systolic pressure–volume point. The end–systolic pressure–volume point for loop E, like those of loops C and D, is on the same line as for the normal individual (diagonal line in illustration). Loop B, however, has an end–systolic pressure–volume point at a higher level (would fall on a end–systolic pressure–volume line that begins at about the same intercept with the abscissa, but has a steeper slope than for normal contractility). Thus loop B represents a pressure–volume loop for increased contractility.

237. **(C)** The actual preload on myocardial fibers is the stretch placed on them at the end of diastole just before the beginning of systole. This stretch determines the resting length of the fibers prior to contraction. For practical purposes the end–diastolic volume is used as a convenient index of preload (the greater the end–diastolic volume, the greater the stretch). The pressure–volume loop with the lowest end–diastolic volume, and therefore the lowest preload, is loop C. *(West, 1991, pp 224–231)*

238. **(D)** The direct source of energy for muscle contraction comes from ATP hydrolysis. The most efficient means of generating new ATP to replace that utilized is through aerobic metabolism (mainly by the Krebs cycle). Aerobic metabolism depends on the supply of oxygen to muscle and cannot immediately rise to supply ATP as fast as it is utilized (period B of illustration). This period is one of an "oxygen deficit." Time is required for sufficient increase in cardiac output and pulmonary ventilation to increase enough to supply oxygen at the rate needed. Between the onset of exercise (at "begin work" in illustration) and the highest level of oxygen supply and consumption (plateau in illustration), energy is mainly supplied by anaerobic depletion of high energy phosphate stores (ATP and CP) and anaerobic glycolysis. Resynthesis of these stores requires that $\dot{V}o_2$ remain above normal for a while after cessation of exercise (after "end work" in illustration). This period of time (period D in illustration) is described as repayment of an "oxygen debt."

239. **(B)** This is the period of oxygen deficit during which part of the energy requirements are being met anaerobically by depletion of high energy phosphates (period B of illustration).

240. **(C)** At the onset of exercise the cardiac output and pulmonary ventilation both begin to rise. However, it takes time for them to reach the highest level necessary to sustain oxygen delivery to the muscles at a sufficient rate. *(McArdle, Katch, and Katch, pp 123–141)*

241. **(B)** The proximal tubule reabsorbs the majority (about two-thirds) of filtered salt and water. This is done in an essentially iso-osmotic manner. Both the luminal salt concentration and the luminal osmolality remain constant (and equal to plasma values) along the entire length of the proximal tubule. Water and salt are reabsorbed proportionally because the water is dependent on and coupled with the active reabsorption of Na^+. The water permeability of the proximal tubule is high and therefore a significant transepithelial osmotic gradient is not possible (a minute gradient of as little as one milliosmole/liter may exist). Sodium is actively transported mainly by basolateral sodium pumps into the lateral intercellular spaces; water follows. *(Vander, pp 90–92)*

242. **(D)** The thick ascending limb of the loop of Henle has very low permeability to water. Since there are no regulatory mechanisms to alter its permeability, it remains poorly permeable to water under all circumstances. Sodium and chloride are transported out of the luminal fluid into the surrounding interstitial spaces (they are reabsorbed). Since water must remain behind (is not reabsorbed), the solute concentration becomes less and less (the luminal fluid becomes more dilute). This is one of the principal mechanisms (along with diminution of ADH secretion) for the production of a dilute, hypo-osmotic urine (e.g., as in water diuresis). *(Vander, pp 94–95,100–105)*

243. **(B)** In addition to ADH's well-known effect on collecting duct permeability to water, it also affects urea permeability. However, there is a slight difference; ADH increases permeability to water throughout the collecting duct, while its action to increase permeability to urea is limited to the medullary portion of the collecting duct. In the presence of ADH, urea can diffuse out of the medullary collecting duct into the interstitium. Much of it enters the lumen of the thin ascending limb of Henle's loop. This luminal urea flows to the distal nephron only to be recycled over and over again. This cycle of urea movement adds considerable solute to the medullary interstitium, thereby helping to maintain its normally high osmolality. *(Vander, p 106)*

244. **(A)** The adrenal cortex has three layers of secretory cells that produce steroid hormones. Aldosterone is a mineralocorticoid hormone that is primarily involved with regulation of sodium and potassium transport and excretion by the kidneys. It is produced by the thin, outermost layer of cortical cells, the zona glomerulosa. Its rate of secretion is mainly controlled by the level of plasma potassium and by angiotensin II. Plasma sodium concentration and ACTH have less prominent influences on aldosterone secretion. *(Guyton, pp 842–846)*

245. **(C)** This is a fairly easy one to answer because the name of the hormone describes its principal function: natriuresis (stimulation of urinary Na^+ excretion). ANP is released from atrial cells in response to increased stretch of atrial walls (e.g., by an increase in blood volume). ANP also has vasodilator effects on arterioles (the principal resistance vessels) and veins (the capacitance vessels). It is thought to play a role in the regulation of blood volume and arterial blood pressure. *(Berne and Levy, pp 421–422)*

246. **(E)** In both types of muscle, muscle fibers are connected together by gap junctions (nexi). Gap junctions appear to have a small gap between adjacent cell membranes (hence their name). Actually, there are some structures within the gap that actually make connections between the two cell membranes. These connections within gap junctions are hexagonal-shaped structures called *connexons*. Each connexon contains a central passageway or pore. These are of particular importance as low-resistance pathways through which currents generated by action potentials can flow and maintain propagation. Layers of cells with gap junctions (and connexons) act like functional syncytiums in that the individual cells are electrically coupled together. Cardiac muscle and smooth muscle are good examples of such electrically coupled cells. This permits a virtually simultaneous contraction of all the cells together when electrically stimulated by an action potential. *(Berne and Levy, pp 61,310,398)*

247. **(A)** When repetitively stimulated, skeletal muscle fibers continue to contract even if immersed in a Ca^{++}-free medium. Thus *all* the Ca^{++} needed for contraction comes from within (from intracellular stores in the sarcoplasmic reticulum). This is not the case with cardiac and smooth muscle. Ca^{++} in the extracellular medium of cardiac fibers is essential for contraction. Removal of extracellular Ca^{++} first results in decreased contractile force and eventually in the absence of contractions. Sustained contraction by smooth muscle is also dependent on extracellular Ca^{++}. Both cardiac and smooth muscle have a sarcoplasmic reticulum

Cardiac + smooth muscle Have ① gap junctions ② extracellular Ca^{++}

that releases Ca^{++} into the myoplasm. However, in addition, both depend upon the entry of Ca^{++} across the sarcolemma from the extracellular side. *(Berne and Levy, pp 292–293,320–321,399–403)*

248. **(A)** The lungs will expand to a higher volume during inhalation as a result of an increase in the translung pressure, or distending pressure (P_{alv} – P_{pl}). Static compliance is measured under conditions of no airflow (stepwise changes in volume with no airflow during measurement of distending pressure). Thus, P_{alv} is ambient atmospheric pressure, or zero reference pressure, and P_{pl} is a negative intrapleural pressure that becomes even more negative with each step increase in volume. With each step increase in volume is a corresponding step increase in distending pressure. Compliance is $\Delta V/\Delta P$. *(Berne and Levy, pp 563–565)*

249. **(D)** The thick filaments (myosin) and the thin filaments (actin) overlap each other and interact by cross-bridges. During normal contractions none of the individual filaments actually shorten in length. Instead, they slide by each other as the muscle sarcomeres shorten. In principle this is similar to what happens when you push an extended telescope together to make it shorter. None of the individual telescope sections become shorter, but the entire telescope does as the sections have increased overlap with each other. *(West, 1991, p 71)*

250. **(C)** The thick and thin filaments of myofibrils that make up both skeletal and cardiac muscle fibers are aligned repetitively in transverse register. This gives rise to the striated appearance of these fibers as seen with a microscope. *(Berne and Levy, p 283)*

251. **(C)** The volume of air remaining in the lungs after a maximal effort to exhale all the air possible (i.e., after your best effort to "empty" your lungs) is the residual volume. This volume cannot be measured directly by a spirometer, which measures only change in volume. Since you cannot voluntarily change your lung volume below the residual volume, the spirometer cannot measure it. Other methods (e.g., body plethysmography, inert gas dilution) must be used to measure residual volume. *(Berne and Levy, pp 557–558)*

252. **(A)** When the dome-shaped diaphragm contracts it becomes more flattened. The lungs, separated from the diaphragm by a very thin layer of fluid (or liquid flim) between pleural membranes, are pulled downward. That is, they follow the movement of the diaphragm as it flattens (just as two wet glass slides tend to stick together). Elastic recoil forces in the lungs tend to resist expansion and pull the lungs in the opposite direction. These opposing forces make the normally negative intrapleural pressure (e.g., the intrapleural pressure at FRC might be –3.5 cm H_2O) even more negative (e.g., perhaps to –7 cm H_2O). *(Berne and Levy, pp 567–568)*

253. **(A)** The product of tidal volume (volume moved in or out with each breath) times the frequency or breathing rate (number of breaths/minute) is the total ventilation per minute (also called minute ventilation). In this case the total ventilation is 600 ml times 12 breaths/minute = 7200 ml/minute. As stated in the problem, the alveolar ventilation (air ventilating the respiratory zone for gas exchange each minute) is 6000 ml/minute. The difference is that part of the total ventilation going only to non-exchanging conducting airways = 1200 ml/minute, or 100 ml per breath at 12 breaths/minute. This 100 ml is the dead space volume. *(West, 1991, pp 524–525,526–527)*

254. **(C)** Either severe chronic lung disease or an overdose of heroin would have caused respiratory acidosis due to abnormally high arterial P_{CO_2} (not low P_{CO_2} which this subject has). A lowlander at high altitude for two weeks would have had both low P_{O_2} and low P_{CO_2} like this subject, but would have had an abnormally low plasma bicarbonate and a more nearly normal pH due to renal compensation in the form of bicarbonate excretion. Acute aspirin overdose in adults usually presents first with a respiratory alkalosis, which includes a low P_{CO_2}, but not a low P_{O_2}. Breathing a low oxygen gas mixture is similar to being at high altitude, but if this is only for a few minutes there will be no time for renal compensation. The hypoxia stimulates hyperventilation, which lowers the P_{CO_2}. The slightly lowered bicarbonate is due to buffering by nonbicarbonate buffers. Decreased P_{CO_2} results in decreased H_2CO_3. Decreased H_2CO_3 results in the following reaction being pulled to the right:

$$HCO_3^- + HBuf \rightarrow Buf^- + H_2CO_3$$

thus lowering the plasma bicarbonate to slightly below normal. Had there been time for renal compensation, the bicarbonate would have been much lower. *(Rose, 1989, pp 580–588)*

BIBLIOGRAPHY

Berne RM, Levy MN, eds. *Physiology.* 3rd ed. St. Louis: Mosby Year Book; 1993

Davenport HW. *The ABC of Acid-Base Chemistry.* 6th ed. Chicago: The University of Chicago Press; 1974.

Davenport HW. *A Digest of Digestion.* 2nd ed. Chicago: Year Book Medical Publishers, Inc.; 1978

Ganong WF. *Review of Medical Physiology.* 14th ed. Los Altos, CA: Lange Medical Publications; 1989

Guyton AC. *Textbook of Medical Physiology.* 8th ed. Philadelphia: WB Saunders Co.; 1991

Johnson LR. *Gastrointestinal Physiology.* 3rd ed. St. Louis: CV Mosby Co.; 1985

Kandel ER, Schwartz JH, and Jessel TM. *Principles of Neural Science.* 3rd ed. New York: Elsevier; 1991.

McArdle WD, Katch FI, and Katch VL. *Exercise Physiology.* 3rd ed. Philadelphia: Lea & Febiger; 1991

Mountcastle VB. *Medical Physiology.* 14th ed. St. Louis: CV Mosby Co.; 1980

Patton HD, Fuchs AF et al. *Textbook of Physiology.* 21st ed. Philadelphia: WB Saunders Co.; 1989

Petersen OH, Maruyama Y. *Nature.* February 1984

Rose DB. *Clinical Physiology of Acid–base and Electrolyte Disorders.* 3rd ed. New York: McGraw-Hill Information Services Co.; 1989

Rose DB. *Pathophysiology of Renal Diseases.* New York: McGraw-Hill Book Co.; 1981

Vander AJ. *Renal Physiology.* 3rd ed. New York: McGraw-Hill Inc.; 1985

West JB, ed. *Best and Taylor's Physiological Basis of Medical Practice.* 12th ed. Baltimore: Williams & Wilkins; 1991

West JB. *Pulmonary Pathophysiology—The Essentials.* 4th ed. Baltimore: Williams & Wilkins; 1992

Subspecialty List: Physiology

Question Number and Subspecialty

128. Capillary exchange
129. Nervous system
130. Excretory function
131. Temperature
132. Nervous system
133. Nervous system
134. Nervous system
135. Nervous system
136. Nervous system
137. Special senses
138. Special senses
139. Nervous system
140. Nervous system
141. Nervous system
142. Nervous system
143. Cardiovascular regulation
144. Gastrointestinal
145. Gastrointestinal
146. Endocrinology
147. Gastrointestinal
148. Endocrinology
149. General physiology
150. Nervous system
151. General physiology
152. General physiology
153. Cardiovascular regulation
154. General physiology
155. Special senses
156. Gastrointestinal
157. Special senses
158. Mechanics of breathing
159. Pulmonary gas exchange
160. Regulation of respiration
161. Excretory function
162. Exercise
163. Temperature
164. Cardiac cycle
165. Cardiac cycle
166. Cardiac cycle
167. Cardiovascular system
168. Endocrinology
169. Endocrinology
170. Endocrinology

171. Blood gas transport
172. Body fluids
173. Excretory function
174. Mechanics of breathing
175. Pulmonary gas exchange
176. Pulmonary gas exchange
177. Body fluids
178. Excretory function
179. Pulmonary gas exchange
180. Pulmonary gas exchange
181. Cardiovascular
182. Fluids and electrolytes
183. Pulmonary gas exchange
184. Pulmonary gas exchange
185. Regulation of respiration
186. Excretory function
187. Excretory function
188. Excretory function
189. Excretory function
190. Exercise
191. Cardiac cycle
192. Circulation in specific organs
193. Circulation in specific organs
194. Regulation of respiration
195. Regulation of respiration
196. Regulation of respiration
197. Sensory mechanisms
198. Sensory mechanisms
199. Sensory mechanisms
200. Nervous system
201. Nervous system
202. Nervous system
203. Nervous system
204. Nervous system
205. Endocrinology
206. Endocrinology
207. Endocrinology
208. Renal
209. Renal
210. Cardiac electrotherapy
211. Cardiac electrotherapy
212. Respiratory/Renal
213. Respiratory/Renal
214. Respiratory/Renal
215. Respiratory/Renal

216. Respiratory/Renal
217. Cardiac cycle
218. Cardiac cycle
219. Cardiac cycle
220. Cardiac cycle
221. Cardiac cycle
222. Cardiac cycle
223. Cardiac cycle
224. Circulation in specific organs
225. General physiology
226. Nervous system
227. Sensory mechanisms
228. Endocrinology
229. Nervous system
230. Nervous system
231. Endocrinology
232. Endocrinology
233. Endocrinology
234. Endocrinology

235. Endocrinology
236. Cardiovascular regulation
237. Nervous system
238. General physiology
239. Special senses
240. Body fluids
241. General physiology
242. General physiology
243. Fluid balance
244. General physiology
245. General physiology
246. General physiology
247. Gastrointestinal
248. Respiratory
249. Muscle/Membrane
250. Muscle/Membrane
251. Respiratory
252. Respiratory
253. Respiratory
254. Respiratory

CHAPTER 3

Biochemistry
Questions

DIRECTIONS (Questions 255 through 305): Each of the numbered items or incomplete statements in this section is followed by answers or by completions of the statement. Select the ONE lettered answer or completion that is BEST in each case.

255. Free purine and pyrimidine bases and nucleosides can be converted to the corresponding nucleoside 5′-monophosphate via salvage pathways. These pathways are important for conversion of certain antimetabolites that are employed for chemotherapy. Which of the following antimetabolites would require salvage for proper function?

   (A) azaserine
   (B) methotrexate
   (C) 5-fluorouracil
   (D) allopurinol
   (E) none of the above

256. In muscle tissue, acetoacetate can be converted to acetoacetyl-CoA by the following reaction:

$$\text{Acetoacetate} + \text{coenzyme A} + \text{ATP} \rightarrow \text{acetoacetyl-CoA} + \text{ADP} + P_i$$

   How many moles of ATP (net) can be derived by muscle on conversion of 1 mol of acetoacetate to CO_2 and water?

   (A) 11
   (B) 12
   (C) 22
   (D) 23
   (E) 24

257. Lactate that is released into the circulation can be converted back to glucose in

   (A) liver
   (B) heart muscle
   (C) erythrocytes
   (D) adipose tissue
   (E) brain

258. All of the following are involved in movement of CO_2 from peripheral tissues to the lungs EXCEPT

   (A) carbamate
   (B) carbonic anhydrase
   (C) CO_2 bound to the iron of hemoglobin (Hb)
   (D) bicarbonate
   (E) dissolved CO_2

259. All of the following are true for smooth muscle, cardiac muscle, skeletal muscle, and macrophages EXCEPT that they

   (A) contain actin
   (B) respond to nervous stimulation
   (C) contain myosin
   (D) have a cytoskeleton
   (E) use ATP for contraction

260. The standard free-energy change ($\Delta G^{\circ\prime}$) for the hydrolysis of phosphoenolpyruvate is −14.8 kcal/mol and that for ATP hydrolysis to ADP and orthophosphate (P_i) is −7.3 kcal/mol. For the production of phosphoenolpyruvate by the reaction

$$\text{ATP} + \text{pyruvate} \rightleftharpoons \text{phosphoenolpyruvate} + \text{ADP} + P_i$$
   the $\Delta G^{\circ\prime}$ is

   (A) +7.5 kcal/mol
   (B) −7.5 kcal/mol
   (C) +22.1 kcal/mol
   (D) −22.1 kcal/mol
   (E) −14.8 kcal/mol

261. The carbohydrate employed in the biosynthesis of nucleic acids is made in which of the following pathways?

   (A) glycolysis
   (B) gluconeogenesis
   (C) urea cycle
   (D) citric acid cycle
   (E) pentose phosphate pathway

262. What is the pH of a buffer solution containing 0.05 mol/L KH_2PO_4 and 0.15 mol/L K_2HPO_4? The pK_1 of phosphoric acid is 1.96 and pK_2 is 6.8.

(A) 4.38

(B) 6.35

(C) 6.80

(D) 7.28

(E) 8.76

263. The ATPase activity required for muscle contraction is located in

(A) myosin

(B) troponin

(C) myokinase

(D) sarcoplasmic reticulum

(E) actin

264. All of the following are allosteric effectors regulating the glycolytic pathway EXCEPT

(A) glucose 6-phosphate

(B) ATP

(C) fructose 6-phosphate

(D) citrate

(E) AMP

265. Which of the following saccharides enters glycolysis at the level of three-carbon intermediates?

(A) lactose

(B) mannose

(C) galactose

(D) maltose

(E) fructose

266. The primary positive control of gluconeogenesis is exerted by

(A) high acetyl-CoA levels

(B) high citrate levels

(C) low citrate levels

(D) low ATP levels

(E) high ATP levels

267. All of the following are involved in the cascade of events leading to glycogenolysis in skeletal muscle EXCEPT

(A) adenylate cyclase

(B) phosphorylase kinase

(C) phosphorylase

(D) protein kinase

(E) glucagon

268. Fluorouracil is a drug that is used in the chemotherapy of several solid tumors. The mechanism of action of fluorouracil is that

(A) it is an inhibitor of ribonucleotide reductase

(B) it is an inhibitor of thymidylate synthase

(C) it is an inhibitor of thymidine kinase

(D) it is an inhibitor of de novo pyrimidine biosynthesis

(E) it is an inhibitor of de novo purine biosynthesis

269. For determination of the K_m of an enzyme, it is necessary to know

(A) the molecular weight of the enzyme

(B) the initial velocity of the enzyme-catalyzed reaction at several different substrate concentrations

(C) the turnover number of the enzyme

(D) the equilibrium constant of the enzyme-catalyzed reaction

(E) the initial velocity of the enzyme-catalyzed reaction at several different enzyme concentrations

270. Which of the following is the single most important force in stabilizing protein tertiary structure?

(A) peptide bonds

(B) disulfide bonds

(C) hydrogen bonds

(D) polar interactions

(E) hydrophobic interactions

271. The $\Delta G^{\circ\prime}$ for the sum of the reactions leading to the activation and transfer of amino acids to tRNA is close to zero.

$$\text{Amino} + \text{ATP} + \text{tRNA} + H_2O \rightleftharpoons \text{aminoacyl-tRNA} + \text{AMP} + 2\,P_i$$

The synthesis of aminoacyl-tRNA is driven by

(A) hydrolysis of pyrophosphate (PP_i)

(B) aminoacyl-tRNA synthetase

(C) hydrolysis of ATP

(D) formation of the phosphate ester of aminoacyl-tRNA

(E) formation of the phosphate ester of an intermediate aminoacyl-AMP

272. Glucose is phosphorylated in liver by either of two enzymes, hexokinase and glucokinase. The K_M of hexokinase or glucokinase for glucose is approximately 1×10^{-5} M and 1×10^{-2} M, respectively. The normal glucose concentration in blood is approximately 135 mg/100 ml (approximately 0.75×10^{-2} M). When the blood glucose level is 75 mg/100 ml, the rate of glucose phosphorylation in liver may change because

(A) the rate of the hexokinase-catalyzed reaction will drop but that of the glucokinase-catalyzed reaction will remain unchanged

(B) the rates of both enzyme-catalyzed reactions will drop

(C) the rates of both enzyme-catalyzed reactions will not be affected much

(D) the rate of the glucokinase-catalyzed reaction will increase but that of the hexokinase-catalyzed reaction will be approximately the same

(E) the rate of the glucokinase-catalyzed reaction will drop but that of the hexokinase-catalyzed reaction will be approximately the same

273. All of the following statements concerning the activation of free fatty acids prior to β oxidation are true EXCEPT that

(A) only long-chain fatty acids are activated

(B) activation occurs within the mitochondrial matrix

(C) activation occurs outside the mitochondrial matrix

(D) the carboxyl groups of fatty acids form thioester linkages with CoA

(E) the activation reaction is made irreversible by the hydrolysis of PP_i

274. The key regulatory enzyme of fatty acid synthesis is

(A) citrate cleavage enzyme

(B) ATP citrate lyase

(C) acetyl-CoA carboxylase

(D) malonyl-CoA decarboxylase

(E) malonyl transacylase

275. All of the following reaction sequences in cholesterol biosynthesis are unique to cholesterol biosynthesis EXCEPT the

(A) formation of 3-hydroxy-3-methylglutaryl CoA from acetyl-CoA

(B) demethylation of lanosterol

(C) cyclization of squalene to form lanosterol

(D) formation of mevalonic acid from 3-hydroxy-3-methylglutaryl-CoA

(E) formation of isoprenoid isomers from mevalonic acid

276. The major site of regulation of cholesterol synthesis is

(A) cyclization of squalene to lanosterol

(B) 3-hydroxy-3-methylglutaryl-CoA synthase

(C) 3-hydroxy-3-methylglutaryl-CoA lyase

(D) 3-hydroxy-3-methylglutaryl-CoA reductase

(E) synthesis of squalene from isoprenoid isomers

277. All of the following are phosphoglycerides found in plasma membranes of mammalian cells EXCEPT

(A) phosphatidyl ethanolamine

(B) sphingomyelin

(C) phosphatidyl inositol

(D) phosphatidyl serine

(E) lecithin

278. In adipocytes, a lack of glucose is known to

(A) cause an inhibition of lipolysis

(B) result in glycerol 3-phosphate synthesis

(C) lead to an inhibition of triacylglycerol synthesis

(D) allow gluconeogenesis to proceed

(E) inhibit ketogenesis

279. Which of the following occurs in the lipidosis known as Tay-Sachs disease?

(A) synthesis of a specific ganglioside is excessive

(B) xanthomas due to cholesterol deposition are observed

(C) phosphoglycerides accumulate in the brain

(D) ganglioside GM_2 is not catabolized by lysosomal enzymes

(E) synthesis of a specific ganglioside is decreased

280. In diabetes, the increased production of ketone bodies is primarily a result of

(A) elevated acetyl-CoA levels in skeletal muscle

(B) a substantially increased rate of fatty acid oxidation by hepatocytes

(C) increased gluconeogenesis

(D) decreased cyclic AMP levels in adipocytes

(E) an increase in the rate of the citric acid cycle

Questions 281 through 283

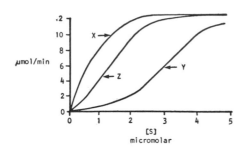

281. Assuming that curve Z represents the plot of an allosteric enzyme with no additions, curve X represents

    (A) an allosteric enzyme with a positive modulator
    (B) a noncompetitively inhibited enzyme
    (C) an allosteric enzyme with an increased K_m
    (D) an allosteric enzyme with a negative modulator
    (E) an irreversibly inhibited enzyme

282. Assuming that all of the curves shown represent the same allosteric enzyme under different conditions, in going from left to right

    (A) the V_{max} is increased
    (B) cooperative binding of substrate is decreasing
    (C) the concentration of a negative modulator is increasing
    (D) the K_m is decreasing
    (E) the concentration of a needed cofactor is increasing

283. The K_m for curve Y is

    (A) 2 µmol/min
    (B) 3 µmol/L
    (C) 5 µmol/L
    (D) 12 µmol/min
    (E) not available in the data given

284. An overdose of insulin in diabetic persons leads to

    (A) hypoglycemia
    (B) glucosuria
    (C) ketonuria
    (D) hyperglycemia
    (E) ketonemia

285. The pituitary prohormone pro-opiocortin is the precursor of all of the following hormones EXCEPT

    (A) thyroid-stimulating hormone (TSH)
    (B) melanocyte-stimulating hormone (MSH)
    (C) adrenocorticotropin (ACTH)
    (D) β-endorphin
    (E) γ-lipotropin

286. Consumption of raw eggs, which contain the protein avidin, could lead to a deficiency resulting in

    (A) an inhibition of decarboxylation reactions
    (B) an inability to form acetylcholine
    (C) a decrease in CoA formation
    (D) an increase in transaminations
    (E) an inhibition of carboxylation reactions

287. Both glutamate transaminase and alanine transaminase require a prosthetic group derived from

    (A) vitamin B_6 (pyridoxine)
    (B) vitamin B_1 (thiamine)
    (C) vitamin B_{12} (cobalamin)
    (D) vitamin B_2 (riboflavin)
    (E) biotin

288. The active form of the cofactor required for oxidative decarboxylation reactions is

    (A) thiamine monophosphate
    (B) thiamine
    (C) thiamine pyrophosphate
    (D) thiamine triphosphate
    (E) hydroxyethyl thiamine prophosphate

289. Which of the following is quantitatively the major contributor to routine clinical measurements of circulating plasma cholesterol concentrations?

    (A) chylomicrons
    (B) low-density lipoproteins (LDLs)
    (C) high-density lipoproteins (HDLs)
    (D) intermediate-density lipoproteins (IDLs)
    (E) very low density lipoproteins (VLDLs)

290. A deficiency in the enzyme galactose 1-phosphate uridyl transferase results in

    (A) low levels of glucose 1-phosphate
    (B) high levels of uridine diphosphate (UDP)-glucose
    (C) high levels of UDP-galactose
    (D) high levels of blood galactose
    (E) high levels of blood glucose

291. Liver conversion of bilirubin to the hydrophilic form secreted in bile involves

    (A) decarboxylation
    (B) conjugation with glucuronic acid

(C) the reduced form of nicotinamine adenine dinucleotide phosphate (NADPH)-dependent reduction to biliverdin

(D) conjugation with glycine

(E) esterification with taurine

292. Activated core oligosaccharides that are transferred to the asparagine of proteins are carried by

(A) guanosine diphosphate (GDP)-mannose

(B) N-acetylglucosamine

(C) dolichol phosphate

(D) N-acetylgalactosamine

(E) UDP-glucose

293. All of the following statements concerning fatty acid synthesis are true EXCEPT that

(A) a decarboxylation takes place

(B) the reductant is NADPH

(C) most of the intermediates are bonded to CoA

(D) a carboxylation takes place

(E) the reactions occur in the cytosol

294. Which of the following is considered to be rate limiting in detoxification of ethanol in alcoholic individuals?   *Alcohol → Acetaldehyde ↓ acetal*

(A) the oxidized form of nicotinamide adenine dinucleotide (NAD+)

(B) the oxidized form of flavin adenine dinucleotide (FAD)

(C) the oxidized form of nicotinamide adenine dinucleotide phosphate (NADP+)

(D) alcohol dehydrogenase

(E) acetaldehyde dehydrogenase

295. Concerning the malate-aspartate shuttle, all of the following are correct EXCEPT that

(A) the shuttle is bidirectional with respect to electron transfer between cytosol and mitochondria

(B) both cytosolic and mitochondrial NADH serve as electron transporters

(C) two ATP are formed for each pair of electrons transferred from cytosolic NADH to mitochondrial electron transport

(D) oxaloacetate is an intermediate

(E) α-ketoglutarate is an intermediate

296. The steps of the pathway for β oxidation of palmitic acid differ from those of the biosynthetic pathway in all of the following respects EXCEPT

(A) acyl group carrier

(B) pyridine nucleotide specificity

(C) effect of citrate

(D) β-hydroxyacyl intermediate

(E) intracellular location

297. Which of the following reactions is the major oxidation reaction of energy metabolism in erythrocytes?

(A) NADPH $\rightleftharpoons$ NADP+

(B) FADH $\rightleftharpoons$ FAD

(C) dihydroxyacetone phosphate + NADH $\rightleftharpoons$ glycerol 3-phosphate + NAD+

(D) pyruvate + NADH $\rightleftharpoons$ lactate + NAD+

(E) acetaldehyde + NADH $\rightleftharpoons$ ethanol + NAD+

298. The affinity of Hb for O_2 is increased by

(A) the formation of salt bridges in Hb

(B) the cross-linking of the β-chains of Hb

(C) lowering of pH

(D) decreases in 2,3-diphosphoglycerate (DPG)

(E) increases in the partial pressure of CO_2

299. An inherited metabolic disorder of carbohydrate metabolism characterized by higher than normal levels of glycolytic intermediates in most cells and a low O_2 affinity of erythrocyte Hb is the result of a deficiency in

(A) pyruvate kinase

(B) hexokinase

(C) aldolase

(D) phosphofructokinase

(E) glucokinase

300. The increased intracellular concentrations of 5-phosphoribosyl-1-pryophosphate (PRPP) and urate in the genetic hyperuricemia called the Lesch-Nyhan syndrome is most likely a consequence of

(A) allopurinol inhibition of xanthine formation

(B) increased purine synthesis

(C) elevated synthesis of hypoxanthine

(D) deficiency of hypoxanthine-guanine phosphoribosyltransferase (HGPRT)

(E) elevated PRPP synthetase activity

301. Although complete blocks of any step of the urea cycle are incompatible with life, inherited partial enzymatic defects have been diagnosed. Mental retardation, episodic vomiting, and lethargy are caused by the diseases. The biochemical hallmark of almost all of these deficiencies is

(A) high blood levels of ammonia

(B) excess accumulation of urea

(C) decreases in aspartate concentrations

(D) gout

(E) increases in the amount of α-ketoglutarate

CARRIER GROUP FOR Fatty Acid syn — ACP
" " " " " Oxid — CoA

302. All of the following are feedback inhibitors of either purine or pyrimidine synthesis EXCEPT

(A) adenosine monophosphate (AMP)
(B) thymidine monophosphate (TMP)
(C) guanosine monophosphate (GMP)
(D) uridine monophosphate (UMP)
(E) cytidine triphosphate (CTP)

303. In the presence of a poison that uncouples oxidative phosphorylation, what would be the net energy yield of the complete oxidation of 1 mol equivalent of glucose in muscle?

(A) 1 mol equivalent ATP
(B) 2 mol equivalent ATP
(C) 3 mol equivalent ATP
(D) 4 mol equivalent ATP
(E) 5 mol equivalent ATP

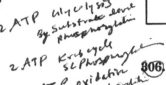
2 ATP Glycolysis By substrate level phosphorylation
2 ATP Krebs cycle SL Phosphoryl
32 ATP oxidative phosphoryl
36

304. In the complete oxidation of glucose by muscle cells, the phosphorus/O_2 ratio is

(A) 2
(B) 3
(C) 4
(D) 36
(E) 38

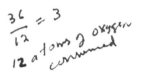
$\frac{36}{12} = 3$
12 atoms of oxygen consumed

305. Which of the following steps is common to both gluconeogenesis and glycolysis?

(A) fructose 6-phosphate to glucose 6-phosphate
(B) pyruvate to oxaloacetate
(C) glucose 6-phosphate to glucose
(D) fructose 1,6-diphosphate to fructose 6-phosphate
(E) oxaloacetate to phosphoenolpyruvate

DIRECTIONS (Questions 306 through 345): Each set of matching questions in this section consists of a list of up to twenty-six lettered options followed by several numbered items. For each item, select the ONE lettered option that is most closely associated with it. Each lettered heading may be selected once, more than once, or not at all.

Questions 306 through 308

For each item described, select the letter in the figure with which it is associated.

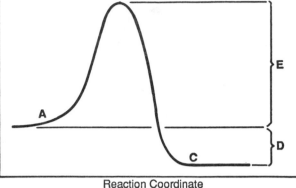

Reaction Coordinate

306. Transition state

307. Energy of activation for the reaction

308. ΔG for the reaction

Questions 309 through 311

For each of the citric acid cycle reactions shown, indicate the statement that applies.

(A) requires a flavoprotein enzyme
(B) requires coenzyme A
(C) requires ATP
(D) yields GTP
(E) yields CO_2

309. Isocitrate → α-ketoglutarate

310. Succinyl-CoA → succinate

311. Succinate → fumarate

Questions 312 through 315

For each reaction described below, choose the enzyme with which it is associated.

(A) glycogen phosphorylase
(B) glycogen synthase
(C) glucose 6-phosphate dehydrogenase
(D) glucokinase
(E) glucose 6-phosphatase

312. Catalyzes a reaction in which inorganic phosphate is a substrate

313. Catalyzes a reaction in which ATP is a substrate

314. Catalyzes a reaction in which UDP-glucose is a substrate

315. Catalyzes a reaction in which glucose is a product

Questions 316 through 319

For each description below, choose the amino acid with which it is associated.

(A) serine
(B) glutamine
(C) glutamate
(D) aspartate
(E) asparagine

316. The common intermediate for the entry of several amino acids into the citric acid cycle

317. A major source of carbon for the one-carbon pool

318. Can be formed by the one-step transamination of an intermediate of the citric acid cycle

319. One-step transamination of it forms a citric acid cycle intermediate

Questions 320 through 322

For each description below, choose the substance with which it is associated.

(A) hydroxyproline
(B) O-phosphoserine
(C) γ-carboxyglutamate
(D) D-valine
(E) cystine

320. Is present in large amounts in keratin

321. Occurs in prothrombin

322. Can be found in collagen

Questions 323 and 324

For each description below, choose the structure with which it is associated.

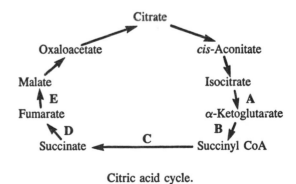

323. Found only in DNA

324. Forms dimers on exposure of DNA to ultraviolet light

Questions 325 and 326

For each step described in the citric acid cycle, choose the lettered point on the diagram with which it is associated.

Citric acid cycle.

325. Step at which flavin nucleotide is reduced

326. Step at which substrate level phosphorylation occurs

Questions 327 and 328

For each description below, choose the correct enzyme based on the data in the table.

Enzyme	K_m (M)	k_{cat} (sec^{-1})
(A) chymotrypsin	5×10^{-3}	100
(B) lysozyme	6×10^{-6}	0.5
(C) carbonic anhydrase	8×10^{-3}	600,000
(D) penicillinase	5×10^{-5}	2000
(E) tyrosyl-tRNA synthetase	1×10^{-5}	40

327. The enzyme with the greatest affinity for its substrate

328. The enzyme with the greatest catalytic efficiency

Questions 329 and 330

For each description below, choose the lettered point in the pathway with which it is associated.

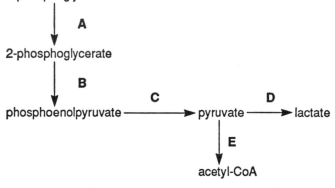

329. ATP is formed by substrate level phosphorylation.

330. Requires NADH

Questions 331 through 333

Within each of the reaction pathways shown below

(A) ATP is consumed
(B) GTP is consumed
(C) ATP is generated
(D) ATP is both consumed and generated
(E) ATP is neither consumed nor generated

331. Glycogen → fructose 6-phosphate

332. Fructose 6-phosphate → glyceraldehyde 3-phosphate

333. Glyceraldehyde 3-phosphate → pyruvate

Questions 334 through 336

For each of the statements below, choose the biosynthetic process that applies.

(A) protein biosynthesis
(B) RNA synthesis
(C) phospholipid synthesis
(D) nucleotide synthesis
(E) cholesterol synthesis

334. Actinomycin D is an inhibitor.

335. Tetracycline is an inhibitor.

336. Methotrexate is an inhibitor.

Questions 337 through 339

For each statement below, choose the process that applies.

(A) transcription in eukaryotes
(B) transcription in prokaryotes
(C) transcription in both eukaryotes and prokaryotes
(D) translation in eukaryotes
(E) translation in prokaryotes

337. Is initiated with formyl-methionyl-tRNA (fMet-tRNA)

338. Is inhibited by α-amanitin

339. Begins at specific sequences on the DNA template

Questions 340 through 342

For each statement below, choose the compound that performs the indicated function.

(A) HDL
(B) bile salts
(C) VLDL
(D) LDL
(E) apoprotein E

340. Carries primarily triacylglycerols

341. Transports cholesterol from peripheral tissues to the liver

342. Transports cholesterol to peripheral tissues

Questions 343 through 345

For each inhibitor listed below, choose the process that is inhibited.

- (A) electron transport dependent on pyruvate or succinate
- (B) electron transfer to O_2 mediated by cytochrome oxidase
- (C) synthesis of ATP by ATP synthase
- (D) electron transport dependent on pyruvate but not succinate
- (E) maintenance of the mitochondrial proton gradient

343. Dinitrophenol

344. Rotenone

345. Antimycin A

DIRECTIONS (Questions 346 through 366): Each of the numbered items or incomplete statements in this section is followed by answers or by completions of the statement. Select the ONE lettered answer or completion that is BEST in each case.

346. The peptide most likely to be found within the intramembrane segment of a transmembrane protein is

- (A) thr-ile-asp-asn
- (B) glu-asp-ser-tyr
- (C) phe-ile-leu-val
- (D) lys-ser-val-asp
- (E) met-cys-glu-arg

347. Which of the following can be synthesized by humans?

- (A) histidine
- (B) leucine
- (C) methionine
- (D) tryptophan
- (E) serine

348. Concerning the biosynthesis of saturated fatty acids, all of the following are correct EXCEPT that the process

- (A) is localized in the cytoplasm
- (B) requires reduced NADH
- (C) is decreased when fatty acid concentrations are elevated
- (D) is controlled by the rate of the reaction catalyzed by acetyl-CoA carboxylase
- (E) increases when the levels of citric acid cycle intermediates are elevated

349. All of the following may characterize sickle cell anemia EXCEPT that

- (A) sickling occurs when there is a high concentration of the deoxygenated form of hemoglobin S
- (B) Hb S is altered by the change of a single amino acid in the β chain
- (C) Hb S has an unchanged electrophoretic mobility relative to normal hemoglobin
- (D) the disease can be diagnosed in fetal DNA by restriction enzyme digestion
- (E) the solubility of deoxygenated Hb S is abnormally low

350. The figure below displays the effect of ATP addition on the activity of phosphofructokinase. This information indicates that

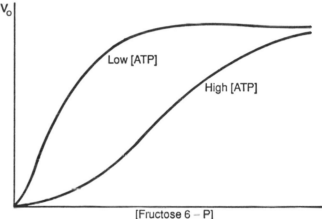

- (A) there is cooperative binding of the substrate, fructose 6-phosphate, to the enzyme in the presence of ATP
- (B) ATP decreases the apparent V_{max} of the reaction
- (C) ATP increases the apparent V_{max} of the reaction
- (D) ATP decreases the apparent K_m of the enzyme
- (E) ATP activates the enzyme

351. The pH of a buffer solution can be determined by

- (A) −log [base]/[acid]
- (B) −log [acid]/[base]
- (C) −log [OH⁻]
- (D) pK + log [base]/[acid]
- (E) pK + log [acid]/[base]

352. UDP-glucose is required for the

(A) synthesis of glucose 6-phosphate
(B) debranching of glycogen
(C) entry of galactose into the glycolytic pathway
(D) entry of fructose into the glycolytic pathway
(E) synthesis of pyruvate

353. All of the following are characteristics of eukaryotic chromosome structure EXCEPT that

(A) the repeating unit of chromosome structure is the nucleosome
(B) histones are small basic proteins that are components of chromatin
(C) the nucleosome core contains 160–240 base pairs of DNA
(D) RNA is an integral component of the nucleosome core
(E) some short DNA sequences may be repeated as many as one million times

354. A major product of the pentose phosphate pathway is

(A) NADPH
(B) fructose 6-phosphate
(C) $FADH_2$
(D) glucose 6-phosphate
(E) NADH

355. GDPCP is an analogue of guanosine triphosphate (GTP) that cannot be hydrolyzed to GDP. All of the following may be expected to be inhibited if GDPCP replaces GTP in a protein synthesizing system EXCEPT

(A) binding of aminoacyl-tRNA to ribosomes
(B) polypeptide chain initiation
(C) polypeptide chain elongation
(D) peptidyl transferase activity
(E) interaction of EF1 or EF-Tu with tRNA

356. The accumulation of an oxygen debt during strenuous physical exercise may be accompanied by

(A) an increase in NAD^+ in muscle
(B) an increase in lactate in blood
(C) a decrease in pyruvate in blood
(D) an increase citrate in muscle
(E) an increase in ATP in muscle

357. Which of the following reagents or enzymes is employed for the determination of the N-terminal amino acid in proteins?

(A) ninhydrin
(B) phenylisothiocyanate
(C) carboxypeptidase
(D) cyanogen bromide
(E) pepsin

358. Which of the following antibiotics is an inhibitor of transcription?

(A) streptomycin
(B) erythromycin
(C) tetracycline
(D) puromycin
(E) rifamycin

359. Carnitine, a zwitterionic compound derived from lysine, is involved in fatty acid metabolism. It is

(A) required for absorption of long chain fatty acids from the intestine
(B) a component of bile salts
(C) a component of coenzyme A
(D) required for transport of long chain fatty acids into mitochondria
(E) required for transport of medium chain fatty acids into mitochondria

360. All of the following are properties of restriction endonucleases EXCEPT that

(A) they recognize specific palindromic sequences in DNA
(B) they cleave only supercoiled DNA
(C) they are produced by bacteria to protect against transformation by foreign DNA
(D) they cleave both strands of DNA at specific sites
(E) they do not degrade the host cell's DNA because the recognition site is methylated

361. The synthesis of all steroid hormones involves all of the following EXCEPT

(A) mono-oxygenases
(B) pregnenolone
(C) vitamin D
(D) molecular O_2
(E) NADPH

362. All of the following are important in the control of de novo purine biosynthesis EXCEPT

(A) stimulation of the conversion of IMP to AMP by GTP
(B) stimulation of the conversion of IMP to GMP by ATP
(C) inhibition of the enzyme xanthine oxidase

(D) availability of 5-phosphoribosyl-1-pyrophos-phate (PRPP)

(E) inhibition of the enzyme PRPP amidotrans-ferase by GMP

363. Which of the following enzyme abnormalities would be expected to lead to hyperuricemia?

(A) xanthine oxidase deficiency

(B) adenosine deaminase deficiency

(C) hypoxanthine-guanine phosphoribosyltrans-ferase (HGPRT) deficiency (Lesch-Nyhan syndrome)

(D) purine nucleoside phosphorylase deficiency

(E) PRPP aminotransferase deficiency

364. Reduced glutathione is known to mediate all the following EXCEPT

(A) react with hydrogen peroxide to detoxify cells

(B) maintain the disulfide bonds of proteins in the reduced state

(C) regenerate from the oxidized form in RBCs by reacting with electrons donated from NADPH to FAD

(D) regenerate from the oxidized form in RBCs by reacting with electrons donated from NADH to FAD

(E) maintain hemoglobin in the ferrous state in RBCs

365. In the presence of arsenate, which of the following may or may not occur during glycolysis?

(A) 1,3-DPG is formed

(B) NADH is formed

(C) P_i reacts with glyceraldehyde 3-phosphate

(D) 3-phosphoglycerate is not formed

(E) pyruvate is not formed

366. Which of the following can be synthesized from di-acylglycerol in one step?

(A) phosphatidyl ethanolamine

(B) phosphatidyl serine

(C) lysophosphatidic acid

(D) phosphatidyl inositol

(E) cardiolipin

DIRECTIONS (Questions 367 through 374): Each set of matching questions in this section consists of a list of up to nine lettered options followed by several numbered items. For each item, select the ONE lettered option that is most closely associated with it. Each lettered heading may be selected once, more than once, or not at all.

Questions 367 through 370

For each description below, choose the compound in-volved.

(A) oligomycin

(B) valinomycin

(C) atractyloside

(D) amytal

(E) antimycin A

(F) dicumarol

(G) cyanide

(H) carbon monoxide

367. Inhibits ATP-ADP translocase

368. Inhibits electron transfer from cytochrome b to cy-tochrome c_1

369. Binds to ATP synthase and inhibits ATP synthe-sis

370. Uncouples oxidative phosphorylation from elec-tron transport by making mitochondria permeable to K^+

Questions 371 through 374

For each reaction below, choose the correct description.

(A) generates GTP

(B) utilizes GTP

(C) stimulated by acetyl CoA

(D) requires NADPH

(E) generates $FADH_2$

(F) yields ATP even in the absence of oxygen

(G) requires $NADP^+$

(H) requires NADH

(I) requires NAD^+

371. oxaloacetate → phosphoenolpyruvate

372. α-ketoglutarate → succinyl CoA

373. glucose 6-phosphate → 6-phosphoglucono-δ-lactone

374. phosphoenolpyruvate → pyruvate

DIRECTIONS (Questions 375 through 378): Each of the numbered items or incomplete statements in this section is followed by answers or by completions of the statement. Select the ONE lettered answer or completion that is BEST in each case.

375. The liver is the only body organ that is capable of

    (A) urea formation

    (B) ganglioside synthesis

    (C) nucleotide synthesis

    (D) medium-chain fatty acid catabolism

    (E) glycogen degradation

376. The cofactor not required for conversion of pyruvate to acetyl-CoA is

    (A) NAD$^+$

    (B) FAD

    (C) thiamine

    (D) biotin

    (E) lipoic acid

377. The disease pellagra can be prevented by a dietary sufficiency of

    (A) vitamin D

    (B) riboflavin

    (C) retinoic acid

    (D) thiamine

    (E) niacin

378. Of the following, which cannot be characterized as a covalently modulated enzyme?

    (A) pepsin

    (B) glycogen synthase

    (C) chymotrypsin

    (D) aspartate transcarbamoylase

    (E) pyruvate kinase

DIRECTIONS (Questions 379 through 381): Each set of matching questions in this section consists of a list of seven lettered options followed by several numbered items. For each item, select the ONE lettered option that is most closely associated with it. Each lettered heading may be selected once, more than once, or not at all.

For each description below, choose the appropriate enzyme or inhibitor.

    (A) fluorodeoxyuridine

    (B) allopurinol

    (C) sulfamethoxazole

    (D) glucose 6-phosphate

    (E) hypoxanthine phosphoribosyltransferase

    (F) adenine phosphoribosyltransferase

    (G) purine nucleoside phosphorylase

379. Deficiency results in hypouricemia

380. Deficiency results in Lesch-Nyhan syndrome

381. Specific inhibitor of thymidylate biosynthesis

Answers and Explanations

255. **(C)** Two distinct pathways for nucleotide biosynthesis exist in most cells. In the de novo pathway, nucleotides are synthesized from smaller precursor molecules, such as amino acids, CO_2, and ammonia. Free nucleic acid bases or nucleosides are not produced as intermediates in this pathway. These latter compounds, however, may be used for the synthesis of nucleotides via the salvage pathways. Free bases and nucleosides become available either through nucleic acid breakdown or diet. Thymidylate can be synthesized in two steps from thymine via the salvage pathways. Thymine is first converted to thymidine by the enzyme thymidine phosphorylase and then to thymidylate by the action of thymidine kinase. 5-Fluorodeoxyuridylate is a potent inhibitor of thymidylate synthase, the enzyme responsible for de novo thymidylate biosynthesis. Inhibition of this enzyme will have a major effect on DNA synthesis, since thymidylate is a precursor employed specifically for DNA synthesis. Cells cannot take up charged compounds, such as nucleotides, from the surrounding environment, and, therefore, the base fluorouracil must be administered rather than fluorodeoxyuridylate. In order to inhibit thymidylate synthase, the fluorouracil must be converted to its corresponding nucleotide by the salvage pathway. *(Stryer, pp 613–616)*

256. **(D)** Under certain conditions (e.g., fasting) acetyl-CoA derived from fatty acid oxidation is diverted from use in the citric acid cycle and employed instead for the formation of acetoacetate and 3-hydroxybutyrate. These compounds are referred to as ketone bodies. The major site of acetoacetate production is the liver, but it can diffuse into the blood, where it can be taken by peripheral tissue. In muscle, a thiokinase enzyme uses 1 mol of ATP to convert acetoacetate to acetoacetyl-CoA. Once produced, acetoacetyl-CoA is cleaved by thiolase to yield 2 mol of acetyl-CoA, which is metabolized via the citric acid cycle to produce 12 mol of ATP/mol of acetyl-CoA. Subtracting the 1 mol of ATP employed in the initial formation of ace-

toacetyl CoA gives a net production of 23 mol of ATP. *(Stryer, pp 478–480)*

257. **(A)** Under anaerobic conditions (e.g., intense exercise), the production of pyruvate via glycolysis exceeds its oxidation by the citric acid cycle. This results in the synthesis of lactate by muscle. Lactate diffuses into the bloodstream and is taken up by the liver, where it is oxidized back to pyruvate. The latter is converted to glucose in the liver via gluconeogenesis. *(Stryer, pp 444–445)*

258. **(C)** In the interior of peripheral tissues, the concentration of CO_2 is high, and the relative O_2 tension is low. As a consequence, O_2 is unloaded from Hb, and CO_2 is taken up. Although some CO_2 is transported as a dissolved gas, most CO_2 is transported as bicarbonate. Bicarbonate is formed by the action of carbonic anhydrase within red blood cells.

$$CO_2 + H_2O \rightleftharpoons HCO_3^- + H^+$$

In addition, CO_2 is carried by Hb as carbamino derivatives. The un-ionized α-amino groups of Hb react reversibly with CO_2.

$$CO_2 + R - NH_2 \rightleftharpoons R - NHCOO^- + H^+$$

The charged carbamates form salt bridges that stabilize the T form of Hb and lower its O_2 affinity. Unlike O_2, CO_2 does not bind to the iron of the heme group. *(Stryer, p 162)*

259. **(B)** All contractile cells contain actin and myosin. In nonmuscle cells, such as macrophages, the contractile elements are important for mobility and shape changes. The mechanisms of contraction seem to be similar, using ATP hydrolysis as a driving force. In all cell types, the cytoskeletons are composed of the contractile filaments. In nonmuscle cells, the cytoskeleton is composed mainly of actin polymerized into a latticework of microfilaments approximately 70 nm thick. Unlike muscle cells, the contraction of nonmuscle cells does not seem to be governed by nervous stimulation. *(Stryer, pp 936–938)*

260. **(A)** During glycolysis, pyruvate is synthesized from phosphoenolpyruvate with the concomitant production of ATP from ADP. The equilibrium of this reaction lies far to the left for the reaction as written:

$$ATP + pyruvate \rightleftharpoons phosphoenolpyruvate + ADP + P_i$$

The standard free-energy change ($\Delta G^{o\prime}$) for the hydrolysis of ATP is −7.3 kcal/mol, whereas the $\Delta G^{o\prime}$ for the phosphorylation of pyruvate to phosphoenolpyruvate is +14.8 kcal/mol (the opposite of the $\Delta G^{o\prime}$ for the hydrolysis of phosphoenolpyruvate). Thus, the calculated $\Delta G^{o\prime}$ for the thermodynamically unfavorable production of phosphoenolpyruvate is +7.5 kcal/mol. *(Stryer, p 316)*

261. **(E)** The carbohydrate moieties in RNA and DNA are ribose and deoxyribose, respectively. A major product of the pentose phosphate pathway is ribose 5-phosphate. The latter is converted to 5-phosphoribosyl-1-pyrophosphate (PRPP), which serves as the donor of ribose in the biosynthesis of nucleotides. *(Stryer, pp 427–430,602–608)*

262. **(D)** Phosphoric acid, H_3PO_4, contains three ionizable hydrogen atoms as indicated in the following equation.

$$H_3PO_4 \rightarrow H_2PO_4^- \rightarrow HPO_4^{2-} \rightarrow PO_4^{3-}$$

pK_2 is the relevant pKa to use in calculating the pH of the solution in this problem because the dissociation involves $H_2PO_4^-$ and HPO_4^{2-}. The pH can be determined by the Henderson-Hasselbalch equation.

$$pH = pKa + \log [salt]/[acid] = 6.8 + \log 0.15/0.05 = 6.8 + \log 3 = 7.28$$

(Stryer, pp 41–42)

263. **(A)** Myosin contains the ATPase activity that hydrolyzes ATP and allows contraction to proceed. The binding of actin to myosin enhances the ATPase activity of myosin. In fact, actin alternatively binds to myosin and is released from myosin as ATP is hydrolyzed. This reaction requires $Mg^{2}+$ and is the driving force of contraction. Although troponin is not directly involved in the ATPase reaction, it binds calcium released by the sarcoplasmic reticulum and in doing so allows conformational changes in tropomyosin and actin to occur, permitting contraction. Myokinase catalyzes the formation of ATP and AMP from two molecules of ADP. *(Stryer, pp 930–932)*

264. **(C)** The allosteric regulatory enzymes of glycolysis are hexokinase, phosphofructokinase, and pyruvate kinase. Of these, phosphofructokinase is the key regulatory enzyme. A high-energy charge or the presence of sufficient citric acid cycle precursors causes the inhibition of phosphofructokinase via accumulation of the negative effectors ATP and citrate. ADP and AMP are positive effectors of phosphofructokinase. Accumulation of glucose 6-phosphate inhibits hexokinase. Pyruvate kinase is inhibited by high ATP levels. Fructose 6-phosphate, the substrate of phosphofructokinase, is not an effector. *(Stryer, pp 359–362)*

265. **(E)** Of the monosaccharides and disaccharides listed in the question, only fructose enters the glycolytic pathway at the level of three-carbon intermediates. Fructokinase catalyzes the phosphorylation of fructose by ATP to fructose 1-phosphate, which is then cleaved to glyceraldehyde and dihydroxyacetone phosphate by aldolase. The glyceraldehyde is phosphorylated to glyceraldehyde 3-phosphate. Thus, two intermediates of glycolysis are formed from one molecule of fructose. In contrast, galactose and mannose enter glycolysis at the level of glucose 1-phosphate and fructose 6-phosphate, respectively. The breakdown products of maltose (i.e., glucose) and lactose (i.e., glucose and galactose) enter glycolysis at the level of six-carbon sugars. *(Stryer, pp 357–359)*

266. **(A)** The first step in gluconeogenesis is the formation of oxaloacetate from pyruvate. The enzyme controlling this step is pyruvate carboxylase, an allosteric enzyme that does not function in the absence of its primary effector, acetyl-CoA, or a closely related acyl-CoA. Thus, a high level of acetyl-CoA signals the need for more oxaloacetate. If there is a surplus of ATP, oxaloacetate will be used for gluconeogenesis. Under conditions of low ATP, oxaloacetate will be consumed in the citric acid cycle. Citrate is the primary negative effector of glycolysis and the primary positive effector of fatty acid synthesis. *(Stryer, p 441)*

267. **(E)** In skeletal muscle, the hormone epinephrine or the neurotransmitter norepinephrine binds to sarcolemma receptors and activates adenylate cyclase. Glucagon, which causes similar effects in the liver, is not specific for muscle. Activated adenylate cyclase forms cyclic AMP from ATP. Cyclic AMP activates protein kinase, which in turn activates phosphorylase kinase. Phosphorylase kinase activates phosphorylase, converting it from the inactive *b* form to the activated *a* form. Both the phosphorylase kinase and phosphorylase itself are activated by phosphorylation mechanisms. Activated glycogen phosphorylase hydrolyzes glycogen, sequentially cleaving off glucose units as glucose 1-phosphate. *(Stryer, pp 462–464)*

268. **(B)** Thymidylate (TMP) is synthesized by methylation of deoxyuridylate (dUMP) at the five-carbon in a reaction catalyzed by thymidylate synthase. TMP is the only precursor for DNA synthesis that is produced separately from the major biosynthetic pathways for purine and pyrimidine ribonucleotides. For this reason, reactions required for TMP biosynthesis are specific targets for drugs that will inhibit DNA synthesis. 5-Fluorouracil is a modified uracil that contains a fluorine attached to the five-carbon. It binds to thymidylate synthase because it is a structural analog of dUMP and forms a covalent complex with the enzyme. This results in complete inactivation of thymidylate synthase. Cells that are rapidly proliferating, such as tumor cells, carry out high levels of DNA synthesis. They, therefore, require larger amounts of TMP than normal cells and, for this reason, are more susceptible to the action of fluorouracil. *(Stryer, pp 614–616)*

269. **(B)** The Michaelis constant (K_m) is determined by measuring the rate of the reaction in the presence of a fixed concentration of enzyme and varying concentrations of substrate. Graphical analysis of such data will provide values for K_m and V_{max}. The turnover number is defined as the number of substrate molecules converted to product per enzyme molecule in a specific period of time. K_m is not related to turnover number. It is also not dependent on the molecular weight of the enzyme. *(Stryer, pp 187–191,199–200)*

270. **(E)** Tertiary structure refers to the three-dimensional arrangement of amino acid residues in a protein. Studies of many proteins reveal that the nonpolar (hydrophobic) amino acid residues are buried in the interior of the protein structure, whereas the polar residues are on the outside in contact with the aqueous environment. The protein folds so as to shield its nonpolar groups from interaction with water molecules. These hydrophobic interactions are the driving force of protein folding. The tertiary structure is further stabilized by hydrogen bonding, polar interactions, and the formation of disulfide bonds. Peptide bonds are only involved in formation of the primary structure of a protein. *(Stryer, pp 29–34)*

271. **(A)** Activation and linking of free amino acids to tRNA are catalyzed by aminoacyl-tRNA synthetases specific for each amino acid. This enzyme, like all others, can only accelerate the time in which a reaction reaches equilibrium. It cannot drive the reaction in a specific direction. During activation, amino acids are linked to AMP.

$$\text{Amino acid} + \text{ATP} \rightleftharpoons \text{aminoacyl-AMP} + \text{PP}_i$$

During transfer, the activated amino acid is linked to a specific RNA.

$$\text{Aminoacyl-AMP} + \text{tRNA} \rightleftharpoons \text{aminoacyl-tRNA} + \text{AMP}$$

Since the free energy of hydrolysis of the ester bonds formed is similar to that of the terminal phosphate of ATP, the $\Delta G^{\circ\prime}$ of the reaction is nearly zero. The reaction is driven by the hydrolysis of pyrophosphate (PP_i).

$$\text{PP}_i + \text{H}_2\text{O} \rightarrow 2\,\text{P}_i$$

The formation of P_i by pyrophosphatase is a common cell mechanism to ensure the irreversibility of an otherwise reversible reaction. *(Stryer, pp 734–735)*

272. **(E)** The rate of an enzymatic reaction is dependent on the concentration of substrate and the K_m and V_{max} of the enzyme. The rate will be maximal when the enzyme is completely saturated with substrate. Binding of substrate to the enzyme is governed by K_m. When substrate concentrations are much greater than K_m (> 100-fold), the enzyme will be nearly saturated with substrate and the reaction will proceed at its maximal rate. Conversely, when the substrate concentration is equal—or nearly equal—to K_m, the reaction rate will not be maximal, but will vary as a function of the substrate concentration as defined by the Michaelis-Menten equation. In the example, the glucose concentration in both cases is much greater than the K_m for hexokinase and, therefore, the hexokinase reaction will always proceed at the maximal rate. For glucokinase, however, the glucose concentration is approximately equal to K_m. Therefore, a drop in glucose levels from 135 mg to 75 mg/100 ml (i.e., from 0.75×10^{-2} M to 0.4×10^{-2} M) will result in a decrease in the rate of the glucokinase-catalyzed reaction. *(Stryer, pp 361,187–191)*

273. **(A)** Long-chain (> 10 carbon atoms) as well as medium-chain (5 to 10 carbon atoms) and short-chain (2 to 4 carbon atoms) fatty acids must be activated before β oxidation, which uses only fatty acids linked to CoA. Long-chain fatty acids are activated outside the mitochondrial matrix and then transported across the inner membrane of mitochondria as acyl carnitine complexes. In contrast, short- and medium-chain fatty acids diffuse across the inner mitochondrial membrane and are activated in the matrix. Fatty acid thiokinase (acyl-CoA synthetase) catalyzes the activation reaction in which the carboxyl group of the free fatty acid forms a thioester linkage with CoA.

$$R\text{-}COO^- + ATP + HS\text{-}CoA \rightleftharpoons R\text{-}CO\text{-}S\text{-}CoA + AMP + PP_i$$

The reaction is made irreversible by the consumption of the equivalent of two high-energy phosphate bonds and the hydrolysis of the resulting PP_i by pyrophosphatase. (Stryer, pp 472–473)

274. **(C)** The formation of the three-carbon CoA thioester malonyl-CoA from acetyl-CoA is the regulatory step of fatty acid synthesis. Acetyl-CoA carboxylase catalyzes this reaction.

$$Acetyl\text{-}CoA + HCO_3^- + ATP \rightleftharpoons malonyl\text{-}CoA + ADP + P_i$$

Citrate, which serves as the means of transport of acetyl-CoA from the mitochondria to the cytosolic site of fatty acid synthesis, is the key allosteric regulator of acetyl-CoA carboxylase. It shifts the enzyme from an inactive protomer to an active filamentous polymer. The end product of the cytosolic fatty acid synthetase complex, palmitoyl-CoA, inhibits the carboxylase. Although acetyl-CoA carboxylase is the prime regulatory enzyme of fatty acid synthesis, it is not a part of the fatty acid synthetase complex, the site where most of the reactions of fatty acid synthesis take place. (Stryer, pp 481–482)

275. **(A)** The first two steps of cholesterol biosynthesis lead to the formulation of 3-hydroxy-3-methylglutaryl-CoA. These are also the first two steps of ketone body synthesis. In ketogenesis, 3-hydroxy-3-methylglutaryl-CoA is cleaved to form acetoacetate and acetyl-CoA. In cholesterol biosynthesis, it is reduced to form mevalonic acid. Although these steps are common to both ketogenesis and cholesterol biosynthesis, they are separate in time and space. Cholesterol biosynthesis occurs in the cytosol of cells from excess acetyl-CoA produced from dietary surplus. In contrast, ketogenesis occurs only in the mitochondria of liver cells from acetyl-CoA derived from β oxidation of fatty acids. Ketogenesis does not occur to any great extent except in states of dietary need, such as fasting and starvation, or under abnormal circumstances, such as an excessively fat-rich diet or diabetes. (Stryer, pp 478–479,554–559)

276. **(D)** Cholesterol is obtained from the diet as well as by de novo synthesis. Although many cells can synthesize cholesterol, the liver is the major site of its production. The rate of cholesterol production is highly responsive to feedback inhibition from both dietary cholesterol and synthesized cholesterol. Feedback regulation is mediated by changes in the activity of 3-hydroxy-3-methylglutaryl-CoA reductase. This enzyme is the first committed step in the production of cholesterol from acetyl-CoA. 3-Hydroxy-3-methylglutaryl-CoA, the substrate of the reductase, also can be synthesized into the ketone body acetoacetate by the action of 3-hydroxy-3-methylglutaryl-CoA lyase. (Stryer, pp 560,564)

277. **(B)** Unlike phosphoglycerides, sphingomyelin lacks a glycerol backbone. Phosphoglycerides are composed of glycerol esterified to two fatty acids by an ester linkage and to a polar group by a phosphate ester linkage. Lecithin is the phospholipid phosphatidyl choline. In contrast, sphingomyelin is composed of one fatty acid esterified to the amino group of sphingosine and a polar group attached to the hydroxyl of sphingosine through a phosphate ester linkage. Choline and ethanolamine are the polar groups of sphingomyelin. All of the lipids listed in the question are important in membrane structure. (Stryer, pp 547–553)

278. **(C)** In contrast to liver cells, adipocytes contain little or no glycerol kinase. Thus, glycerol produced from lipolysis is not used to any great extent as a source of glycerol 3-phosphate, the central substrate for esterification of fatty acids into triacylglycerols. The major source of glycerol 3-phosphate in adipocytes is dihydroxyacetone phosphate, which is derived from glycolysis of glucose. A lack of glucose, such as that which occurs in diabetes or fasting, would inhibit triacylglycerol synthesis and favor lipolysis. Ketogenesis and gluconeogenesis do not occur in adipocytes. (Stryer, pp 471–472)

279. **(D)** In the genetic disorder known as Tay-Sachs disease, ganglioside GM_2 is not catabolized. As a consequence, the ganglioside concentration is elevated many times higher than normal. The functionally absent lysosomal enzyme is β-N-acetylhexosaminidase. The elevated GM_2 results in irreversible brain damage to infants, who usually die before the age of 3 years. Under normal conditions, this enzyme cleaves N-acetylgalactosamine from the oligosaccharide chain of this complex sphingolipid, allowing further catabolism to occur. The cause of most lipidoses (lipid storage diseases) is similar. That is, a defect in catabolism of gangliosides causes abnormal accumulation. (Stryer, p 554)

280. **(B)** In fasting or diabetes, lipolysis predominates in adipocytes because of the inability of these cells to obtain glucose, which is normally used as a source of glycerol 3-phosphate. Glycerol 3-phosphate is necessary for the esterification of fatty acids into triacylglycerides. Circulating fatty acids become the predominant fuel source, and β oxidation in the liver becomes substantially elevated.

This leads to an increased production of acetyl-CoA. Since glucose use in diabetes is reduced, gluconeogenesis is increased in the liver. This predisposes oxaloacetate and makes the citric acid cycle unavailable for heightened use of acetyl-CoA. As a consequence, acetyl-CoA is diverted to the formation of ketone bodies. *(Stryer, pp 478–480)*

281–283. (281-A, 282-C, 283-B) The curve to the left of curve Z on the reaction velocity vs. substrate concentration plot shown in the question has a lower K_m. This can be easily demonstrated since $K_m = \frac{1}{2} V_{max}$ and all the curves shown have the same V_{max}. Thus, curve X demonstrates higher reaction velocities at lower substrate concentrations than the other curves shown. Curve X represents a positively modulated reaction velocity of the same enzyme represented by curve Z. In contrast, curve Y represents a plot of the same enzyme shown in curve Z in the presence of a negative modulator.

In going from left to right in the figure that accompanies the question, the reaction velocity per unit substrate concentration decreases in those areas of the curves where V_{max} is not being approached. The K_m of the curves to the right increases, indicating a decreased affinity for substrate. Most likely, this would be because of an increase in inhibitory modulator concentrations or a decrease in positive modulator concentrations. The V_{max} is similar in all of the curves shown, and either an increase in a needed cofactor or positive cooperativity would push the curves from right to left.

Since $K_m = \frac{1}{2} V_{max}$ the apparent K_m for curve Y in the question is 3 μmol/L. The V_{max} of all the curves shown is 12 μmol/min. A line drawn horizontally from one-half that value on the *y* axis to curve Y and from that point vertically to the *x* axis will give the apparent K_m. *(Stryer, pp 187–195, 239–243)*

284. (A) Untreated diabetes leads to high blood glucose levels (hyperglycemia) and glucosuria, as glucose exceeds the kidney threshold and spills into the urine. At the same time that blood glucose levels are high, the lack of insulin leads to a favoring of lipolysis and consequent ketogenesis by the liver. The high level of ketogenesis by the liver produces ketonemia (high blood levels of ketone bodies) and ketonuria (ketone bodies in the urine). Insulin injections help to reduce these symptoms and allow diabetic persons to live relatively normal lives. However, insulin injections when blood glucose levels are low, as well as overdoses of insulin, can cause severe hypoglycemia (low blood levels of glucose). If blood glucose levels fall below 80 mg/100 ml, insulin shock occurs. When blood levels fall below 20 mg/100 ml, convulsions and coma occur because of the deprivation of glucose

to the brain. IV glucose injections can reverse insulin shock. *(Stryer, pp 641–642)*

285. (A) Pro-opiocortin can give rise to five peptide hormones of the anterior pituitary. ACTH and β-lipotropin, a prohormone, are formed by cleavage of pro-opiocortin. α-Melanocyte-stimulating hormone (α-MSH) is a cleavage product of ACTH, whereas β-endorphin and γ-lipotropin are cleavage products of β-lipotropin. β-MSH is a cleavage fragment of β-endorphin. This is summarized below.

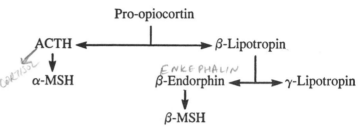

TSH is a hormone of the anterior pituitary that is not derived from pro-opiocortin. *(Stryer, pp 993–994)*

286. (E) Biotin serves as an intermediate carrier of CO_2 during carboxylations catalyzed by acetyl-CoA carboxylase, propionyl carboxylase, and pyruvate carboxylase. This vitamin is present in the prosthetic groups of these enzymes. Biotin is made from intestinal bacteria and is also obtained from a wide variety of foods. Avidin, a protein present in egg whites, tightly binds biotin in the gut, preventing its absorption. In individuals who consume large quantities of raw eggs, this leads to a toxic reaction due to biotin's role in carboxylation reactions. *(Stryer, pp 481–482)*

287. (A) The α-amino group of many amino acids is transferred to α-ketoglutarate to form glutamate, which is then oxidatively deaminated to ammonium ion. A similar transamination reaction yields alanine from pyruvate during degradation of amino acids. The prosthetic group of all transaminases is pyridoxal phosphate (PLP), which is derived from pyridoxine. During transamination, the aldehyde group of PLP forms a Schiff's-base linkage with the α-amino group of amino acids, ultimately transferring the amino group to either a α-ketoglutarate or pyruvate. *(Stryer, pp 495–499)*

288. (C) Vitamin B_1 is obtained as thiamine from pork, yeast, whole grains, and nuts. Its active form in enzymatic reactions is thiamine pyrophosphate (TPP), a form to which it is converted in the body. During decarboxylation, substrates form a hydroxyethyl-TPP intermediate, which is then oxidized to an acetyl group before being transferred off of TPP. A deficiency of thiamine leads to beriberi, a wasting disease with nervous system damage and edema. *(Stryer, pp 379–382)*

289. **(B)** LDLs are the primary carriers of blood cholesterol. Routine plasma lipid measurements are carried out after a 12-hr fast. In this way, the major endogenous plasma lipoproteins, VLDLs, and the major exogenous plasma lipoproteins (chylomicrons) have been cleared from the blood of normal individuals. LDLs, which are the end products of VLDL delipidation, and HDLs, which are protein rich, are the only lipoproteins circulating after a 12-hr fast. LDLs are rich in cholesterol, being composed of about 45 percent cholesterol or cholesterol esters. In both dietary and familial hypercholesterolemia, circulating LDL levels are increased. *(Stryer, pp 560–561)*

290. **(D)** A deficiency in galactose 1-phosphate uridyl transferase causes galactosemia, a disease characterized by high blood levels of galactose, defective growth, mental retardation, and in some cases death. Early diagnosis and treatment with a galactose-free diet reverse most clinical symptoms. Galactose is formed by the hydrolysis of lactose and is normally formed into glucose. First, galactose is phosphorylated to galactose 1-phosphate by galactokinase. The uridyl transferase reaction transfers UDP from UDP-glucose to the phosphorylated galactose. UDP-galactose is then converted to UDP-glucose by UDP-galactose-4-epimerase. *(Stryer, pp 357–359)*

291. **(B)** After hydrolysis of the apoprotein of Hb in old erythrocytes in the spleen, the heme group is degraded. First, the α-methene bridge is cleaved to form biliverdin, a linear tetrapyrrole, which is green. The mono-oxegenase called heme oxygenase catalyzes the reaction, which requires molecular O_2 and the reduced form of NADPH. A methene bridge carbon is released. The enzyme biliverdin reductase catalyzes the reduction by NADPH of the central methene bridge carbon of biliverdin to form bilirubin, which is red. After these reactions, bilirubin is transported to the liver complexed to serum albumin. There, each bilirubin molecule is conjugated via UDP-glucuronate to two glucuronates to form bilirubin diglucuronide. These six-carbon, carboxylated derivatives of glucose are attached to the propionated side chains of bilirubin, making it more soluble before its excretion in the bile. Unlike bile pigments, the bile acids are conjugated to glycine or taurine. *(Stryer, pp 596–597)*

292. **(C)** Carbohydrates attached to asparagine residues have a common inner-core structure. Such a block of oligosaccharides is built up and carried to the asparagine of proteins on a lipid carrier. That carrier is dolichol phosphate, an aliphatic chain composed of isoprene units. *N*-acetylglucosamine is the sugar residue directly bonded to dolichol phosphate and then transferred to the asparagine side chain. *(Stryer, pp 773–774)*

293. **(C)** Except for the initial formation of malonyl-CoA by the carboxylation of acetyl-CoA, most of the reactions of fatty acid synthesis occur on the cytosolic fatty acid synthetase complex. The intermediates are attached to the complex by the sulfhydryl group of the acyl carrier protein (ACP). When malonyl-ACP is condensed with acyl-ACP, the carbon atom derived from bicarbonate is decarboxylated as CO_2. The β-ketoacyl intermediate formed is reduced in the presence of NADPH to a β-hydroxyacyl, which then is dehydrated to form an enoyl. The enoyl is reduced by NADPH to a saturated acyl in the final step of each round of elongation. *(Stryer, pp 481–487)*

294. **(A)** During ethanol clearance in any individual, including alcoholic persons, ethanol is first converted to acetaldehyde by the action of alcohol dehydrogenase and then to acetate by the action of acetaldehyde dehydrogenase. Both of these enzymes require the oxidized form of NAD$^+$ to function. During alcohol oxidation, the level of the reduced form of nicotinamide adenine dinucleotide (NADH) increases greatly in the liver, leading to an overload of the shuttle normally used to regenerate NAD$^+$. This causes the level of NAD$^+$ to be the bottleneck in the removal of alcohol from the body. The levels of alcohol dehydrogenase may be somewhat higher than normal in chronically alcoholic persons. Nevertheless, NAD$^+$ is still the rate-limiting factor in the oxidation of ethanol. *(Stryer, pp 362–364)*

295. **(C)** In contrast to the glycerol 3-phosphate shuttle operating in skeletal muscle, in the heart and liver the bidirectional malate-aspartate shuttle transfers the electrons of cytoplasmic and mitochondrial NADH between the two cell compartments reversibly. The pathway is complex, with glutamate, aspartate, malate, and α-ketoglutarate serving as diffusible carriers. Mitochondrial and cytosolic oxaloacetate and NADH also serve as electron transporters. In contrast to the glycerol 3-phosphate shuttle, which yields only two ATP per pair of electrons derived from cytosolic NADH, the malate-aspartate shuttle yields three ATP per cytosolic NADH. This occurs because NADH and not the reduced form of flavin adenine dinucleotide (FADH) is the mitochondrial carrier of electrons. *(Stryer, pp 417–418)*

296. **(D)** Except for the fact that the carrier groups for fatty acid synthesis (ACP) and β oxidation (CoA) are different, the attached intermediates are similar. In each group of reactions, the enzymatic steps result in acyl, enoyl, β-hydroxyacyl, and β-ketoacyl intermediates being formed or degraded. The enzymatic steps differ in that fatty acid synthesis is carried out in the cytosol using NADPH as a reductant. Biosynthesis is stimulated by citrate. β oxidation occurs in the mitochondrial matrix using flavin adenine dinucleotide (FAD) and NAD$^+$ as pyridine nucleotide acceptors of electrons. Citrate levels are low during fatty acid oxidation. *(Stryer, pp 472–488)*

297. (D) Glycolysis is the only major source of ATP in erythrocytes, since they lack mitochondria. In order for glycolysis to continue uninterrupted, NADH must constantly be reoxidized to NAD$^+$ so that glyceraldehyde 3-phosphate may be oxidized. Conversion of pyruvate to lactate by lactate dehydrogenase accomplishes this. The excess lactate diffuses into the liver, where it is converted to glucose via gluconeogenesis. *(Stryer, pp 444–445)*

298. (D) Increases in either hydrogen ion concentration (lowered pH), CO_2 partial pressure, or 2,3-DPG all lead to a decreased affinity of Hb for O_2. Conversely, decreases in these factors lead to an increased affinity of O_2 for Hb. A decrease in pH changes the charge on histidine residues in Hb, favoring the release of O_2. Binding of DPG to deoxyhemoglobin causes the cross-linking of the β chains, leading to a stabilization of the deoxygenated form of Hb and a lowered affinity for O_2. CO_2 binds to the un-ionized α-amino groups on the terminal ends of Hb. This results in charged carbamino derivatives, which form salt bridges. The salt bridges further reduce the affinity of Hb for O_2. *(Stryer, pp 156–157,160–163)*

299. (A) In persons with a deficiency in pyruvate kinase, glycolytic intermediates are high because the terminal step is blocked. 2,3-DPG, which is formed from the glycolytic intermediate 1,3-DPG by a mutase, accumulates in RBCs. 2,3-DPG is a regulator of O_2 transport that acts by stabilizing the structure of deoxyhemoglobin. Thus, an increase in 2,3-DPG levels leads to a low O_2 affinity in persons with pyruvate kinase deficiency. Just the opposite effect has been observed in individuals with hexokinase deficiency. Deficiencies of any of the other enzymes listed in the question would not result in accumulations of glycolytic intermediates that would lead to increases in 2,3-DPG. *(Stryer, pp 361–362,368–370)*

300. (D) The biochemical deficiency of the enzyme HGPRT results in mental retardation and compulsive self-destructive behavior. This X-linked recessive disease also results in gout because of elevated levels of urate. However, unlike gout alone, allopurinol treatment of patients with Lesch-Nyhan syndrome does not increase the rate of synthesis of purines because it does not lower the level of PRPP. In genetically normal individuals, HGPRT allows the salvage synthesis of guanosine 5′-monophosphate (GMP) or inosine 5′-monophosphate (IMP) from guanine or hypoxanthine plus PRPP. The relationship between salvage pathways of purine synthesis and de novo pathways is not yet understood. *(Stryer, pp 620–623)*

301. (A) Partial defects of enzymes of the urea cycle commonly lead to hyperammonemia, since the synthesis of urea in the liver is the major route of ammonia (NH_4^+) removal. The high levels of NH_4^+ are toxic. It is thought that the increased concentration of ammonia ions depletes α-ketoglutarate levels by shifting the equilibrium of glutamate dehydrogenase toward glutamate and glutamine formation.

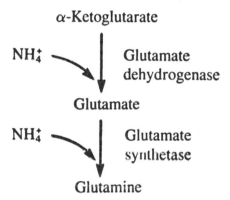

The decrease of α-ketoglutarate adversely affects the citric acid cycle, leading to a decrease in ATP levels. Development and function of brain tissue are highly vulnerable to low ATP levels. Deficiencies of urea cycle enzymes also lead to decreased amounts of urea and increases in the concentrations of certain cycle intermediates preceding the lesion. In mild forms of hyperammonemia, low-protein diets may allow clinical improvement by lowering blood NH_4^+ levels. Gout, which results from elevated levels of urate in the serum, is not related to the urea cycle. It is often caused by partial deficiencies of the enzyme HGPRT, a purine salvage pathway enzyme. *(Stryer, pp 500–502)*

302. (B) The nucleotide thymine, unlike all the other nucleotides, is synthesized at the level of a deoxyribonucleoside monophosphate by the methylation of deoxyuridylate (dUMP) to deoxythymidylate (dTMP). The enzyme thymidylate synthetase catalyzes this reaction. Thus, TMP as such is not a product of the pathway of thymine synthesis. In contrast, all other nucleotides are synthesized as ribose phosphates. CTP is derived from uridine triphosphate (UTP) and is a feedback inhibitor of aspartate transcarbamoylase, the enzyme catalyzing the formation of carbamoyl aspartate, the precursor of UMP. In turn, UMP is the feedback inhibitor of the formation of carbamoyl phosphate, the precursor of carbamoyl aspartate. In purine nucleotide biosynthesis, the formation of PRPP from ribose 5-phosphate, as well as the conversion of PRPP to phosphoribosylamine, is inhibited by AMP, GMP, and IMP. The conversion of IMP to adenylosuccinate, the AMP precursor, is inhibited by AMP. The conversion of IMP to xanthylate, the GMP precursor, is inhibited by GMP. *(Stryer, pp 602–609,613–614)*

303. **(D)** Under normal aerobic conditions, 36 net ATP are formed from the complete oxidation of glucose. Glycolysis yields 2 net ATP from substrate level phosphorylation, the citric acid cycle yields 2 ATP [as guanosine triphosphate (GTP)] from substrate level phosphorylation, and oxidative phosphorylation yields 32 ATP. In the presence of an uncoupling agent, such as dinitrophenol, substrate level phosphorylation still proceeds. Thus, 4 net ATP are produced. *(Stryer, pp 421–422)*

304. **(B)** The net reaction for the complete oxidation of glucose is as follows:

$$\text{Glucose} + 36\ \text{ADP} + 36\ \text{P}_i + 36\ \text{H}^+ + 6\ \text{O}_2 \rightarrow 6\ \text{CO}_2 + 36\ \text{ATP} + 42\ \text{H}_2\text{O}$$

The phosphorus/O_2 ratio is 3, since 36 ATP are formed and 12 atoms of oxygen are consumed. Of the 36 ATP, only 4 (net) are not formed by oxidative phosphorylation. These include the 2 net ATP derived from substrate level phosphorylation in glycolysis and the 2 ATP equivalents formed as GTP from succinyl-CoA in the citric acid cycle. *(Stryer, pp 420–421)*

305. **(A)** Glucose phosphate isomerase catalyzes the reversible conversion of fructose 6-phosphate to glucose 6-phosphate in both glycolysis and gluconeogenesis. In fact, most of the steps of glycolysis are simply reversed in gluconeogenesis. However, the three regulatory steps in the conversion of glucose to pyruvate are not reversible. These steps are (1) glucose → glucose 6-phosphate, which is catalyzed by hexokinase, (2) fructose 6-phosphate → fructose 1,6-diphosphate, which is catalyzed by phosphofructokinase, and (3) phosphoenolpyruvate → pyruvate, which is catalyzed by pyruvate kinase. The reversal of these steps in gluconeogenesis requires the enzymes glucose 6-phosphatase and fructose diphosphatase for the formation of glucose and fructose 6-phosphate, respectively. The formation of phosphoenolpyruvate from pyruvate is more complicated in that the four following

steps are involved: (1) pyruvate carboxylase catalyzes the conversion of pyruvate to oxaloacetate, (2) oxaloacetate is reduced to malate by mitochondrial malate dehydrogenase, (3) malate is reconverted to oxaloacetate by extramitochondrial malate dehydrogenase, and (4) oxaloacetate is transformed to phosphoenolpyruvate by GTP-dependent phosphoenolpyruvate carboxykinase. *(Stryer, pp 438–440)*

306–308. **(306-B, 307-E, 308-D)** The transition state is an unstable intermediate in a reaction pathway between reactants and products. It is usually the intermediate of highest free energy. The energy of activation designated $\Delta G^{\neq}$) of any reaction is the difference in free energy between the ground state of the reactants and the transition state. There is a relationship between the rate of a reaction of its $\Delta G^{\neq}$: the larger the $\Delta G^{\neq}$, the slower the reaction. The free energy change of a reaction (ΔG) is given by the difference in free energy between the ground states of the products and reactants (i.e., $G_{prod} - G_{reac}$). A negative value for ΔG indicates that the reaction will proceed spontaneously without the input of any energy. It does not, however, indicate anything about the rate of the reaction. *(Stryer, pp 180–184)*

309–311. **(309-E, 310-D, 311-A)** The reactions of the citric acid cycle are shown in the figure below. *(Stryer, p 378)*

312–315. **(312-A, 313-D, 314-B, 315-E)** Glycogen phosphorylase catalyzes the sequential release of glucose from glycogen. The glycosidic bond between the two terminal glucose residues is split by inorganic phosphate. The reaction is

$$\text{Glycogen}_{(n)} + \text{P}_i \rightarrow \text{glucose 1-phosphate} + \text{glycogen}_{(n-1)}$$

Glucokinase catalyzes the reaction 1st *step in glycolysis.*

$$\text{Glucose} + \text{ATP} \rightarrow \text{glucose 6-phosphate} + \text{ADP}$$

This enzyme in liver provides the glucose 6-phosphate necessary for glycogen synthesis. The addition of glucose units to a growing glycogen chain is catalyzed by glycogen synthase in the following reaction.

$$\text{Glycogen}_{(n)} + \text{UDP-glucose} \rightarrow \text{glycogen}_{(n+1)} + \text{UDP}$$

An activated derivative of glucose, UDP-glucose, serves as the glucosyl donor in this reaction. Glucose 6-phosphatase catalyzes the reaction.

$$\text{Glucose 6-phosphate} + \text{H}_2\text{O} \rightarrow \text{glucose} + \text{P}_i$$

The enzyme functions primarily in the liver to release free glucose into the blood for uptake by other tissues, chiefly brain and muscle. Glucose 6-phosphate dehydrogenase catalyzes the conversion of glucose 6-phosphate to 6-phosphoglucono-δ-lactone. It requires NADP⁺ as a cofactor. *(Stryer, pp 361,428,451,454,456)*

316–319. **(316-C, 317-A, 318-D, 319-D)** The carbon skeletons of glutamine, proline, arginine, and histidine enter the citric acid cycle at the level of α-ketoglutarate. All of these amino acids are converted to the common intermediate glutamate, which is oxidatively deaminated by glutamate dehydrogenase to yield α-ketoglutarate. In the formation of glycine from serine, the side chain β-carbon of serine is transferred to tetrahydrofolate to form methylenetetrahydrofolate. The reaction is catalyzed by serine transhydroxymethylase, which is a pyridoxal phosphate enzyme. This is the major source of one-carbon units for tetrahydrofolate derivatives. Transamination of oxaloacetate by glutamate results in the formation of aspartate from oxaloacetate and α-ketoglutarate from the glutamate skeleton. In turn, asparagine is produced by the amidation of aspartate with ammonium ion. During amino acid degradation, asparagine is hydrolyzed by asparaginase to aspartate. Transamination of α-ketoglutarate by aspartate forms oxaloacetate and glutamate. *(Stryer, pp 503–505,578–583)*

320–322. **(320-E, 321-C, 322-A)** Keratins contain as much as 14 percent cystine, the disulfide form of the amino acid cysteine. Hair and nails, as well as the cytoskeletal elements known as intermediate filaments, are composed of fibrous keratin proteins. Functional prothrombin contains γ-carboxylated glutamate, which results from a vitamin K-dependent posttranslational modification of nascent prothrombin. Agents that competitively block vitamin K action, such as warfarin and dicumarol, act as anticoagulants. Proline is modified to hydroxyproline by a posttranslational mechanism in collagen synthesis. The reducing agent ascorbic acid is needed for the hydroxylation reaction. Scurvy, a disease caused by dietary insufficiency of vitamin C (ascorbate), is characterized by abnormal collagen that cannot properly form fibers because of the lack of hydroxylated proline residues. Phosphorylation and dephosphorylation of serine are control mechanisms for the regulation of enzyme activity via protein kinase and phosphatase reactions that are under the control of hormonal mechanisms. D-Valine is not a biologically active amino acid. Only L-amino acids are effective in mammalian systems. *(Stryer, pp 250–252,261–268,459–460,938–940)*

323–324. **(323-A, 324-A)** The variable part of nucleic acids is their sequence of bases. The base thymine, shown in **A** in the question, is found only in DNA. The base uracil, shown in **E**, replaces thymine in RNA. Uracil lacks the C-5 methyl group present in thymine. All of the other purines and pyrimidines shown in the question are common to both DNA and RNA (**B**, cytosine; **C**, adenine; **D**, guanine). Exposure to ultraviolet light, particularly in the skin, causes a cross-linking of adjacent thymine bases in DNA via bonding between each C-5 and C-6 atom. A specific repair mechanism composed of ultraviolet-specific endonuclease, DNA polymerase I (including its 5′ ⇌ 3′ exonuclease activity) and DNA ligase replace the affected area. In the autosomal recessive skin disease known as xeroderma pigmentosum, the endonuclease is functionally absent. *(Stryer, pp 72,86,677–679)*

325–326. **(325-D, 326-C)** The reduced flavin nucleotide FADH is produced at only one point in the citric acid cycle, at the conversion of succinate to fumarate. This reaction is catalyzed by succinate dehydrogenase. In contrast, NADH is formed during the two decarboxylation steps (labeled **A** and **B** on the figure that accompanies the question) and during the conversion of malate to oxaloacetate. Substrate level phosphorylation occurs during the formation of succinate from succinyl-CoA. In this step, GDP is phosphorylated to GTP using the energy of the CoA-thioester bond. *(Stryer, pp 374–379)*

327–328.   (327-B, 328-C) Under most enzymatic conditions K_m is a measure of the affinity of the enzyme for its substrate. A low K_m value indicates tight binding of substrate to enzyme; a high value denotes weak binding. In the enzymes listed in the question, lysozyme has the lowest K_m and, thus, the greatest affinity for its substrate. k_{cat}, the catalytic rate constant, is the rate of the enzymatic reaction when the enzyme is fully saturated with substrate. In many cases, this is the turnover number of the enzyme. A high value for k_{cat} indicates that the enzyme converts its substrate to product very rapidly. The overall catalytic efficiency of an enzyme is, therefore, determined by the expression k_{cat}/K_m. The higher the value for this expression, the greater the catalytic efficiency of the enzyme. Of the enzymes listed in the problem, carbonic anhydrase has the highest value for k_{cat}/K_m and, therefore, the greatest catalytic efficiency. *(Stryer, pp 190–191)*

329–330.   (329-C, 330-D) Most ATP is synthesized in the mitochondria via oxidative phosphorylation. A small amount of ATP, however, can be formed outside the mitochondria by phosphoryl group transfer from a high-energy compound directly to ADP. Phosphoenolpyruvate is a high-energy compound, and its phosphate group is transferred to ADP, yielding ATP and pyruvate. This reaction is catalyzed by pyruvate kinase. Under anaerobic conditions, such as pertains in muscle during vigorous exercise, pyruvate formed during glycolysis accumulates because of the inactivity of the citric acid cycle. The pyruvate is instead reduced to lactate in a reaction catalyzed by lactate dehydrogenase. This reaction requires NADH as a cofactor. *(Stryer, pp 355–357,363–364)*

331–333.   (331-D, 332-C, 333-B) The first three reaction sequences are distinct parts of the glycolytic pathway. The precursor for formation of fructose 6-phosphate can be either glucose or glycogen. In the first instance, 1 mol of ATP is consumed to generate glucose 6-phosphate, which is converted to fructose 6-phosphate. In muscle, however, glycogen can be broken down via a phosphorolysis reaction involving inorganic phosphate and catalyzed by glycogen phosphorylase. The product is glucose 1-phosphate, which is converted to glucose 6-phosphate and metabolized via the glycolytic pathway. Thus, the phosphorylated sugar intermediate is generated from glycogen without expenditure of an ATP. Fructose 6-phosphate is converted to fructose 1,6-biphosphate in a reaction that uses ATP. In the conversion of glyceraldehyde 3-phosphate to pyruvate, 2 mol of ATP are generated. Pyruvate may be used for the synthesis of glucose by gluconeogenesis. Four moles of ATP (and 2 mol of GTP) are consumed in the conversion of pyruvate to glucose via the gluco-

neogenic pathway. *(Stryer, pp 349–357,438–442,451–454)*

334–336.   (334-B, 335-A, 336-D) Actinomycin D binds specifically to DNA and prevents its use as a template for RNA synthesis. It inhibits the growth of rapidly growing cells and is used for the treatment of certain cancers. Tetracycline binds to bacterial ribosomes and interferes with the binding of aminoacyl-tRNA. It has no effect on eukaryotic ribosomes and is, therefore, a potent antibiotic. Methotrexate is an inhibitor of dihydrofolate reductase and several steps in the de novo purine biosynthetic pathway. It, therefore, blocks the synthesis of thymidylate (TMP) and purines. It is widely used in the chemotherapy of a variety of cancers. *(Stryer, pp 614–616,715,759)*

337–339.   (337-E, 338-A, 339-C) Protein biosynthesis (translation) is always initiated at an AUG codon (at GUG on rare occasions), which codes for methionine. A special initiator, tRNA, which is charged with methionine, recognizes the initiation codon. In prokaryotes the α-amino group on the methionine is blocked by formylation. This is not the case for eukaryotic initiator tRNA. The enzymes that mediate RNA biosynthesis (transcription) are referred to as RNA polymerases. In eukaryotes, there are three different RNA polymerases that are responsible for the transcription of ribosomal RNA, messenger RNA or transfer and 5S RNA, respectively. B contrast, a single RNA polymerase, is responsible for the transcription of all RNA species in prokaryotes. The enzyme responsible for mRNA synthesis in eukaryotes is RNA polymerase II. This enzyme is specifically inhibited by α-amanitin. RNA synthesis in all organisms begins at a specific nucleotide position. RNA polymerase binds to the DNA template at a specific sequence called a promoter. In prokaryotes, the promoter consists of two sequence elements that occur at 10 and 35 nucleotides before the transcription start site. Similar sequences comprise eukaryotic promoters but, in general, are found 25 and between 40 and 100 nucleotides upstream of the transcription start site. *(Stryer, pp 704–705,716–718,752–753)*

340–342.   (340-C, 341-A, 342-D) Triacylglycerols are transported in the blood by chylomicrons and VLDLs. The endproducts of VLDL delipidation are LDLs, which are rich in cholesterol. LDLs are taken up by peripheral tissues via specific LDL receptors. In this manner, LDLs are responsible for delivering cholesterol to peripheral tissues. HDLs are protein-rich lipoproteins that are important in the transport of cholesterol from peripheral tissues to the liver for excretion as bile. Bile salts are polar derivatives of cholesterol and are its major breakdown products. Lipoproteins, such as HDL and LDL, contain a variety of proteins that are referred to as apoproteins, one of which is apoprotein E. It is a constituent of chylomicrons, VLDL and IDL. *(Stryer, pp 559–564)*

343–345. **(343-E, 344-D, 345-A)** Mitochondrial electron transport (ET) is tightly coupled to oxidative phosphorylation (ATP synthesis) at three sites along the ET chain: NADH-Q reductase → QH_2, cytochrome b → cytochrome c_1 and cytochrome oxidase → O_2. At each of these steps a proton gradient is generated across the inner mitochondrial membrane and one molecule of ATP is synthesized by the flow of a pair of electrons. The oxidation of many substrates, including pyruvate, is coupled to NAD^+ reduction and the electrons enter the ET chain via NADH. Rotenone specifically inhibits ET from NADH to coenzyme Q. In contrast, succinate oxidation coupled to FAD^+ reduction (yielding $FADH_2$) and these electrons enter the ET chain at coenzyme Q, past the block produced by rotenone. As a result, rotenone does not affect electron transport dependent on succinate. Antimycin A specifically blocks electron flow between cytochromes b and c_1. Thus, it inhibits electron transport dependent on succinate. Dinitrophenol dissipates the proton gradient across the inner mitochondrial membrane and uncouples ET from oxidative phosphorylation. It has no effect on electron transport or the enzyme ATP synthase. The energy produced during ET, which normally is utilized to establish the proton gradient, is dissipated as heat in the presence of dinitrophenol. *(Stryer, pp 412–413,421–422)*

346. **(C)** Membranes consist of a bilayer structure composed of both lipid and protein. The protein components of a membrane can be classified as either integral or peripheral. For integral membrane proteins, some portion of the molecule is embedded within the lipid bilayer. By contrast, peripheral membrane proteins are loosely associated with the membrane surface. Transmembrane proteins traverse the lipid bilayer and are a type of integral protein. These proteins are tightly bound to the lipid portion of the membrane via hydrophobic interactions between nonpolar amino acid sidechains and nonpolar lipids. The segments of proteins present within the membranes will contain a high degree of nonpolar residues. *(Stryer, pp 292–293,303–304)*

347. **(E)** Humans have the capacity to synthesize 11 of the 20 common amino acids required for protein synthesis. The remaining nine amino acids must be supplied in the diet. These latter amino acids are referred to as essential amino acids. They are: histidine, isoleucine, leucine, lysine, methionine, phenylalanine, threonine, tryptophan, and valine. Of the amino acids listed in the question, only ser-

ine is a nonessential amino acid, which can be synthesized by humans. *(Stryer, p 578)*

348. **(B)** The cofactor for fatty acid biosynthesis is NADPH. Fatty acid biosynthesis takes place in the cytoplasm. The committed step in the process is formation of malonyl-CoA in a reaction catalyzed by acetyl-CoA carboxylase. Citrate stimulates the activity of this enzyme, resulting in increased fatty acid biosynthesis. Elevated fatty acid levels, primarily that of palmitoyl-CoA, is a negative regulator of the process. *(Stryer, pp 481–485,490–491)*

349. **(C)** In sickle cell anemia, patients suffer from hemolytic anemia due to the presence of sickled erythrocytes in the venous circulation. Sickle cell anemia is a genetic disease that is caused by a single base change in the gene for β-globin. This change results in a single amino acid substitution of valine for glutamic acid at position 6 in the β-globin protein. The single base change in the DNA results in the loss of a restriction enzyme digestion site that allows the disease to be diagnosed by fetal DNA testing. The amino acid change is from a highly polar amino acid (glu) to a non-polar amino acid (val) and leads to a change in the electrophoretic mobility of Hb S. The amino acid substitution also results in aggregation of deoxygenated Hb S. This aggregation does not occur with the oxygenated form. Thus, the solubility of deoxygenated Hb S is lower than normal and precipitation of the aggregates causes sickling of the red cells. *(Stryer, pp 163–170)*

350. **(A)** The kinetic plot shown in the figure is characteristic of an allosteric enzyme. The curve, in the presence of high [ATP], has a sigmoid shape (S shape), which indicates that substrate binding to the enzyme is cooperative. This indicates that the binding of one substrate molecule enhances the binding of subsequent substrate molecules to the enzyme. Allosteric enzymes have binding sites for molecules other than the substrate. Binding of such compounds will modify the activity of the enzyme and are called allosteric effectors. In the figure, the maximum velocity is ultimately achieved at both low and high [ATP], and thus V_{max} is not affected by ATP. The curve is shifted to the right, which indicates that the apparent K_m is increased (not decreased) in the presence of high [ATP]. ATP is a negative effector of phosphofructokinase and inhibits the activity of the enzyme. *(Stryer, pp 193,239–243,359–361)*

351. **(D)** The pH of a buffer solution can best be calculated by the Henderson-Hasselbalch equation:

$$pH = pK + \log [base]/[acid]$$

The pK of an acid is the pH at which it is half-dissociated. If the molar proportions of the basic and acidic forms of the buffer, as well as the pK, are known, this equation can be used to calculate pH. For example, for a solution of acetic acid (pK = 4.8) containing 0.1 mol/L of acetic acid and 0.2 mol/L of acetate ion, the pH can be calculated as follows:

$$pH = 4.8 + \log 0.2/0.1 = 4.8 = \log 2 = 4.8 + 0.3 = 5.1$$
(Stryer, pp 41–42)

352. **(C)** UDP-glucose is an activated form of glucose, which is synthesized from glucose 1-phosphate and UTP in a reaction catalyzed by the enzyme UDP-glucose pyrophosphorylase. The utilization of galactose by the glycolytic pathway requires its conversion to glucose 1-phosphate. Galactose is first phosphorylated to galactose 1-phosphate in a reaction requiring ATP and catalyzed by the enzyme galactokinase. Galactose 1-phosphate is then utilized as follows:

galactose 1-phosphate + UDP-glucose → UDP-galactose + glucose 1-phosphate

Glucose 1-phosphate is isomerized to glucose 6-phosphate by the enzyme phosphoglucomutase and glucose 6-phosphate enters glycolysis. UDP-glucose is regenerated from UDP-galactose by action of the enzyme UDP-galactose-4-epimerase. Glucose 6-phosphate is formed from glucose and ATP and fructose enters glycolysis by conversion to fructose 1-phosphate. Neither of these processes requires UDP-glucose. Similarly, debranching of glycogen and synthesis of pyruvate do not require UDP-glucose. *(Stryer, pp 357–359)*

353. **(D)** Eukaryotic chromatin is comprised of repeating units called nucleosomes. These are composed of between 160 and 240 base pairs of DNA and two molecules each of the histones H2A, H2B, H3, and H4. Histones are small basic proteins that bind very tightly to DNA, and the eight histone molecules form a protein core around which the DNA is wound. This arrangement is one factor that allows the packing of large amounts of DNA into the nucleus. RNA is not part of the essential nucleosome structure. The eukaryotic genome contains some DNA sequences that are repeated up to one million times. These are referred to as repetitive sequences. Some of these may serve a structural function in the chromosome; e.g., centromeres contain highly repetitive DNA sequences. *(Stryer, pp 824–829,834–836)*

354. **(A)** In the pentose phosphate pathway, NADPH is generated as glucose 6-phosphate is oxidized to ribose 5-phosphate. The first step of the pathway, the conversion of glucose 6-phosphate to 6-phos-

phogluconolactone, is catalyzed by the enzyme glucose 6-phosphate dehydrogenase. NADP$^+$ is a cofactor for this reaction, which is regulated by its availability. Elevated concentrations of NADPH inhibit the reaction and thus inhibit the pathway. *(Stryer, pp 427–431)*

355. **(D)** In general, GTP serves as the energy source for protein synthesis on the ribosome. Binding of aminoacyl-tRNA to the ribosomal A site is mediated by formation of a ternary complex between tRNA, elongation factor EF-Tu (or EF1 in eukaryotes), and GTP. The GTP is hydrolyzed concomitant with tRNA binding to the ribosome. Similarly, binding of the specific initiator tRNA, met-tRNA$_i$, to the ribosome involves the participation of the initiation factor IF2 (eIF2 in eukaryotes) and GTP. Hydrolysis of GTP is a necessary step for formation of productive initiation complexes on the ribosome. Polypeptide chain elongation proceeds after peptide bond formation via the process of translocation, which is also mediated by a protein factor (EF-G or EF2) and requires GTP hydrolysis. The actual formation of the peptide bond is catalyzed by the peptidyl transferase activity of the ribosome and does not require any non-ribosomal protein factors or GTP hydrolysis. *(Stryer, pp 754–758)*

356. **(B)** During strenuous physical exercise, the rate of production of pyruvate via glycolysis exceeds the capacity of the citric acid cycle to utilize it and pyruvate accumulates. NADH also accumulates and glycolysis cannot continue unless NAD$^+$ is regenerated. This is accomplished by the conversion of pyruvate to lactate by lactate dehydrogenase, which uses NADH as a cofactor and produces NAD$^+$. Pyruvate and lactate diffuse out of muscle into blood and are taken up by the liver, where pyruvate is converted to glucose. *(Stryer, pp 444– 445)*

357. **(B)** An important step in the elucidation of protein structure is determination of the amino acid sequence. The initial step in this process usually is identification of the N-terminal amino acid. This can be accomplished by chemical means through the use of several possible reagents, including phenylisothiocyanate. This reagent reacts with the free α-amino group at the N-terminus of a protein to yield modified amino acids, which can be identified by a variety of techniques. Ninhydrin reacts with amino acids to give a blue color and can be used for measurement of protein concentration. Cyanogen bromide cleaves peptide bonds whose carboxyl function is donated by methionine. Carboxypeptidase is an enzyme that sequentially removes amino acids from the C-terminal of proteins. Trypsin is a proteolytic enzyme that cleaves peptide bonds whose carboxyl function is donated by lysine or arginine. *(Stryer, pp 50–57)*

358. **(E)** Rifamycin (rifampicin) is an inhibitor of transcription. It specifically blocks initiation of transcription by interfering with formation of the first phosphodiester bond in the RNA chain. The other antibiotics listed are all inhibitors of protein synthesis. *(Stryer, pp 714–715,759–760)*

359. **(D)** Fatty acids are activated to the coenzyme A derivatives at the outer mitochondrial membrane but are oxidized inside the mitochondria. Long chain fatty acyl-CoA molecules do not cross the mitochondrial membrane. A special transport system involving carnitine is utilized for movement of the activated fatty acids into the mitochondria. The fatty acyl moiety is transferred from the CoA to carnitine in a reaction catalyzed by carnitine acyltransferase I. Acyl carnitine thus formed is shuttled across the inner mitochondrial membrane where the fatty acyl group is transferred back to a coenzyme A molecule within the mitochondrial matrix. The latter reaction is catalyzed by carnitine acyltransferase II. Medium chain fatty acyl CoAs can cross the mitochondrial membrane and do not require the carnitine transport system for entry into the mitochondria. *(Stryer, pp 473–474)*

360. **(B)** Restriction endonucleases are enzymes produced by bacteria that recognize a specific nucleotide sequence in DNA and cleave the phosphodiester bonds of both DNA strands. In bacteria, these enzymes serve the protective function of preventing transformation by the uptake of foreign DNA. The recognition sites for the enzymes possess a two-fold axis of rotational symmetry, i.e., the sites are palindromes. The DNA in the host cell is protected from digestion because the recognition site is modified by methylation. Restriction enzymes cleave DNA regardless of its higher order structure and do not require that the DNA be supercoiled. These enzymes are widely used in the application of recombinant DNA technology. *(Stryer, pp 118–119,858–859)*

361. **(C)** The synthesis of all steroid hormones involves formation of progesterone from cholesterol. An intermediate in this conversion is pregnenolone. These reactions, as well as many of the reactions leading from progesterone to other steroid hormone derivatives, require the action of monooxygenases (or mixed-function oxygenases). These enzymes mediate hydroxylation reactions necessary for synthesis of the steroid hormones. These reactions involve the incorporation of oxygen atoms from molecular oxygen, using the reductive potential of NADPH. Vitamin D is a steroid that is formed from cholesterol (more specifically, 7-dehydrocholesterol) by the action of ultraviolet light. It does not play a role in steroid hormone biosynthesis. *(Stryer, pp 565–569)*

362. **(C)** The initial step in purine nucleotide biosynthesis is the formation of phosphoribosylamine from PRPP and glutamine. This reaction is catalyzed by PRPP amidotransferase and is the committed step in purine biosynthesis. The reaction is regulated by feedback inhibition by AMP and/or GMP. Since PRPP is a substrate in this reaction, the rate of purine biosynthesis is governed by the availability of PRPP. The initial purine nucleotide product of the de novo pathway is IMP. This compound serves as a branch point in the synthesis of AMP and GMP. In one branch of the pathway, IMP is converted to AMP and requires GTP, whereas in the other branch of the pathway, IMP is converted to GMP in reactions requiring ATP. The reciprocal requirements of one purine nucleotide for the synthesis of the other serves to insure that relatively balanced amounts of both are produced. Xanthine oxidase is involved in the degradation of purines and plays no role in the biosynthesis. *(Stryer, pp 602–607)*

363. **(C)** Any condition that results in elevated levels of purine nucleotides is likely to cause hyperuricemia. HGPRT is a salvage pathway enzyme that catalyzes the condensation of hypoxanthine or guanine with PRPP to yield IMP or GMP. In this way, purine bases, which become available in the diet or by virtue of nucleic acid degradation, can be recycled into the corresponding nucleotides and used for nucleic acid biosynthesis. If this salvage is blocked, the purine bases are degraded further to uric acid. Xanthine oxidase, adenosine deaminase, and purine nucleoside phosphorylase are all purine degradative enzymes. The absence of any of these enzymes would prevent the formation of uric acid. PRPP amidotransferase is the enzyme that catalyzes the committed step in purine biosynthesis. Its absence would result in lower levels of purines and would not result in elevated uric acid levels. *(Stryer, pp 602–604,618–623)*

364. **(D)** Reduced glutathione is an antioxidant. It is regenerated by the transfer of electrons from NADPH to oxidized glutathione via FAD. This reaction, which transfers the electrons to a disulfide bridge of glutathione, is catalyzed by glutathione reductase. In erythrocytes, the reduced form of glutathione maintains the cysteine residues of Hb and other RBC proteins in a reduced state. It also plays a role in cell detoxification by reacting with organic peroxides and hydrogen peroxides. *(Stryer, pp 436–438)*

365. **(A)** Arsenate replaces the P_i that normally reacts with glyceraldehyde 3-phosphate to form 1,3-DPG. Instead, an unstable intermediate, 1-arseno-3-phosphoglycerate, is produced and immediately hydrolyzes to 3-phosphoglycerate. NADH is formed as usual. Thus glycolysis proceeds in the presence of arsenate, but the ATP usually produced in the conversion of 1,3-DPG to 3-phosphoglycerate is lost. Since glycolysis proceeds, pyruvate is formed. *(Stryer, p 368)*

366. (A) Although CDP-diacylglycerol can be the activated intermediate in the synthesis of phosphoglycerides, diacylglycerol itself can be used in salvage pathways. In the latter reactions, ethanolamine is activated to CDP-ethanolamine, which can then be esterified to diacylglycerol in one step. A similar pathway is available for synthesis of phosphatidyl choline, but not for phosphatidyl serine or phosphatidyl inositol. Lysophosphatidic acid is glycerol esterified to a fatty acid at the 1′ position and to phosphate at the 3′ position. It is an intermediate in the synthesis of diacylglycerols. Cardiolipin is diphosphatidyl glycerol. *(Stryer, pp 547–550)*

367–370. (367-C, 368-E, 369-A, 370-B) ATP and ADP do not diffuse freely across the inner mitochondrial membrane. A specific transport protein, ATP-ADP translocase, concomitantly mediates the exit of ATP from and the entry of ADP into mitochondria. This protein is specifically inhibited by atractyloside. Antimycin A blocks electron transport from cytochrome b to cytochrome c_1. The energy available from electron transport is coupled to the synthesis of ATP by proton flow through ATP synthase. This multi-subunit protein complex consists of a portion (designated F_1), which catalyzes the synthesis of ATP and a segment (F_0), which contains the proton channel. Oligomycin binds to the stalk between F_1 and F_0 and prevents utilization of the proton gradient for ATP synthesis. Valinomycin is an antibiotic that binds K^+ very tightly and interferes with oxidative phosphorylation because the mitochondria use the energy of electron transport to accumulate K^+ rather than for synthesis of ATP. Amytal blocks electron transfer within the NADH-Q reductase complex. Cyanide and carbon monoxide block electron transfer from cytochrome oxidase to O_2. Dicumarol, a derivative of coumarin, is an anticoagulant, due to its function as a vitamin K antagonist. *(Stryer, pp 251,412–415,418–419,964–968)*

371–374. (371-B, 372-I, 373-G, 374-F) One of the key steps in gluconeogenesis is the conversion of pyruvate to phosphoenolpyruvate. This cannot be accomplished by the simple reversal of the pyruvate kinase reaction of glycolysis. Rather, pyruvate is first converted to oxaloacetate, which in turn is decarboxylated and phosphorylated to phosphoenolpyruvate. The latter reaction is catalyzed by phosphoenolpyruvate carboxykinase and requires GTP. α-Ketoglutarate is oxidatively decarboxylated to succinyl CoA during the citric acid cycle in a reaction catalyzed by the α-ketoglutarate de-

hydrogenase complex. The reaction requires NAD^+ as a cofactor and generates NADH. The initial step in the pentose phosphate pathway is the conversion of glucose 6-phosphate to 6-phosphoglucono-δ-lactone and is catalyzed by glucose 6-phosphate dehydrogenase. The reaction requires NADP+ and generates NADPH, which is one of the major products of the pathway. The last step of glycolysis is the production of pyruvate from phosphoenolpyruvate in a reaction catalyzed by pyruvate kinase. The reaction proceeds with the production of a mole of ATP and is not dependent on mitochondrial oxidative phosphorylation. Therefore, ATP is produced even in the absence of oxygen. *(Stryer, pp 355,382–383,428,439)*

375. (A) The amino groups of amino acids are converted to urea for excretion via the urea cycle. The liver is the only organ capable of carrying this out. The human liver produces some 20 to 30 g of urea each day. Synthesis of gangliosides, which are components of all mammalian plasma membranes, can be carried out in all cells. Nucleotide biosynthesis is also carried out by most cells, as is utilization of medium-chain fatty acids as an energy source. Glycogen can be degraded not only in the liver but also chiefly in muscle. *(Stryer, pp 500–502)*

376. (D) Formation of acetyl-CoA from pyruvate is catalyzed by the enzymes of the pyruvate dehydrogenase complex.

$$\text{pyruvate} + \text{CoA} + \text{NAD}^+ \rightarrow \text{acetyl-CoA} + \text{CO}_2 + \text{NADH}$$

As can be seen from the reaction, the stoichiometric cofactors are CoA and NAD^+. In addition, pyruvate dehydrogenase requires thiamine pyrophosphate, dihydrolipoyl transacetylase requires lipoic acid, and dihydrolipoyl dehydrogenase requires FAD. Biotin is not required for these reactions. *(Stryer, pp 379–382)*

377. (E) Niacin (nicotinic acid) is required for the synthesis of NAD^+. Its deficiency results in pellagra, a disease characterized by psychic disturbances, diarrhea, and dermatitis. A diet rich in niacin will prevent the disease. *(Stryer, pp 617–618)*

378. (D) Aspartate transcarbamyolase is an allosteric enzyme that is regulated by noncovalent modification. Binding of ATP to the enzyme inhibits its activity. By contrast, the activities of the other enzymes are modulated by covalent modification. Pepsin and chymotrypsin are derived from proteolytic cleavage of the zymogens pepsinogen and chymotrypsinogen. The zymogen forms are not active. Glycogen synthase and pyruvate kinase activity are modulated by reversible phosphorylation. Both enzymes are less active in the phosphorylated form and are activated by dephosphorylation. *(Stryer, pp 243–247,359–362,462–463)*

379–381. **(379-G, 380-E, 381-A)** Purine nucleoside phosphorylase catalyzes the conversion of guanosine and inosine to guanine and hypoxanthine, respectively. Guanine is then converted to xanthine and both xanthine and hypoxanthine are substrates for xanthine oxidase yielding uric acid. A deficiency in purine nucleoside phosphorylase will prevent the production of uric acid and will result in hypouricemia. The major effect of this enzyme deficiency, however, is immunodeficiency. Lack of the salvage pathway enzyme hypoxanthine phosphoribosyl transferase results in Lesch-Nyhan syndrome, which is characterized by severe behavioral disorders. It also results in significantly elevated levels of uric acid production. Thymidylate synthase catalyzes the methylation of deoxyuridylate (dUMP) to thymidylate. Fluorodeoxyuridylate is a substrate analogue of dUMP and specifically inhibits the activity of thymidylate synthase. Allopurinol is an inhibitor of xanthine oxidase. Sulfamethoxazole is an inhibitor of folate biosynthesis in bacteria. Since humans do not possess the capacity to synthesize folate, sulfamethoxazole is employed as an antibiotic. Glucose 6-phosphatase catalyzes the conversion of glucose 6-phosphate to glucose in the liver. A deficiency of this enzyme results in glycogen storage disease. Since glucose 6-phosphate is not converted to glucose, it is employed as a substrate in the pentose phosphate pathway. This results in higher than normal amounts of ribose 5-phosphate which, in turn, drives increased levels of purine biosynthesis. As a result, a deficiency of this enzyme leads to hyperuricemia. Adenine phosphoribosyl transferase is a salvage pathway enzyme that converts adenine to AMP. *(Stryer, pp 606,613–615,620–623)*

BIBLIOGRAPHY

Lehninger AL. *Biochemistry.* 2nd ed. New York: Worth Publishers, Inc; 1977

Stryer L. *Biochemistry.* 3rd ed. San Francisco: WH Freeman and Co; 1988

Subspecialty List: Biochemistry

Question Number and Subspecialty

255. Nucleotide metabolism
256. Energy metabolism
257. Integration of metabolism
258. Blood
259. Muscle contraction
260. Thermodynamics
261. Integration of metabolism
262. pH
263. Muscle contraction
264. Carbohydrate metabolism
265. Carbohydrate metabolism
266. Carbohydrate metabolism
267. Carbohydrate metabolism
268. Nucleotide metabolism
269. Enzymes
270. Proteins
271. Molecular biology
272. Enzymes
273. Lipids
274. Lipids
275. Lipids
276. Lipids
277. Lipids
278. Lipids
279. Lipids
280. Lipids
281. Enzymes
282. Enzymes
283. Enzymes
284. Integration of metabolism
285. Hormones
286. Vitamins
287. Vitamins
288. Vitamins
289. Lipids
290. Carbohydrate metabolism
291. Small molecule metabolism
292. Proteins
293. Lipids
294. Carbohydrate metabolism
295. Energy metabolism
296. Lipids
297. Carbohydrate metabolism
298. Blood
299. Carbohydrate metabolism
300. Nucleotide metabolism
301. Amino acid metabolism
302. Nucleotide metabolism
303. Energy metabolism
304. Energy metabolism
305. Carbohydrate metabolism
306. Thermodynamics
307. Thermodynamics
308. Thermodynamics
309. Carbohydrate metabolism
310. Carbohydrate metabolism
311. Carbohydrate metabolism
312. Carbohydrate metabolism
313. Carbohydrate metabolism
314. Carbohydrate metabolism
315. Carbohydrate metabolism
316. Amino acid metabolism
317. Amino acid metabolism
318. Amino acid metabolism
319. Amino acid metabolism
320. Protein
321. Protein
322. Protein
323. Molecular biology
324. Molecular biology
325. Energy metabolism
326. Energy metabolism
327. Enzymes
328. Enzymes
329. Carbohydrate metabolism
330. Carbohydrate metabolism
331. Carbohydrate metabolism
332. Carbohydrate metabolism
333. Carbohydrate metabolism
334. Molecular biology
335. Molecular biology
336. Molecular biology
337. Molecular biology
338. Molecular biology
339. Molecular biology
340. Lipids
341. Lipids
342. Lipids

343. Energy metabolism
344. Energy metabolism
345. Energy metabolism
346. Membranes
347. Amino acid metabolism
348. Lipids
349. Blood
350. Enzymes
351. pH
352. Carbohydrate metabolism
353. Molecular biology
354. Carbohydrate metabolism
355. Molecular biology
356. Carbohydrate metabolism
357. Proteins
358. Molecular biology
359. Lipids
360. Molecular biology
361. Lipids
362. Nucleotide metabolism
363. Nucleotide metabolism
364. Carbohydrate metabolism
365. Carbohydrate metabolism
366. Lipids
367. Energy metabolism
368. Energy metabolism
369. Energy metabolism
370. Energy metabolism
371. Carbohydrate metabolism
372. Carbohydrate metabolism
373. Carbohydrate metabolism
374. Carbohydrate metabolism
375. Integration of metabolism
376. Vitamins
377. Vitamins
378. Proteins
379. Nucleotide metabolism
380. Nucleotide metabolism
381. Nucleotide metabolism

CHAPTER 4

Microbiology
Questions

DIRECTIONS (Questions 382 through 490): Each of the numbered items or incomplete statements in this section is followed by answers or by completions of the statement. Select the ONE lettered answer or completion that is BEST in each case.

382. Protective strategies for prevention of the septic shock syndrome could include all of the following EXCEPT

   (A) anticachectin antibody
   (B) core polysaccharide-specific antibody
   (C) lipid A-specific antibody
   (D) antibody to terminal polysaccharides of O antigen
   (E) pharmacologic antileucotriene agents

383. Staphylococcal scalded skin syndrome is related to the organism's ability to produce

   (A) α-toxin
   (B) lipase
   (C) exfoliatin
   (D) hyaluronidase
   (E) coagulase

384. Of the following, the virus that is most resistant to chemical and physical agents is the one that causes

   (A) mumps
   (B) measles
   (C) influenza
   (D) serum hepatitis
   (E) polio

385. For viruses, the burst size is

   (A) the interval of time between infection and release of progeny virus
   (B) the average number of progeny viruses released per infected cell
   (C) the interval between infection and the appearance of intracellular progeny viruses

   (D) the average number of viruses that infect a cell
   (E) the number of viruses per unit volume of suspension

386. All of the following are stages of conjugation EXCEPT

   (A) effective pair formation
   (B) plasmid or chromosome mobilization
   (C) recombination
   (D) competency
   (E) transfer of a unique strand of DNA

387. Ticks are the arthropod vector of

   (A) Tsutsugamushi disease
   (B) Rocky Mountain spotted fever
   (C) murine typhus
   (D) epidemic typhus
   (E) bubonic plague

388. The plasma membrane receptor for influenza virus is

   (A) an unsubstituted protein
   (B) a glycolipid
   (C) a glycoprotein
   (D) a mucopolysaccharide
   (E) a nucleic acid

389. All of the following contribute directly to the intracellular killing of microbes by neutrophils EXCEPT

   (A) myeloperoxidase–hydrogen peroxide–halide system
   (B) oxygen metabolites
   (C) lysozyme and other hydrolytic enzymes
   (D) iron chelating proteins, such as lactoferrin
   (E) catalase

390. Which of the following statements concerning the Ouchterlony diagram below is true?

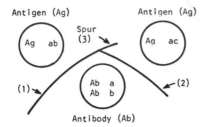

(A) Line 1 will contain Ag ab and Ab b only.
(B) Line 2 will contain Ag ac and Ab b.
(C) The spur will contain Ab a and Ag ab.
(D) The spur will contain Ag ac and Ab a.
(E) The spur will contain Ag ab and Ab b.

391. The base pair substitution that results in the change of a purine for a pyrimidine is a

(A) transformant
(B) transition
(C) transversion
(D) transposition
(E) frame shift

392. Transformation of bacteria can be blocked by

(A) RNAse in the medium
(B) DNAse in the medium
(C) antiserum against bacteriophage
(D) bacteriophage that adsorb to sex pili
(E) preventing cell-to-cell contact between donor and recipient cultures

393. A lysogenic cell refers to a bacterial cell that

(A) is susceptible to a virulent phage
(B) is resistant to lysozyme
(C) is resistant to lysis
(D) carries a prophage
(E) excretes lysozyme

394. The antibody induced by which of the following parts of an influenza virus is most protective?

(A) envelope
(B) neuraminidase
(C) hemagglutinin
(D) nucleic acid
(E) internal protein

395. Chlamydiae and rickettsiae are correctly described as

(A) spread by the bite of an infected arthropod
(B) resistant to the usual broad-spectrum antibiotics
(C) containing either RNA or DNA but not both
(D) obligate parasites of living cells
(E) dividing solely by binary fission

396. In the following diseases, the etiologic agents are initially introduced to the host in the form of spores EXCEPT

(A) tetanus
(B) infant botulism
(C) anthrax
(D) gas gangrene
(E) diphtheria

397. A genetic test of function that depends on the interaction of the products of genes is

(A) suppression
(B) postreplication repair
(C) recombination
(D) host-induced modification
(E) complementation

398. Ultraviolet light

(A) disrupts the bacterial cell membrane
(B) removes free sulfhydryl groups
(C) is a common protein denaturant
(D) causes the formation of pyrimidine dimers
(E) acts as an alkylating agent

399. Members of the genera *Rhizobium* and *Azotobacter*

(A) are involved in nitrogen fixation
(B) grow best at a pH of 3.5 to 4.0
(C) are thermophilic
(D) contain capsules composed of D-glutamic acid
(E) adhere to human cells

400. Penicillin would be LEAST effective in treating which of the following diseases?

(A) syphilis
(B) gonorrhea
(C) pneumococcal pneumonia
(D) mycoplasmal pneumonia
(E) streptococcal pharyngitis

401. In coccidioidomycosis, which of the following is a poor prognostic sign?

(A) conversion to positive skin test
(B) positive precipitin titer
(C) decreased precipitin titer

(D) increasing complement fixation titers

(E) decreasing complement fixation titers

402. All of the following diseases are associated with herpes viruses EXCEPT

(A) central nervous system diseases

(B) congenital infections

(C) venereal diseases

(D) skin rashes

(E) scrapie

403. A rising titer of antistreptolysin O indicates a diagnosis of

(A) acute rheumatic fever

(B) glomerulonephritis

(C) a recent streptococcal infection

(D) scarlet fever

(E) erysipelas

404. Secretory IgA consists of IgA dimer, secretory component (SC), plus

(A) paraprotein

(B) J chain

(C) SC epitope

(D) γ chain

(E) ε chain

405. The antiphagocytosis property of group A streptococci is associated with

(A) M protein

(B) hyaluronidase

(C) streptolysin O

(D) streptolysin S

(E) DNAse

406. The mutagen 5-bromouracil (5-BU) preferentially causes

(A) frame shift mutations

(B) transitions

(C) transversions

(D) deletions

(E) recombinations

407. Antigens can best be processed for presentation by

(A) macrophages

(B) Kupffer cells

(C) B cells

(D) young erythrocytes

(E) suppressor T cells

408. All of the following substances affect lymphocytes EXCEPT

(A) migration inhibitory factor (MIF)

(B) interleukin 1

(C) transfer factor

(D) interleukin 2

(E) blastogenic factor

409. One of the first events that occurs after poliovirus infects a cell is

(A) hydrolysis of viral DNA

(B) synthesis of viral DNA

(C) hydrolysis of viral protein

(D) hydrolysis of host DNA

(E) cessation of host cell macromolecular biosynthesis

410. Damage to DNA caused by bifunctional alkylating agents that damage both strands of DNA is repaired by

(A) photoreactivation

(B) excision repair

(C) direct repair

(D) recombination of postreplication repair

(E) microinsertion

411. Patients with X-linked infantile agammaglobulinemia are known to

(A) exhibit profound deficiencies of cell-mediated immunity

(B) have very low quantities of immunoglobulin in their serum

(C) have normal numbers of B lymphocytes

(D) have a depletion of lymphocytes in the paracortical areas of lymph nodes

(E) be particularly susceptible to viral and fungal infections

412. During a routine pelvic examination, a woman is found to have a tender, open lesion on the vagina. The patient states that she had similar lesions 12 months previously. The causative agent is most likely to be

(A) echovirus

(B) coxsackievirus

(C) rubella virus

(D) herpes simplex virus

(E) measles virus

413. Antibodies against acetylcholine neural receptors are thought to be involved in the pathogenesis of

(A) myasthenia gravis
(B) multiple sclerosis
(C) acute idiopathic polyneuritis
(D) Guillain-Barré syndrome
(E) postpericardiotomy syndrome

414. A 7-month-old child is hospitalized for a yeast infection that does not respond to therapy. The patient has a history of acute pyogenic infections. Physical examination reveals that the spleen and lymph nodes are not palpable. A differential WBC count shows 95 percent neutrophils, 1 percent lymphocytes, and 4 percent monocytes. A bone marrow specimen contains no plasma cells or lymphocytes. X-ray reveals absence of a thymic shadow. Tonsils are absent. These findings are most compatible with

(A) multiple myeloma
(B) severe combined immunodeficiency disease
(C) X-linked agammaglobulinemia
(D) Wiskott-Aldrich syndrome
(E) chronic granulomatous disease

415. The figure below represents the

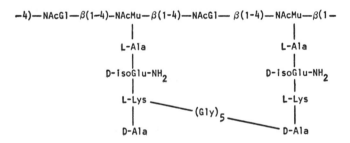

(A) O antigen of *Salmonella typhimurium*
(B) peptidoglycan of *Staphylococcus aureus*
(C) C substance of *Streptococcus pneumoniae*
(D) peptidoglycan of *Mycoplasma pneumoniae*
(E) H antigen of *S. typhimurium*

416. A stage of competence of recipient cells is necessary for

(A) complementation
(B) transduction
(C) transformation
(D) conjugation
(E) transposition

417. Enteroviruses are the causative agents of all of the following diseases EXCEPT

(A) aseptic meningitis
(B) gastrointestinal infections
(C) myocarditis
(D) pleurodynia
(E) shingles

418. A rabbit is repeatedly injected with a hapten. Two weeks later, its serum is subjected to a gel diffusion assay with the hapten and a carrier protein. It would be expected that

(A) no precipitin line will be present
(B) a line of identity between the serum and carrier protein will be detected
(C) a line of identity between serum and both the carrier and the hapten will be present
(D) a line of partial identity between serum, carrier, and hapten will be detected
(E) a line of nonidentity between serum, carrier, and hapten will be detected

419. All of the following are components of R plasmids EXCEPT

(A) R determinant
(B) the pilus
(C) RTF component
(D) insertion sequences
(E) antibiotic resistance genes

420. Skeletal muscle, cardiac, and central nervous system involvement occurs with which of the following?

(A) *Wuchereria bancrofti*
(B) *Onchocerca volvulus*
(C) *Enterobius vermicularis*
(D) *Trichinella spiralis*
(E) *Necator americanus*

421. The infectiveness of *Chlamydia trachomatis* has been related to its

(A) elementary body (EB)
(B) capsule
(C) cell wall
(D) reticulate body (RB)
(E) phagosome

422. All of the following viruses have hemagglutinin in their viral envelope EXCEPT

(A) rubeola virus
(B) influenza B virus
(C) Parainfluenza virus 3
(D) rubella virus
(E) human papovavirus

423. The Vi or virulence antigen of *Salmonella* serotype *typhi* is

(A) the polysaccharide capsule
(B) the core polysaccharide of the lipopolysaccharide molecule
(C) the flagellar antigen
(D) a plasmid encoded exotoxin
(E) the lipid A portion of the LPS molecule

424. Muscle pains, eosinophilia, facial edema, and gastrointestinal upsets are classic symptoms of clinical

(A) hookworm infection
(B) trichinosis
(C) toxoplasmosis
(D) onchocerciasis
(E) pediculosis

425. High-molecular-weight substances that possess both immunogenicity and specificity are termed

(A) simple haptens
(B) determinant groups
(C) adjuvants
(D) antigens
(E) complex haptens

426. A laboratory test used to identify *Staphylococcus aureus* is based on the clotting of plasma. The microbial product that is responsible for this activity is

(A) coagulase-reactive factor
(B) coagulase
(C) prothrombin
(D) thrombin
(E) thromboplastin

427. The Weil-Felix reaction is correctly described as

(A) useful in the diagnosis of rickettsial diseases
(B) based on the agglutination of species of *Salmonella* by the patient's convalescent serum
(C) a test to detect antiviral antibodies
(D) based on scrotal swelling in a male guinea pig infected with the organism
(E) positive for Q fever when *Proteus* OXK is agglutinated

428. The most common cause of meningitis in children in the age range of 6 months to 5 years is

(A) *Haemophilus influenzae* type B
(B) pneumococcus
(C) meningococcus

(D) *Escherichia coli*
(E) *Streptococcus agalactiae*

429. The most common medium used for the cultivation of fungi is

(A) tellurite medium
(B) SS agar
(C) Lowenstein–Jensen medium
(D) selenite F medium
(E) Sabouraud's glucose agar

430. Congenital rubella syndrome is most prominent in an infant when a pregnant woman becomes infected

(A) during the first trimester of pregnancy
(B) one week before a full-term delivery
(C) one month before a full-term delivery
(D) hours before childbirth
(E) during the third trimester of pregnancy

431. The causative agents for the following infections are dimorphic fungi EXCEPT

(A) sporotrichosis
(B) candidiasis
(C) cryptococcosis
(D) histoplasmosis
(E) blastomycosis

432. A burn patient developed a wound infection, and a bacteriologic culture of the site indicates a gram-negative rod that was oxidase positive and produced a bluish green pigment. The organism was relatively resistant to antibiotics but susceptible to ticarcillin, gentamicin, and tobramycin. The organism is likely to be identified as

(A) *Escherichia coli*
(B) *Klebsiella pneumoniae*
(C) *Proteus mirabilis*
(D) *Serratia marcescens*
(E) *Pseudomonas aeruginosa*

433. Acute glomerulonephritis is a sequela of a previous infection by

(A) any M type of group A streptococci
(B) a few M types of group A streptococci
(C) only lysogenic group A streptococci
(D) all of the Lancefield groups of streptococci
(E) only encapsulated strains of *Streptococcus pneumoniae*

434. *Cryptococcus neoformans* differs from other pathogenic fungi in that it

    (A) has a capsule
    (B) is an intracellular parasite
    (C) has septate hyphae
    (D) reproduces by binary fission
    (E) is dematiacious

435. *Diphyllobothrium latum* causes anemia by

    (A) its blood-sucking activities
    (B) the production of a toxin that affects hematopoiesis
    (C) competition with the host for vitamin B_{12}
    (D) occlusion of the common bile duct
    (E) inhibition of the absorption of iron

436. Which of the following zoonotic diseases is usually transmitted to humans by the bite of an arthropod vector?

    (A) anthrax
    (B) brucellosis
    (C) salmonellosis
    (D) plague
    (E) leptospirosis

437. The greatest amount of chromosomal DNA can be transferred by

    (A) Hfr × F⁻ mating
    (B) F′ × F⁻ mating
    (C) plasmid transfer
    (D) transportation of transposable elements
    (E) specialized transduction

438. The specific biochemical reaction that describes the mechanism of action of diphtheria toxin is the

    (A) inhibition of acetylcholine release
    (B) glycosylation of mRNA
    (C) inhibition of oxidative phosphorylation
    (D) ADP-ribosylation of elongation factor 2 (EF-2)
    (E) activation of adenylcyclase

439. All of the following are true statements about *Streptococcus pneumoniae* EXCEPT that

    (A) colonies form readily on blood agar
    (B) colonies are beta hemolytic
    (C) organisms may be isolated in small numbers from normal human throat cultures
    (D) colonies are inhibited by optochin
    (E) organisms are bile soluble

440. The substance responsible for the adherence of *Streptococcus mutans* to smooth surfaces is

    (A) peptidoglycan
    (B) lipoteichoic acid
    (C) glucose
    (D) fructan
    (E) dextran

441. The best method for assessing the total number of B lymphocytes is

    (A) quantitative immunoglobulin levels
    (B) Fc receptor assay
    (C) E rosette assay
    (D) surface immunoglobulin (sIg) assay
    (E) phytohemagglutinin A (PHA) mitogenicity

442. Functional assessment of T lymphocytes includes

    (A) E rosette assay
    (B) surface immunoglobulin (sIg) evaluation
    (C) transformation of lymphocytes by phytohemagglutinin A (PHA)
    (D) serum immunoglobulin determination
    (E) enumeration of θ-bearing cells

443. Lyme disease

    (A) is transmitted by mites
    (B) is caused by *Leptospira interrogans*
    (C) is a disease in which the serum levels of IgM correlate with disease activity
    (D) has not been associated with arthritis
    (E) does not respond to tetracycline treatment early in the acute illness

444. A gram-negative bacterium is isolated from a patient's cerebrospinal fluid (CSF). It grows on enriched chocolate agar but does not grow on blood agar except adjacent to a streak of staphylococci. The organism most probably is

    (A) *Neisseria meningitidis*
    (B) *Neisseria gonorrhoeae*
    (C) *Haemophilus influenzae*
    (D) *Streptococcus pneumoniae*
    (E) *Listeria monocytogenes*

445. A common cause of pneumonia in children that is becoming increasingly common in adults with chronic obstructive pulmonary disease is

    (A) *Streptococcus pneumoniae*
    (B) *Streptococcus pyogenes*
    (C) *Klebsiella pneumoniae*
    (D) *Haemophilus influenzae*
    (E) *Staphylococcus aureus*

446. The most common cause of bacterial meningitis in newborns is

(A) *Staphylococcus aureus*

(B) *Escherichia coli*

(C) *Streptococcus pyogenes*

(D) *Neisseria meningitidis*

(E) *Streptococcus pneumoniae*

447. *Helicobacter pylori*

(A) is found usually in the oral cavity

(B) produces an abundant amount of coagulase

(C) appears to be important in the pathogenesis of peptic ulcer

(D) is an obligate intracellular parasite

(E) does not induce specific antibodies in gastritis patients

448. Immunoglobulin class, which passes the placental barrier in human beings, is

(A) IgM

(B) IgD

(C) IgE

(D) IgA

(E) IgG

449. Chagas disease is correctly described by each statement below EXCEPT

(A) caused by *Trypanosoma cruzi*

(B) transmitted to man by large reduviid (kissing) bugs

(C) characterized by fever, lymphadenitis, facial edema, and myocardiopathy

(D) animal reservoirs include cats, dogs, rats, opossums, and armadillos

(E) infection occurs by regurgitation of the organism into the wound through the insect's proboscis

450. If *Salmonella typhimurium* is grown exponentially with a generation time of 20 minutes and has reached a density of 2×10^4 colony forming units (cfu) per ml, then its density in cfu/ml in 60 additional minutes will be

(A) 2×10^6

(B) 8×10^4

(C) 1.6×10^5

(D) 3.2×10^4

(E) 4×10^5

451. Viruses are attractive vectors for gene therapy because

(A) they infect cells with a much higher efficiency as compared to chemical or physical means of gene transfer

(B) the genes inserted into viruses may be expressed in a regulated way

(C) adenovirus vectors may be used to target gene transfer into cells of the respiratory tract

(D) retrovirus vectors can be produced in large quantities from producer cell lines

(E) all of the above

452. An experiment is performed in which a lawn bacteria is plated onto a nutrient plate and "replica plated" to four media, each containing an antibiotic. Results are shown below.

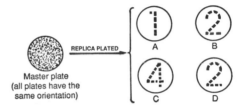

Master plate
(all plates have the same orientation)

Which of the following statements is true concerning the interpretation of this experiment?

(A) Plates B and D likely contain the same antibiotics.

(B) Lamarckian theory is supported.

(C) Plates B, C, and D all contain different antibiotics.

(D) The replica plate technique is an inappropriate method to answer questions about spontaneous mutation.

(E) Mutation is not likely to occur in bacteria.

453. Skin may be best disinfected by washing with

(A) isopropyl alcohol

(B) soap

(C) mercurochrome

(D) 1% hydrogen peroxide

(E) 1% solution of iodine in 70% ethanol

454. X-linked agammaglobulinemic patients are most likely to present with repeated infections involving

(A) viruses

(B) fungi

(C) intracellular bacteria

(D) extracellular bacteria

(E) *pneumocystis carinii*

455. Recent experiments in gene therapy have taken the approach of expressing TNF (tumor necrosis factor) in TIL (tumor infiltrating lymphocytes). We hope that this approach will

(A) generate high serum levels of endotoxin
(B) allow the TIL to return to the tumor and produce local, high levels of TNF
(C) stimulate T cell proliferation
(D) lyse tumor cells due to retrovirus infection
(E) stimulate NK cell activity

456. The uptake of iron is facilitated in many bacteria by the production of

(A) ionophores
(B) matrix proteins (porins)
(C) enzyme II
(D) heat stable protein (HPr)
(E) siderophores

457. Which of the following applies to transformation by *Streptococcus pneumoniae?*

(A) Donor cells autolyse, releasing DNA fragments and competence factor.
(B) Competence factor induces recipient cells to synthesize a special battery of proteins required for transformation.
(C) Transformation is also important in *Haemophilus influenzae* and *Neisseria gonorrhoeae.*
(D) Transformation is inhibited by DNAse.
(E) all of the above

458. Which of the following structural features is NOT true of retroviruses?

(A) lipid envelope
(B) double-stranded RNA genome
(C) virus-associated reverse transcriptase
(D) genome is in a protein core
(E) replication via a DNA intermediate

459. A hemagglutination assay was performed with a sample of influenza virus. A fixed number of chicken red blood cells were mixed with increasing dilutions of the influenza virus. The results of the assay are shown below. The hemagglutination titer of the virus was

1:20   1:40   1:80   1:160   1:320
Dilution

(A) 20
(B) 40
(C) 80
(D) 160
(E) 320

460. All of the following antibiotics may cause misreading of mRNA and block the functioning of the initiation complex during protein biosynthesis EXCEPT

(A) kanamycin
(B) amikacin
(C) erythromycin
(D) gentamicin
(E) streptomycin

461. An extrachromosomal element that can replicate either autonomously in the cell cytoplasm or as an integral part of the cell chromosome is a(n)

(A) plasmid
(B) transposon
(C) episome
(D) competence factor
(E) Hfr

462. A 24-year-old construction worker, who has had four injections of the DPT vaccine (diphtheria, pertussis, and tetanus) in his first year of life and boosters at ages 5 and 19, received a deep laceration while excavating a building's foundation. The preferred method of treatment would be

(A) an aminoglycoside antibiotic
(B) human tetanus immune globulin, because it will stimulate his anamnestic response
(C) equine tetanus immune globulin, because it will passively immunize him
(D) tetanus toxoid, because it will stimulate his anamnestic response
(E) none of the above

463. Bacterial chromosome replication

(A) does not begin at the replication site
(B) is unidirectional
(C) is not semiconservative
(D) does not require protein synthesis
(E) does not involve mitosis

464. The structure below represents

Zidovudine (azidothymidine)

(A) azidothymidine (AZT), which inhibits the AIDS virus reverse transcriptase
(B) dideoxyinosine, which inhibits poliovirus replication
(C) idoxuridine, which inhibits herpes virus thymidine kinase
(D) acyclovir, which inhibits the herpes virus encoded DNA polymare
(E) enviroxine, which inhibits rhinoviruses

465. Nitrogen fixation

(A) is catalyzed mainly by nitrogenase
(B) is encountered mainly in *Clostridium*
(C) has not been observed in *Azotobacter*
(D) has been observed only in *Rhizobium*
(E) is encountered in bacteria that use CO_2 as their sole source of carbon

466. Pili of *Neisseria gonorrhoeae* are known to

(A) be responsible for the absence of secretory IgA in urethral exudates
(B) impart resistance to intracellular killing on piliated strains
(C) have endotoxic properties
(D) be organelles of attachment
(E) be composed of lipopolysaccharides

467. Which of the following nonpathogenic organisms may cause clinical disease in an immunosuppressed patient?

(A) *Pneumocystis carinii*
(B) varicella virus
(C) *Toxoplasma gondii*
(D) *Streptococcus pneumoniae*
(E) *Saccharomyces cerevisiae*

468. Which of the following is an antifungal agent?

(A) ketoconazole
(B) chloramphenicol

(C) methicillin
(D) streptomycin
(E) penicillin

469. A disease in which activated macrophages play a *key role* is

(A) diphtheria
(B) pneumococcal pneumonia
(C) furunculosis
(D) tuberculosis
(E) botulism

470. Which of these viruses have a segmented, double-stranded RNA genome?

(A) reoviruses
(B) papovaviruses
(C) influenza viruses
(D) arenaviruses
(E) rhabdoviruses

471. Lymphocytes leaving fetal liver or bone marrow will be rich in

(A) sheep cell rosetting factors
(B) idiotype determinants
(C) OK8 or LEU1 determinants
(D) cytotoxic potential
(E) cell surface TdT

472. Q fever is an acute infectious disease of worldwide occurrence that

(A) is caused by *Rickettsia akari*
(B) stimulates the production of *Proteus* agglutinins
(C) involves a rash that spreads from the trunk to the extremities
(D) is acquired by inhaling dust containing infected animal excreta
(E) is usually acquired by tick bites

473. A gardener pricked his toe while cutting rose bushes. Four days later a pustule that changed to an ulcer developed on his toe. Then 3 modules formed along the local lymphatic drainage. The most likely agent is

(A) *Trichophyton rubrum*
(B) *Aspergillus fumigatus*
(C) *Candida albicans*
(D) *Sporothroix schenkii*
(E) *Cryptococcus neoformans*

474. The genome of this virus is a circular molecule of DNA having the structure diagrammed below.

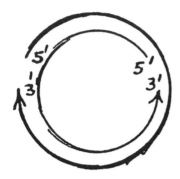

    (A) papilloma virus
    (B) hepatitis A virus
    (C) Epstein-Barr virus
    (D) J.C. virus
    (E) hepatitis B virus

475. A 19-year-old girl has smooth, annular, scaly, erythematous, vesicular lesions on her leg. Assuming that you suspect tinea corporis, what would be the most suitable laboratory diagnostic approach?

    (A) silver staining of tissue scrapping
    (B) acid-fast staining on the vesicular fluid
    (C) culture of the vesicular fluid on agar
    (D) digestion of tissue biopsies with 10–20% KOH
    (E) serology for *Blastomyces dermatitidis*

476. The cause of antigenic drift of influenza viruses is

    (A) mixing of the double-stranded DNA genome
    (B) reassortment of genome segments during mixed infections
    (C) phenotypic mixing
    (D) accumulated point mutations in the hemagglutinin gene
    (E) phenotypic masking

477. A 46-yr-old cattle rancher develops a low-grade fever 5 days after his 20th high school reunion, which included a rabbit hunt. Standard febrile agglutinin titrations reveal low levels of antibodies to the following organisms: *Francisella tularensis, Brucella suis, Brucella abortus, Salmonella typhi,* and *Proteus* OX-19. The differential diagnosis should include

    (A) tularemia
    (B) brucellosis
    (C) typhoid fever

    (D) Rocky Mountain spotted fever
    (E) all of the above

478. The "virus" responsible for this disease may be just infectious protein with no nucleic acid.

    (A) subacute sclerosing panencephalitis
    (B) distemper
    (C) progressive multifocal leukoencephalopathy
    (D) progressive multifocal leukoencephalopathy
    (E) Creutzfeldt-Jacob disease
    (F) dengue

479. Plasmid encoded genes specify

    (A) multiple drug resistance
    (B) enterotoxins of *Escherichia coli*
    (C) bacteriocins
    (D) exotoxin production
    (E) all of the above

480. The cellular oncogene involved in the chromosomal translocation that is characteristic of many Burkitt's lymphomas is

    (A) *V-abl*
    (B) *V-ras*
    (C) *C-myc*
    (D) *V-fms*
    (E) *V-src*

481. All of the following viral genomes are replicated in the cytoplasm EXCEPT

    (A) reoviruses
    (B) picornaviruses
    (C) poxviruses
    (D) paromyxoviruses
    (E) herpes viruses

482. Congenital syphilis can best be detected by

    (A) x-rays
    (B) use of Wassermann Complement fixation test
    (C) dark-field examination
    (D) FTA-ABS IgM test
    (E) silver nitrate staining of spirochetes

483. A positive purified protein derivative (PPD) skin test may indicate that the individual tested has

    (A) inactive tuberculosis
    (B) been exposed to *Mycobacterium tuberculosis*
    (C) received BCG vaccine
    (D) active tuberculosis
    (E) all of the above

484. Amantadine is often useful in the treatment of infections by

(A) herpes simplex virus
(B) rabies virus
(C) Epstein-Barr virus
(D) influenza virus
(E) rhinovirus

485. Immunologic suppression for transplantation may occur by

(A) lymphoid irradiation
(B) antilymphocyte globulin
(C) cyclosporine
(D) steroids
(E) all of the above

486. The genome of this virus is a linear double-stranded DNA molecule in which the complementary strands are covalently crosslinked at the termini of the genome.

(A) herpes simplex virus
(B) varicella-zoster virus
(C) adenovirus
(D) SV40
(E) vaccinia virus

487. Immune complexes appear to be involved in the pathogenesis of

(A) poststreptococcal glomerulonephritis
(B) the Arthus reaction
(C) glomerulonephritis of systemic lupus erythematosus
(D) serum sickness
(E) all of the above

488. Desirable properties of a vector plasmid for use in molecular cloning include

(A) high copy number
(B) selectable phenotype
(C) autonomous replication
(D) single sites for restriction enzymes
(E) all of the above

489. *Legionella pneumophila*

(A) can survive for months in tap water at 25°C
(B) is the major cause of legionellosis in humans
(C) is not usually demonstrable in gram stains of clinical specimens
(D) has been found in air-conditioning systems
(E) all of the above

490. A patient is complaining of a sore throat. Physical examination of the throat indicates a severe redness and an exudate; lymphadenopathy is also evident. This triggers key thoughts of

(A) throat culture
(B) bacitracin discs
(C) blood agar
(D) penicillin
(E) all of the above

DIRECTIONS (Questions 491 through 508): Each set of matching questions in this section consists of a list of up to nine lettered options followed by several numbered items. For each item, select the ONE lettered option that is most closely associated with it. *Each lettered heading may be selected once, more than once, or not at all.*

Questions 491 and 492

For each parasitic organism listed below, choose the mode by which it is usually transmitted to humans.

(A) ingestion of infective egg
(B) ingestion of cyst stage
(C) ingestion of animal tissue that contains the larva
(D) penetration of skin by infective larva
(E) ingestion of adult form

491. *Entamoeba histolytica*

492. *Schistosoma mansoni*

Questions 493 through 495

For each of the components described below, choose the letter on the diagram that represents the portion of the immunoglobulin molecule with which it is associated.

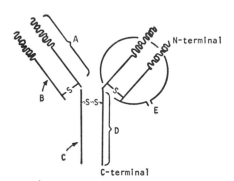

493. Fab fragment

494. Complement-binding area

495. Constant region of the light chain

Questions 496 through 498

For each descriptive term below, choose the letter on the figure that represents the corresponding phase of antigen clearance in vivo.

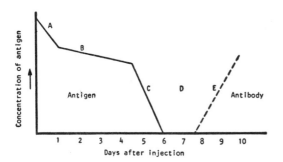

496. Immune elimination

497. Metabolic clearance

498. Equilibration phase

Questions 499 and 500

   (A) pili
   (B) endotoxin
   (C) calcium dipicolinate
   (D) heat-stable protein (HPr)
   (E) H antigen

499. Participation in bacterial conjugation

500. Spore component

Questions 501 through 503

Two triple auxotrophic strains of *Escherichia coli*, Trp⁻ Lys⁻ His⁻ Pro⁺ Pan⁺ Bio⁺ and Trp⁺ Lys⁺ His⁺ Pro⁻ Pan⁻ Bio⁻, are allowed to conjugate in liquid medium for 30 min. After dilution of the broth, the bacteria are plated onto a complete medium. After 24 hr of growth, six replicas are made, each into a plate containing minimal medium and additional nutrient or nutrients as indicated in the figure below. For each of the following genotypes of the colony, choose the mutant strain with which it is associated.

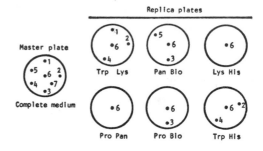

   (A) Trp⁻
   (B) Trp⁻ Lys⁻
   (C) Bio⁻
   (D) Pan⁻ Bio⁻
   (E) Trp⁻ Lys⁻ Bio⁻

501. The genotype of colony 1

502. The genotype of colony 4

503. The genotype of colony 5

Questions 504 through 505

   (A) Graves' disease
   (B) systemic lupus erythematosus (SLE)
   (C) thrombocytopenia
   (D) myasthenia gravis
   (E) rheumatoid arthritis

504. Association with antibodies to acetylcholine receptors

505. Association with HLA-DR4

Questions 506 through 508

   (A) Adenovirus
   (B) Rhabdovirus
   (C) measles virus
   (D) mumps virus
   (E) J.C. virus
   (F) Bunyavirus
   (G) Varicella-zoster virus
   (H) cytomegalovirus
   (I) molluscum contagiosum virus

506. Etiologic agent or "shingles"

507. Transmitted by anthropoids

508. Bullet-shaped, enveloped virus

Answers and Explanations

382. **(D)** Multiplication of a given gram-negative bacterium within the blood stream leads to release of its specific endotoxin that produces the septic shock syndrome. The endotoxin is composed of three regions. Region I contains the nonspecific, nontoxic, O antigen. Thus, administration of antibodies to the terminal polysaccharide of the O antigen, that already are present in the blood stream, is not likely to constitute an effective protective strategy for prevention of the septic shock syndrome. Region II of the endotoxin contains the core polysaccharide that is linked to the region III, or lipid, moiety of the endotoxin. The toxicity of the endotoxin resides mostly in the lipid A moiety. Therefore, administration of specific antibody to lipid A and its associated core-linked polysaccharide should assist in prevention of the septic shock syndrome. Cachectin plays a pivotal role in the pathophysiology of sepsis and by itself can produce the septic shock syndrome in experimental animals. Conversely, animals that have been previously immunized against cachectin will survive an otherwise lethal dose of endotoxin. A well-known effect of endotoxin is that it induces vasodilation, hypotension, and increased permeability. This action is prolonged by leucotrienes. Thus, administration of antileucotriene agents should be indicated in septic shock syndrome. *(Joklik et al, pp 86–87,390)*

383. **(C)** Staphylococcal scalded skin syndrome is an intoxication in which exfoliation, produced by phage group II organisms growing somewhere in the body (usually the gut), obtain access to the blood stream. The resultant toxemia is evidenced by changes in the integrity of the integument: The skin separates at the stratum granulosum because of the effect of the toxin on the desmosomes located there. This causes the skin to appear to float. It has no resilience and will stay wrinkled if pushed in one direction (Nikolsky's sign). *(Joklik et al, pp 406–411)*

384. **(D)** Hepatitis B virus is practically indestructible; hence the need for the use of disposable syringes, needles, and other equipment that may carry the pathogen. This agent has taken on particular significance in the dental profession, where cold sterilization with disinfectant solutions is commonly practiced. The virus is not inactivated by most of the agents used. It is now recommended that dentists be vaccinated against hepatitis B. The increased use of self-injected drugs by a segment of our society has greatly increased the occurrence of hepatitis B in the population and, thus, has also increased the danger of transmission by any procedures that involve skin puncture or bleeding. *(Jawetz et al, p 454)*

385. **(B)** The term burst size is defined as the average number of progeny viruses released per infected cell. *(Joklik et al, pp 790–795)*

386. **(D)** The stages of conjugation are as follows: (1) specific pair formation, in which the donor and recipient make contact through the F pili, (2) effective pair formation with cell-to-cell contact, (3) chromosome mobilization, (4) transfer of a unique strand of DNA to the recipient cell, which leads to (5) formation of partial diploids, or merozygotes (entire recipient chromosome and partial chromosome from the donor), and (6) genetic recombination, in which the donor chromosome replaces segments of the recipient chromosome. Competency is a condition that is necessary for transformation of cells and is *not* a stage of conjugation. *(Joklik et al, pp 136–145)*

387. **(B)** Rocky Mountain spotted fever is spread from its reservoir in nature (e.g., rodents, dogs) to humans by the bite of infected ticks, primarily the wood tick *(Dermacentor andersoni)* in the western USA and the dog tick *(Dermacentor variabilis)* in the eastern areas. Tsutsugamushi disease is spread by mites, epidemic typhus is spread by human body lice, and endemic (murine) typhus and bubonic plague are transmitted by rat fleas. There is no vector in Q fever, which is acquired by inhalation of infectious particles. *(Joklik et al, pp 705–713)*

388. (C) Viral infection is initiated with the attachment of the viral hemagglutinin to a specific host cell membrane glycoprotein (mucopeptide) receptor. The viral particles then fuse with the membrane, and the nucleocapsid enters the cell to begin the replicative cycle. The virus enters the eclipse phase, during which no viral material can be detected in the cell by conventional procedures. During this time viral proteins and nucleic acids are being produced. The next phase is assembly, when mature virus is manufactured. Release follows, and the cycle is repeated in a new cell. (*Joklik et al, pp 824–827*)

389. (E) The increased metabolic activity associated with the phagocytosis of microbes by neutrophils results in the formation of such oxygen metabolites as the superoxide radical O^-_2, H_2O_2, which may be lethal for many microorganisms. H_2O_2 in the presence of cofactors, such as myeloperoxidase, and the halides chlorine, iodine, or bromine result also in microbial death. Nonoxidative mechanisms, such as the action of lactoferrin, lysozyme, and other hydrolytic phagocytic enzymes, may be directly lethal for various microorganisms. Catalase is an enzyme that degrades H_2O_2 to O_2 and H_2O. Thus, since it destroys an antimicrobial agent, it cannot contribute to the intracellular killing of microbes by neutrophils. (*Joklik et al, pp 350–351*)

390. (E) In the Ouchterlony diagram that accompanies the question, each antibody will react with its homologous determinant group on the antigen molecule. Thus, both antibodies a and b will react with antigen ab, but only antibody a will react with antigen ac. Antibody b will diffuse through the line of precipitate formed by antibody a and antigen ac to precipitate with antigen ab, forming the spur at position 3. Line 1 will contain both antibodies. The spur (3) will contain antibody b, not antibody a. Line 2 will contain antigen ac and antibody a only. (*Joklik et al, p 785*)

391. (C) A transformant is a recipient cell that is transformed by naked DNA and gains new properties in the process of transformation. A transition refers to a base pair substitution that results in the substitution of a purine for a purine or a pyrimidine for a pyrimidine. A transversion is a base pair substitution that results in the substitution of pyrimidines for purine and vice versa (AT → CG). Transposition is the process in which a transposon is translocated from one position to another in a replicon or is transferred to a different replicon. A frame shift mutation generates shifts in the reading frame of the transcribed DNA by insertion or deletion of a single nucleotide. On translation of the transcribed DNA (containing the insertion or deletion), the reading frame is shifted, and a nonfunctional protein is produced. (*Joklik et al, pp 126–127*)

392. (B) Transformation is the transfer of genetic information from one bacterial cell to another by the introduction of naked DNA into a bacterial cell. Transformation is not affected by RNAse in the medium, since DNA is resistant to RNAse. However, DNAse in the medium destroys the transforming material (DNA), and hence transformation of bacteria can be blocked by DNAse. Antiserum against bacteriophage is not effective in blocking transformation because bacteriophage are not involved in transformation. Antiserum to bacteriophage will block transfer of genetic information by transduction. In contrast to transformation, transfer of genetic information by conjugation requires effective pair formation or cell-to-cell contact. In some bacteria, the sex pili are involved in cell-to-cell contact, and bacteriophage that bind to the tips of the pili block effective pair formation. Therefore, bacteriophage that adsorb to sex pili block conjugation but do not affect transformation. As already stated, transformation does not require cell-to-cell contact, and prevention of cell-to-cell contact between donor and recipient cultures does not hinder transformation. (*Joklik et al, pp 136–138*)

393. (D) When a temperate bacteriophage infects a susceptible bacterium, the phage may enter either the lytic cycle or the lysogenic cycle of replication. If the phage enters the lytic cycle, the phage replicates, the cell is lysed, and viable progeny phage are released. With the lysogenic cycle, the bacteriophage DNA integrates into the host chromosome, where it is maintained until the lytic cycle is induced. The integrated viral DNA is referred to as a prophage, and the bacterial cell carrying the prophage is referred to as a lysogenic bacterium, or a lysogen. (*Joklik et al, pp 923–928*)

394. (C) The attachment of influenza virus to host cells occurs through a reaction of the hemagglutinin with a receptor on the membrane. Thus, antibody that blocks this reaction will prevent the disease. Antineuraminidase antibodies reduce viral spread and can diminish the severity of the disease. (*Joklik et al, pp 824–827*)

395. (D) Chlamydiae and rickettsiae are the largest of the obligate intracellular parasites. They are bacteria-like in that they have a cell wall, contain both DNA and RNA, and are susceptible to certain antibiotics (e.g., tetracyclines and chloramphenicol). Most rickettsiae are spread by arthropod vectors; chlamydiae are spread by direct contact or by the respiratory route. In addition, chlamydiae divide by binary fission and by an unequal divisional process involving elementary and reticulate body formation. *(Joklik et al, pp 701–713, 719–729)*

396. **(E)** The causative agents of tetanus, botulism, gas gangrene, anthrax, and diphtheria are *Clostridium tetani, Clostridium botulinum, Clostridium perfringens, Bacillus anthacis,* and *Corynebacterium diphtheriae,* respectively. Spore formation is a property that is found in bacteria belonging to the genus *Clostridium* and genus *Bacillus. (Joklik et al, pp 491,615,637,652)*

397. **(E)** Genetic complementation is a genetic tool that is employed to determine whether two mutants lacking the same functions have mutations in the same location on the genes. If the genetic information from one of the mutants is introduced into the other mutants and the resulting diploid organism regains the ability to synthesize the proper end product, one may conclude that the two mutations are located in regions of distinct genetic function. The two types of genetic complementation are intragenic (within the same gene) and intergenic (within different genes) complementation. Intragenic complementation requires an end product that is an oligomeric polypeptide with two or more identical subunits. For example, one mutant may have a mutation that causes a conformational change in the subunit that makes the enzyme inactive. On association with another mutationally altered subunit due to a mutation in the same gene at a different location, the restraints may cancel out to produce an active enzyme. In this case, the peptide subunits coded for by two genes from two mutants can complement each other and produce an active protein. With intergenic complementation, two nonidentical gene products from two mutants complement each other. For example, introduction of a P⁻ Lys⁺ phage (unable to replicate) into a bacterium containing a P⁺ Lys⁻ phage (unable to produce lysozyme) will result in release of viable progeny from the bacterium. Suppression is a method in which a second mutation corrects the damage done by the first mutation. The remainder of the choices listed in the question are not genetic tests of function. *(Jawetz et al, p 386)*

398. **(D)** The germane mode of action of ultraviolet light on microorganisms is related to its absorption by the DNA. This absorption leads to the formation of covalent bonds between adjacent pyrimidine bases. These pyrimidine diamers alter the form of the DNA and thus interfere with normal base pairing during the synthesis of DNA. Disruption of the bacterial cell membrane, removal of free sulfhydryl groups, protein denaturation, and addition of alkyl groups to cellular components are induced by detergents, heavy metals, heat or alcoholic compounds, and ethylene oxide or formaldehyde, respectively. *(Joklik et al, pp 190–197)*

399. **(A)** Members of the genera *Rhizobium* and *Azotobacter* produce nitrogenase, which converts atmospheric N_2 to NH_4^+. The reduction of N_2 to NH_4^+ by nitrogenase permits the assimilation of NH_4^+ into amino acids and other cellular components. Members of the genera *Rhizobium* and *Azotobacter* grow best at a pH close to 7.0 and will not grow at temperatures of 50 to 60°C, at which thermophilic bacteria thrive. Capsules may be present in *Rhizobium* and *Azotobacter,* but they do not contain D-glutamic acid, which is the key component of the *Bacillus anthracis* capsule. Attachment to human cells of members of the genera *Rhizobium* and *Azotobacter* is not known to occur. *(Joklik et al, p 54)*

400. **(D)** Mycoplasma organisms do not have a cell wall and are therefore resistant to penicillin. Other forms of bacteria that lack a cell wall are spheroplasts and protoplasts, which are formed from gram-negative and gram-positive bacteria, respectively, through the action of penicillin or by other procedures that remove the cell wall or interfere with its formation. The remaining organisms listed in the question are all susceptible to the action of penicillin, although certain strains of the gonococcus have acquired a β-lactamase-producing plasmid. Tetracyclines, erythromycin, and the aminoglycosides are effective antibiotics for the treatment of mycoplasmal infections. *(Joklik et al, pp 735–736)*

401. **(D)** Complement-fixing antibodies tend to appear relatively late in coccidioidomycosis. With chemotherapeutic treatment they will persist longer than the precipitins detected in the serum of affected patients. In disseminated disease the titers may increase dramatically, which is a poor prognostic sign. Conversion to skin test negativity would also be a poor prognostic sign, as it can signal the terminal anergy that may occur when the system is overloaded with antigen. Precipitins normally decrease with time, so decreased precipitin titers would have no particular prognostic significance. *(Joklik et al, p 1096)*

402. **(E)** A severe form of encephalitis may be produced by herpesvirus type 1, and is thought to be the result of a lesion in the temporal lobe. Herpesvirus type 2 may be transmitted to the newborn during passage through an infected birth canal. Severely infected infants who survive may have permanent brain damage. Genital herpes caused by herpesvirus type 2 is characterized by vesiculoulcerative lesions of the penis, cervix, vulva, vagina, or perineum and may be transmitted venereally. Vesicles and skin rashes are also caused by the varicella-zoster virus (herpesvirus type 3). Scrapie is a degenerative central nervous disease of sheep. The causative agent has been associated with a proteinaceous material devoid of detectable amounts of nucleic acid, and it is called prion instead of virus. *(Joklik et al, pp 957, 1065–1067)*

403. **(C)** All of the conditions listed in the question are of streptococcal etiology; therefore, a rise in antistreptolysin O would occur in all of these. The only valid diagnostic conclusion regarding patients with a rising antistreptolysin O titer is that a recent streptococcal infection has occurred. Two of the diseases listed, scarlet fever and erysipelas, are distinguished on the basis of clinical signs. The former is a generalized, febrile disease with an associated sore throat and scarlatinal rash, whereas the latter is a local cellulitis that occurs in the subcutaneous tissues and may radiate locally, involving draining lymphatics. Rheumatic fever and glomerulonephritis are postinfection sequelae of group A streptococcal infections. The organisms cannot be isolated from the patient at the time the disease is developing. As the diseases involve different organs, the symptoms will be correspondingly diverse. *(Joklik et al, p 422)*

404. **(B)** Polymeric forms of IgM and IgA are held together by a 15,000-dalton polypeptide chain called the J chain. It does not share antigenic determinants or amino acid sequences with H or L chains. The J chain is S-S bonded to the heavy chains in the polymeric forms of these immunoglobulins. *(Joklik et al, pp 224–227)*

405. **(A)** Group A streptococci produce two antiphagocytic surface components, hyaluronic acid and M protein, which interfere with ingestion. The streptolysins and DNAse are able to kill phagocytic cells by membrane disruption (streptolysin O) or by leukotoxicity exhibited only after phagocytosis. Other streptococcal extracellular products that may have a deleterious effect on leukocytes include DNAse, proteinase, and RNAse. Hyaluronidase and streptokinase are virulence factors that may play a role in the organism's spread through the body. *(Joklik et al, pp 421–423)*

406. **(B)** The base analog 5-BU causes transitions or subtransitions of AT for GC (or vice versa) to occur in the DNA of cells or viruses. 5-BU is a thymine analog, and on DNA replication, the 5-BU can be incorporated into the new DNA in place of the normal thymine base. Once incorporated, the 5-BU may undergo transient internal rearrangement (tautomerization) from the keto state to the enol state, in which it pairs with guanine instead of adenine. In subsequent replications, the cytosine will be paired with the guanine

and the AT will be replaced by a GC. Transversions, which are caused by mutagens, such as the alkylating agent ethylethane sulfonate, result in the substitution of a pyrimidine for a purine and vice versa (AT → GC). Frame shift mutations are induced by acridine derivatives. The acridines shift the reading frame by intercalating between successive base pairs of DNA. The shift of the reading frame produces a nonfunctional protein. Deletions in DNA are induced by agents such as nitrous acid, bifunctional alkylating agents, and irradiation. These agents cause cross-links between complementary DNA strands, and on DNA replication the DNA around the cross-links is not replicated, while the segments on each side replicate and join together. Finally, recombinations are not considered a type of mutation. *(Joklik et al, p 130)*

407. **(A)** There is evidence that antigens must be metabolically processed by macrophages before they can be recognized by the T helper cells. For example, T helper cells from F_1 hybrids between two inbred strains ($P_1 \times P_2$) that have been sensitized on antigen-pulsed macrophages from one parent (P_1) will proliferate in response to a second challenge of the antigen only if F_1 macrophages or macrophages from P_1 are present. Kupffer cells, young erythrocytes, or suppressor T cells from P_1 are not considered as inducers of T helper cell proliferation. B cells may be involved in antigen processing but are not the best antigen processors. *(Levinson and Jawetz, pp 278–279)*

408. **(A)** Mediators affecting lymphocytes include the following: interleukin 1 (IL-1), which potentiates mitogenic responses of T cells and thymocytes, interleukin 2 (IL-2), which promotes and maintains the proliferation of T lymphocytes, transfer factor, which prepares nonsensitive lymphocytes to respond to specific antigens and to the transfer of delayed hypersensitivity, and the blastogenic factor, which is involved in lymphocyte proliferation. The MIF does not affect lymphocytes, but it inhibits the migration of macrophages from an antigen reaction site. *(Jawetz et al, p 117)*

409. **(E)** One of the early steps in viral infections is the cessation of host cell synthesis of macromolecules. Cellular nucleic acids are not degraded, but chromosomal breaks may occur. Polyribosomes are disaggregated, favoring a shift to viral synthetic processes. The virus first directs the synthesis of new proteins (which may require a brief burst of mRNA synthesis), then viral nucleic acids are synthesized, and assembly and release occur. In poliovirus, the viral nucleic acid is tRNA, which thus serves as its own messenger. *(Joklik et al, p 851)*

410. **(D)** Excision repair follows damage by bifunctional alkylating agents or ultraviolet (UV) irradiation. With excision repair, a specific endonuclease makes a nick adjacent to the damaged base or dimers. Next, the altered bases are excised from the DNA, DNA polymerase I fills the gap, and the two strands are ligated. Bifunctional alkylating agents [e.g., mechlorethamine (nitrogen mustard) and mitomycin] cause cross-links between the complementary strands of DNA. These cross-links are removed by two steps. First the altered base on one strand is removed, and then the altered base on the opposite strand is removed. Photoreactivation is a method of repairing DNA that has been damaged by UV light. Exposure of bacterial cells to UV light results in the formation of pyrimidine dimers in the DNA. Subsequent exposure to light in the visible region of the spectrum induces an enzyme that cleaves the dimers and restores the original pyrimidine bases. Direct repair is synonymous for photoreactivation. Postreplication repair or recombination repair may occur in bacteria that are incapable of excision repair or photoreactivation. In this type of repair, replication of the DNA occurs, and the new strands contain gaps corresponding to areas of pyrimidine dimers. Multiple crossovers between the daughter strands restore the intact molecule. Since bifunctional alkylating agents cross-link DNA, DNA damaged by this method cannot replicate. Therefore, this is not an acceptable method for repair. *(Joklik et al, pp 130–133)*

411. **(B)** Bruton's hypogammaglobulinemia is a B cell immunodeficiency disorder. Affected patients are deficient in B cells in the peripheral blood and in B-dependent areas of lymph nodes and spleen. Most of the serum immunoglobulins are absent, and the IgG level is <200 mg/L. Recurrent pyogenic infections usually begin to occur at 5 to 6 months of age, when maternal IgG has been depleted. *(Joklik et al, pp 329–330)*

412. **(D)** Recurrent vesiculating lesions in the genital region suggest herpesvirus type II, although type I is seen in some cases. The remaining organisms listed in the question either are not recurring or do not produce vesicular lesions. Rubella and measles are associated with maculopapular rashes that do not progress to vesicles. Coxsackievirus and echovirus produce a wide variety of diseases, including meningitis, encephalitis, upper respiratory tract infections, and enteritis. A macular rash may accompany some of these conditions, but its presence has no particular diagnostic significance. *(Joklik et al, pp 956–957)*

413. **(A)** Antiacetylcholine receptor antibodies are found in more than 90 percent of myasthenia gravis patients. If the clinical symptoms are suggestive of myasthenia gravis, this finding alone is often considered diagnostic. Multiple sclerosis patients tend to have high levels of measles virus antibodies in their spinal fluid. However, the role of this agent in the disease is undetermined. Guillain-Barré syndrome (also called acute idiopathic polyneuritis) is a demyelinating disease of peripheral nerves. It commonly occurs after a viral infection or an injection, such as influenza immunization. The disease seems to be caused by a T cell response to nervous tissue. *(Joklik et al, pp 321–997)*

414. **(B)** The patient described in the question has a profound deficiency of both the B cell and T cell components of the immune response (i.e., severe combined immunodeficiency disease). The dramatic absence of lymphocytes and lymphoid tissue would not be found in any of the other conditions listed. Patients with acquired immunodeficiency syndrome (AIDS) may have a similar immune function deficit (absence of effective B and T cell responses); however, they will have adequate lymphoid tissues. The cells are present, perhaps in diminished numbers, but are not mature and functional. *(Joklik et al, pp 333–338)*

415. **(B)** The figure that accompanies the question represents the peptidoglycan of *S. aureus*. Although the general features of this structure are essentially the same in all bacteria possessing a cell wall (the mycoplasmas lack a cell wall), species-specific variations are present. Variations in the cell walls of other species may occur in the amino acids of the tetrapeptide attached to *N*-acetylmuramic acid or in the cross-linking peptide bridge. Both the C substance from *S. pneumoniae* and the O antigen from *S. typhimurium* are carbohydrates and do not contain peptides. The H antigen of *S. typhimurium* is composed of a small basic protein of approximately 20,000 daltons. *(Joklik et al, pp 77–85)*

416. **(C)** Competent cells are necessary for the uptake of naked DNA. Therefore, recipient cells need to be in a state of competency for transformation to occur. A protein called competence factor is produced by bacterial cultures during a brief period of the growth cycle. This protein increases competency of noncompetent bacterial cells when added to the cell culture. Additionally, one can artificially induce competence in a cell culture by making the cell envelope more permeable to DNA by exposure to calcium chloride. Transduction, conjugation, and transposition do not require competent cells for exchange of genetic information from a donor (F+, Hfr) to a recipient cell (F–). Transduction requires infection of a cell by a phage that is carrying chromosomal genes. Transposition is the translocation of genetic information from a plasmid to a chromosome (or vice versa) by a transposon. Complementation involves the interaction of gene products (proteins) and does not require competent cells. *(Joklik et al, pp 136–137)*

417. **(E)** The enterovirus group includes such RNA-containing viruses as the poliomyelitis virus, the coxsackieviruses, which cause pleurodynia, aseptic meningitis, myocarditis, or diarrhea in neonates, and the echoviruses types 4,6,9,11,14,16, 18, and others, which have been associated with aseptic meningitis. Shingles is caused by the DNA-containing herpesvirus type 3. *(Jawetz et al, pp 143,983–985)*

418. **(A)** By definition, a hapten is a substance of low molecular weight that by itself does not elicit the formation of antibodies. However, when attached to a carrier protein, antibody production becomes feasible. The hapten–carrier approach has been employed to produce antibodies against penicillin, steroids, nucleotides, lipids, and even 2,4-dinitrophenol. Since the rabbits have been repeatedly injected with the hapten only, their serum cannot be expected to have antibodies against the hapten. Thus, when the rabbit serum is subjected to the gel diffusion assay with the hapten and a carrier protein that was not used to complex the hapten during immunization, no antigen–antibody precipitin lines of either identity, partial identity, or nonidentity can be expected. *(Joklik et al, pp 207,213,219,223,237)*

419. **(B)** R plasmids are large plasmids composed of two functionally distinct parts: (1) the RTF and (2) the resistance determinant (R determinant). The RTF constitutes the major part of the R plasmid and contains the genes for autonomous replication and conjugation. The R determinant contains the genes for antibiotic resistance. The RTF and R determinant usually exist together in the cell as one unit. However, the IS elements at the boundaries of these two parts promote crossover and allow the R determinant and the RTF to dissociate. When the R determinant and the RTF are in the same cell, they may associate and dissociate, and the R determinant may be exchanged with a different RTF. The pilus is not a component of the R plasmid but is an appendage of the bacterial cell. *(Joklik et al, pp 147–149,182)*

420. **(D)** *T. spiralis* can damage many tissues, such as skeletal muscle, cardiac muscle, or nervous tissue. Myositis is the most prominent feature of trichinosis. However, myocarditis with congestive heart failure and neurologic symptoms also is often encountered. *W. bancrofti* attacks the lymphoid system, leading to what is known as filariasis, lymphangitis, hydrocele, or elephantiasis. *O. volvulus* is responsible for dermatologic nodules and

rashes, and ocular onchocerciasis frequently results in visual impairment or blindness. *E. vermicularis* causes anal itching (pruritis) and occasional abdominal discomfort in children, and it is thought to be the most commonly encountered helminth parasite in the United States. *N. americanus* attacks the lungs, producing hemorrhages and pneumonitis. *(Joklik et al, pp 1188,1196, 1202–1205)*

421. **(A)** *C. trachomatis* can be found in two forms, a small spherical body 0.2 to 0.4 μm, the EB, which is the infective form, and a large 0.6 to 1.0 μm circular-oval structure, the RB. The EB is responsible for binding and entrance of *C. trachomatis* to the host cells. The EB has a cell wall, but no known capsule, that allows it to survive for brief periods in the extracellular environment. *(Joklik et al, pp 719,724–727)*

422. **(E)** The viral envelopes of rubeola, influenza B, parainfluenza, and rubella viruses all possess hemagglutinins on their viral envelopes. The human papovavirus is not known to have hemagglutinins. Hemagglutinins are glycoproteins occurring as spikes on viral envelopes and serve as points of attachment to host cells. Five major hemagglutinin types for influenza virus have been identified: H swine, H0, H1, H2, and H3. Influenza virus mutates its hemagglutinin types (antigenic drift), and this accounts for the loss of immunity to influenza virus that has led to influenza virus epidemics. *(Joklik et al, pp 766–767)*

423. **(A)** The Vi antigen of *Salmonella* serotype *typhi* is believed to act as a capsule, composed of polysaccharide, that prevents phagocytosis, or the intracellular destruction of *S. typhi* by the phagocytes. For example, studies with human volunteers have shown that *S. typhi* mutants lacking Vi antigen are less virulent than those that contain Vi antigen. *(Joklik et al, pp 560–561)*

424. **(B)** Trichinosis is acquired by ingestion of *Trichinella spiralis* larvae in undercooked meat (usually pork). The larvae quickly excyst and invade the mucosal epithelium, where they mature into adult worms by the second day of infection. Mating ensues, and the fertilized eggs develop into minute larvae. By the sixth day of infection, the larvae migrate into the intestinal lymphatics or mesenteric venules and are disseminated throughout the body. The pathologic changes associated with this disease occur in the gastrointestinal tract (associated with the presence of the adult worms), lungs, skeletal muscles, heart, CNS, eyes, and other organs where the larvae take up residence and become encysted. The severity of symptoms is related to the number of worms, the size, age, and immunologic status of

the host, and the tissues invaded. The primary symptoms of hookworm are mainly intestinal. Anemia may occur as a consequence of severe infection. *Toxoplasma* infections usually are asymptomatic in adults but may produce serious CNS disease in the developing fetus. *Onchocerca* larvae develop into adult worms in subcutaneous tissue and cause tumorlike nodules. Microfiliarial forms may migrate through the eyes and cause blindness. Pediculosis is an infestation with the human body louse, *Pediculus humanus*. *(Joklik et al, p 1202)*

425. **(D)** Antigens have the ability to induce an immune response (immunogenicity) and also react specifically with the products of that response, either humoral antibodies or specifically sensitized lymphocytes. Determinant groups are the portions of the antigen molecule that determine its specificity. Haptens are partial, or incomplete, antigens. They have specific reactivity but are not immunogenic by themselves. Adjuvants are substances that have the ability to enhance the immune response to antigens without necessarily being antigenic themselves. For example, *Bordetella pertussis* will cause the host to produce large amounts of IgE antibodies to antigens that normally would not induce the production of this antibody at all. Similarly, mycobacterial presence in a vaccine will encourage the development of cell-mediated immunity to other antigens in the vaccine. *(Joklik et al, p 207)*

426. **(B)** In a laboratory test used to identify *S. aureus,* coagulase reacts with a prothrombin-like compound in plasma to produce an active enzyme (a complex of thrombin and coagulase) that converts fibrinogen to fibrin. This activity of the staphylococcal organism has a very high correlation with the organism's virulence, although coagulase-negative organisms may also cause disease, which are usually less severe. The necessity for a relatively accurate test to predict virulence stems from the presence of nonpathogenic staphylococci as indigenous flora of many areas of the human body. Another test that is used to identify a pathogenic isolate is the production of DNAse. This assay is somewhat more easily performed than is the coagulase test. Consequently, many laboratories have switched to the DNAse agar plate test. *(Joklik et al, p 407)*

427. **(A)** The Weil-Felix reaction, which is based on the agglutination of differing strains of *Proteus vulgaris* by serum from patients with rickettsial diseases, is a useful diagnostic test. Another test, rarely used in diagnosis of rickettsial diseases today, is the Neill-Mooser reaction, in which viable murine typhus organisms are injected into laboratory animals. Scrotal swelling is the end point of this test. Q fever does not induce the production of *Proteus* agglutinins. OXK agglutination suggests a diagnosis of scrub typhus. *(Joklik et al, pp 703–704)*

428. **(A)** *H. influenzae* type B is responsible for 70 percent of the bacterial meningitides in children between the ages of 2 months and 5 years. The pneumococcus causes meningitis in debilitated adults. Meningococcal meningitis occurs sporadically in all age groups and takes on epidemic proportions in military populations. *E. coli* and *S. agalactiae* cause meningitis in neonates, who acquire the infection during passage through the birth canal. *(Jawetz et al, p 238)*

429. **(E)** Cultivation of fungi requires a medium that is adjusted to the optimal pH of growth for fungi, that is, a pH of 4.0 to 5.0. Such a medium is the one developed by Sabouraud. The SS medium is a medium used to isolate bacterial species belonging to the genus *Salmonella* or *Shigella*. Selenite medium is employed to enrich the number of *Salmonella* species that may be present in small numbers in fecal or other clinical specimens. Tellurite medium is used for the selective isolation of *Corynebacterium diphtheriae*, which is not as sensitive to the concentration of tellurite incorporated into the medium as the other bacteria that may be encountered in specimens submitted for the microbiologic diagnosis of diphtheria. Lowenstein-Jensen medium is used for the cultivation of *Mycobacterium tuberculosis* and other mycobacteria. *(Jawetz et al, pp 220,272,310)*

430. **(A)** The route of infection of rubella virus is the respiratory tract, with spread to lymphatic tissue and then to the blood (viremia). Maternal viremia is followed by infection of the placenta, which leads to congenital rubella. Many organs of the fetus support the multiplication of the virus, which does not seem to destroy the cells but reduces the rate of growth of the infected cells. This leads to fewer than normal numbers of cells in the organs at birth. Therefore, the earlier in pregnancy infection occurs, the greater the chance for the development of abnormalities in the infected fetus. A vast percentage of maternal infections that occur during the first trimester of pregnancy result in such fetal defects as pulmonary stenosis, ventricular septal defect, cataracts, glaucoma, deafness, mental retardation, and other maladies. *(Joklik et al, pp 1016–1017)*

431. **(C)** A common feature of the cytology of the fungi is their ability to exist in a yeastlike form as well as filaments, or hyphae, depending on the temperature (25°C or 37°C) or environment in which they are grown. This ability to exist in either the yeastlike or hyphae form is known as dimorphism. Cryptococcosis is meningitis caused by *Cryptococcus neoformans,* which, when cultured on Sabouraud's agar at either 25°C or 37°C, appears as a budding yeast with a large capsule. Sporotrichosis, candidiasis, histoplasmosis, and blastomycosis are all caused by dimorphic fungi. *(Jawetz et al, pp 309–326)*

432. **(E)** *P. aeruginosa* is a gram-negative, oxidase-positive, aerobic rod that produces a green-blue pigment called pyrocyanin. This microorganism has been associated frequently with wound infections in burn patients, and it is considered as the second leading cause of burn infections after *Staphylococcus aureus. P. aeruginosa* tends to develop resistance to various antibiotics. However, it may respond to ticarcillin, gentamicin, tobramycin, piperacillin, or azlocillin. *E. coli, K. pneumoniae, P. mirabilis,* and *S. marcescens* may cause urinary or pulmonary tract infections but are not considered leading causes of burn infections. Furthermore, these bacteria are oxidase negative and do not produce blue-green pigments. *(Jawetz et al, pp 225–226)*

433. **(B)** There are two nonsuppurative sequelae of group A streptococcal disease, rheumatic fever and acute glomerulonephritis. Although rheumatic fever can follow pharyngeal infection with practically any group A streptococcal organism, the majority of nephritogenic strains belong to only six or seven M types. Types 1, 4, 12, 25, and 49 are the most commonly associated with acute glomerulonephritis. The preceding streptococcal infection need not be restricted to the upper respiratory tract to trigger this condition, and streptococcal erysipelas is a frequent cause. *(Joklik et al, pp 425–426)*

434. **(A)** *C. neoformans* is the only encapsulated yeast that is pathogenic for humans. Visualization of a capsule around yeast cells in an India ink preparation of spinal fluid is diagnostic for cryptococcal disease, although soluble capsular antigen could also be detected by countercurrent immunoelectrophoresis or latex agglutination. This organism is considered to be an opportunistic pathogen, as over 80 percent of the individuals who become clinically ill are immunosuppressed in some way or have compromised respiratory functions. The organism is abundant in pigeon excreta-contaminated soil, which is most probably the source of human infections. *(Joklik et al, pp 1144–1147)*

435. **(C)** *D. latum,* also known as the fish or broad tapeworm, is the biggest worm and can reach 10 m in size. Humans acquire the infection by eating raw fish containing the larvae of the tapeworm. The worm attaches to the small intestine and causes abdominal discomfort. Nausea, diarrhea,

weight loss, and pernicious anemia can result. The anemia is induced by the tapeworm's tendency to compete with humans for vitamin B_{12}, which it easily accumulates from the intestinal contents. *(Joklik et al, pp 1206–1207)*

436. **(D)** Plague, a zoonotic disease caused by the bacillus *Yersinia pestis,* is transmitted to humans from its animal reservoir (rats in urban plague; squirrels and other wild animals in sylvatic plague) by fleas (e.g., *Xenopsylla cheopis,* the rat flea). Anthrax is an industrial disease, usually acquired by wool and leather workers. The spores contaminate the hides and raw wool and are inhaled by the workers during processing. Brucellosis and salmonellosis are acquired by ingestion of contaminated foods. Humans may develop leptospirosis if they come in contact with groundwater that has been contaminated with the urine from rodents who are harboring the agent in their normal flora or in a subclinical infection. This disease occurs usually in campers and hunters. Veterinarians are particularly prone to develop zoonotic infections because of their constant contact with infected animals. *(Joklik et al, pp 586–590)*

437. **(A)** Hfr × F⁻ mating results in the transfer of the greatest amount of chromosomal DNA as compared to F′ × F⁻ mating, specialized transduction, or transposition. Incorporation of the F plasmid into the chromosome produces an Hfr or high frequency of recombination bacterium. When the Hfr bacterium encounters an F⁻ recipient bacterium, the donor bacterial chromosome is mobilized and is transferred to the F⁻ cell. Theoretically, given enough time, the entire donor bacterial chromosome and the F factor can be transferred to the F⁻ recipient. Hfr cells can revert to F⁺ cells by excision of the F plasmid from the bacterial chromosome. Occasionally, the excision is imprecise, and the F plasmid carries a segment of chromosomal DNA adjacent to the integration site of the F plasmid. The resulting F′ hybrid plasmid can then introduce the chromosomal DNA into F⁻ cells with high efficiency. The amount of chromosomal DNA that is transferred by this procedure can vary but is usually not as much as that transferred by Hfr × F⁻ mating. Specialized transduction is the transfer of chromosomal DNA adjacent to the site of integration of a temperate phage in the bacterial chromosome. A very limited amount of DNA is transferred by specialized transduction because of the limited size of the phage capsid. Plasmid transfer is not a common method of transfer of chromosomal DNA, since plasmids other than the F factor rarely integrate into the bacterial chromosome. Plasmid transfer of chromosomal markers occurs only if a transposon transfers chromosomal DNA to the plasmid. Transposons can transfer chromosomal DNA, but the amount of chromosomal DNA transferred is limited to the DNA adjacent to IS elements of the transposon. *(Joklik et al, pp 139–141)*

438. **(D)** There are two portions of the diphtheria toxin molecule; the B fragment is responsible for bringing the molecule into proximity of a mammalian cell, whereas the A fragment is the proenzyme that, when activated by mild proteolysis, will catalyze the ADP-ribosylation of EF-2, thus blocking protein synthesis. Certain strains of pseudomonads also have a toxin with similar biologic activity. Botulinum toxin inhibits acetylcholine release in the peripheral nervous system. Choleragen and the enterotoxin from certain strains of *Escherichia coli* activate adenylcyclase. *(Joklik et al, pp 488–491)*

439. **(B)** *S. pneumoniae* is a gram-positive lancet-shaped diplococcus that may be present in small numbers in the human throat. This microorganism is lysed by 10 percent bile salts, such as desoxycholate at pH 7.0, and it is inhibited by optochin (ethyl hydrocuprein hydrochloride). When it is grown on blood agar, it converts the hemoglobin of the red blood cells to methemoglobin, so that there is a green coloration around the colonies of *S. pneumoniae,* which is called alpha hemolysis. Beta hemolysis refers to the complete breakdown of the hemoglobin of the red blood cells around the colonies of *Streptococcus pyogenes* but not of *S. pneumoniae. (Joklik et al, pp 432–435)*

440. **(E)** High-sucrose diets are cariogenic because the *S. mutans* organisms use sucrose as a substrate for the synthesis of dextran, which causes the organisms to adhere to the teeth in the form of plaques of microbial colonies. This is the first step in the development of caries and also is an important component in the initiation of peridontal disease. *(Joklik et al, pp 684–687)*

441. **(D)** Quantitative immunoglobulin levels reflect the secretory activity of B lymphocytes and could be misleading as to the actual number of such cells; for example, in multiple myeloma or other B cell malignancies, one would expect to find a marked hypergammaglobulinemia. B cells are not the only cells that have receptors for the Fc fragment of immunoglobulin. Phagocytic cells also have such receptors and thus could be included in an Fc receptor assay. E rosetting is a property of T lymphocytes, as is PHA mitogenic response; hence neither of these assays would be appropriate for the enumeration of B lymphocytes. *(Joklik et al, pp 244–245)*

442. **(C)** The E rosette assay measures the number of T lymphocytes and does not indicate their functional status. Enumeration of θ-bearing cells also would not give any information of their functional status. Both sIg and serum immunoglobulin determinations would measure B cell functions. PHA induces mitosis in thymus-derived lymphocytes (T cells). The mitosis is detected in the assay by measuring the amount of radioactive thymidine that is incorporated into the T cells during a 24-hr period of incubation with this nucleotide. *(Joklik et al, p 245)*

443. **(C)** Lyme disease is a recently discovered illness caused by *Borrelia burgdorferi,* which is transmitted to humans by tick bites. The disease produces a unique annular skin lesion called erythema chromicum migrans (ECM). Certain patients develop neurologic and cardiovascular symptoms and arthritis. Diagnosis of the disease may be assisted by correlating the serum levels of IgM with Lyme disease activity because these patients develop IgM antibodies to *B. burgdorferi* 3 to 6 weeks after infection. *(Jawetz et al, p 285)*

444. **(C)** The organisms of the genus *Haemophilus* are small, gram-negative, nonmotile, nonsporeforming bacilli with complex growth requirements. *H. influenzae* requires a heat-stable factor found in blood (X factor), which can be replaced by hematin, and nicotinamide adenine dinucleotide (V factor), which can be added to the medium as a supplement or can be supplied by other microorganisms, such as staphylococci (satellite phenomenon). *(Jawetz et al, pp 237–238)*

445. **(C)** *K. pneumoniae* is present in 5 to 10 percent of healthy adults and frequently occurs as a secondary pathogen in the lungs of patients with chronic pulmonary disease. It causes about 3 percent of all acute bacterial pneumonias, primarily acting as an opportunistic pathogen in individuals whose respiratory system is in some way compromised. It is an important pathogen because of its resistance to many of the antibiotics commonly employed in the treatment of pneumonia, and it usually develops into a pulmonary abscess as a complication of the pneumonic process. The major virulence factor of this pathogen is an antiphagocytic capsule. The organism is gram negative and has a lipopolysaccharide endotoxin that also contributes to its virulence. Other diseases caused by *K. pneumoniae* include bronchitis, bronchiectasis, and urinary tract infections. *(Joklik et al, pp 548–549)*

446. **(B)** *E. coli* is the most frequent cause of meningitis in neonates, who acquire the organism during birth. Group B streptococci also are an important cause of this disease in this age group. The remaining organisms listed in the question cause meningitis in all age groups on a relatively sporadic basis, with the exception of *N. meningitidis,* which can become epidemic in closed populations such as army training camps. *(Joklik et al, pp 544–548)*

447. **(C)** *Helicobacter pylori* is a newly discovered curved and spiral-shaped gram negative bacterium found in the human gastric mucosal layer. Evidence now shows that *H. pylori* is associated with the pathogenesis of peptic ulcer. It is found in almost all patients with duodenal ulcers, and more than 80% with stomach ulcers. *H. pylori* produces an abundant amount of urease. It does not produce coagulase, which is elaborated by *Staphylococcus aureus*. It is not an obligate intracellular parasite because it can be cultured on a number of artificial media in 2–7 days. Patients infected with *H. pylori* develop IgM, IgG, and IgA, which can be used in the diagnosis of *H. pylori*. *(Jawetz et al, pp 234–235)*

448. **(E)** There are five known classes of immunoglobulins: IgG, IgA, IgM, IgD, and IgE. IgG is the major immunoglobulin that is found in human serum and the only one that has been shown to pass the placental barrier in human beings. IgG has a molecular weight of 140,000–160,000. IgA is the major immunoglobulin of extracellular secretions, has a molecular weight of 160,000–440,000, has modest agglutinating capacity, and its carbohydrate content is 2–3 times higher (7.5%) than that of IgG. IgM possesses higher agglutinating and complement fixing capacity than IgG. IgM has a molecular weight of 900,000. Carbohydrates constitute 7–11% of the total weight of IgM. IgD constitutes a minor portion of serum immunoglobulins (1%). It contains higher amounts of carbohydrate (13%) than the other immunoglobulins, but it is an important B cell receptor. No other biological functions have been described for IgD. IgE is the immunoglobulin that has been associated with anaphylactic hypersensitivity. IgE has a molecular weight of 190,000–200,000, contains 11–12% carbohydrate, and constitutes 0.002% of the total serum immunoglobulin. *(Joklik et al, pp 224–225)*

449. **(E)** Chagas' disease, or American trypanosomiasis, is caused by *Trypanosoma cruzi*, which is transmitted to humans by various species of reduviid bugs that are also known in the United States as the kissing bugs. Cats and dogs serve as the main reservoir of infection for humans. Rats and other wild animals also serve as reservoirs of Chagas' disease. American trypanosomiasis is characterized by fever, lymphadenitis, facial edema, and myocardiopathy. In contrast to the transmission of *T. gambiense* or *T. rhodesiense*, *T. cruzi* is not transmitted to humans by bites of the kissing bugs. Transmission of *T. cruzi* to humans

occurs when infected feces of the kissing bugs are rubbed into the broken skin or the conjunctiva. *(Jawetz et al, pp 339–340)*

450. **(C)** Bacterial multiplication occurs by a process known as binary fission. That is, each cell enlarges and then divides into two cells. The time required for bacteria to divide is known as the generation time. The stated generation time of *Salmonella typhimurium* is 20 minutes. Thus, within 60 minutes *Salmonella typhimurium* will have undergone 3 divisions. Therefore, the number of colony forming units per ml (cfu/ml), if we start with 2×10^4, will proceed as follows: 4×10^4 in 20 minutes; 8×10^4 in 40 minutes; 1.6×10^5 in 60 minutes. *(Joklik et al, pp 62–64)*

451. **(E)** The concept of gene therapy is based on the assumption that definitive treatment for any genetic disease should be possible by directing treatment to the site of the defect itself, the mutant gene, and not to the secondary effects of that mutant gene. Since there are many hereditary diseases that are caused by defects in a single gene, there are many potential applications of this type of therapy to the treatment of human diseases. In addition, gene therapy may be useful for acquired diseases such as cancer or infectious diseases. One of the problems encountered in gene therapy is the need of introducing the desired gene into the host cells. Viruses with weak pathogenic potential, capable of entering into host cells, have been found to be useful gene carriers. They are attractive vectors in gene therapy for the following reasons: They infect cells with a much higher efficiency as compared to chemical or physical means of gene transfer. The genes inserted introviruses may be expressed in a regulated way. Adenovirus vectors may be used to target gene transfer into cells of the respiratory tract. Retrovirus vectors can be produced in large quantities from producer cell lines. *(Jawetz et al, pp 95–104)*

452. **(A)** Mutation occurs in bacteria as in all other cells. After the initial observation that bacterial populations contain mutants (such as a mutant that is resistant to an antibiotic), the question is posed as to whether the mutation is *directed* (induced by the antibiotic) or *random* (spontaneous). This question is most easily answered by the use of the *replica plate technique*. A velveteen pad is used to press over the colonies of the master plate and then pressed to plates A,B,C,(D). When the bacteria are replica plated to plates A,B,C,D containing a given antibiotic, the resistant colonies always appear in the same places. This is indeed the case in plates B and D, which contain the same antibiotic. This implies that resistant colonies existed before exposure to antibiotic.

Hence mutation is spontaneous. The Lamarckian theory states that acquired characteristics may be transmitted to descendants. *(Boyd and Hoerl, p 120)*

453. **(E)** Disinfection is defined as the destruction of pathogenic microorganisms. Isopropyl alcohol at 70% concentration has been used for skin disinfection because it denatures microbial proteins and enzymes that the microbes need to function. At unspecified concentrations, its action cannot be predicted. The most effective skin disinfectant currently in use is a solution of 1% iodine in 70% ethanol. Iodine oxidizes the free sulfhydryl groups of enzymes. This leads to enzyme inactivation. 70% ethanol acts as a protein denaturant. Mercurochrome easily loses its disinfective properties by extraneous organic material or unclean skin surfaces. Soap removes mechanically pathogenic and nonpathogenic bacteria, but it does not kill necessarily pathogenic bacteria. 3% hydrogen peroxide has a modest disinfective action. However, it is not as effective as 1% solution of iodine in 70% ethanol. *(Jawetz, et al, pp 46–47)*

454. **(D)** Individuals who have been diagnosed as X-linked agammaglobulinemic lack B lymphocytes and are not able to produce immunoglobulins. They have T cells that are the key players in cell mediated immunity associated with graft rejection, with intracellular parasites, viruses, and fungi. *Pneumocystis carinii* is now considered a fungus, causing infections in immuno-compromised patients, such as AIDS. The lack of immunoglobulins in X-linked agammaglobulinemia renders individuals susceptible to a succession of infectious diseases caused by extracellular bacteria. These infections may be partially controlled by the injection of specific gamma globulin as a supportive therapy. *(Joklik et al, pp 329–330)*

455. **(B)** Tumor necrosis factor (TNF) is a mediator of endotoxin induced shock and is involved in inflammation. It is also cytotoxic to certain tumor cells. Recent experiments in gene therapy have taken the approach of expressing TNF in tumor infiltrating lymphocytes (TIL), with the hope of allowing the TIL to return to the tumor and produce a high concentration of TNF and kill the tumor cells. TNF does not stimulate T cell proliferation or natural killer (NK) cell activity. NK cells can destroy tumor cells. However, they cannot be stimulated by TNF. *(Joklik et al, p 86)*

456. **(E)** The uptake of iron by bacteria is facilitated by low molecular weight compounds such as catechols and hydroxamates, the best examples of which are enterobactin and ferrichrome, respectively. Ionophores are compounds that destroy the selective permeability of the cytoplasmic membrane. Valinomycin is an example of an ionophore. Matrix proteins or porins are protein channels. They are found in the outer membrane of the cell wall of gram negative bacteria. Porins are just the right size to permit entry into the bacterial cell of compounds smaller than 600–700 daltons. Enzyme II and the heat stable protein HPr are components of the phosphoenol phosphopyruvate system, which is required for the transport of sugars into the cell. *(Joklik et al, pp 57–61)*

457. **(E)** There are different ways by which transfer of genes can occur in bacteria. One of these mechanisms of bacterial gene transfer is transformation, which involves passage of DNA from the donor to the recipient cell without the aid of a bacteriophage, cell donor-cell recipient contact, or a bacterial pilus. During transformation in *Streptococcus pneumoniae*, donor cells autolyse, releasing DNA fragments and competence factor. The competence factor induces recipient cells to synthesize a special set of proteins required for transformation. Transformation is inhibited by DNAse because this enzyme digests DNA and thus destroys its biological function. Transformation is an important mechanism of gene transfer in *Streptococcus pneumoniae, Streptococcus sanguis, Neisseria gonorrhoeae, Haemophilus influenzae,* and *Bacillus subtilis. (Joklik et al, pp 136–137)*

458. **(B)** Retroviruses are single stranded, linear, positive polarity RNA viruses 90–120 nm in diameter. The RNA is surrounded by an inner protein envelope with an icosahedral symmetry and an outer envelope that contains lipid and glycoprotein spikes, which serve to attach the virus to the host cells. Retroviruses have been associated with leukemia, sarcoma, mammary tumors, and especially with AIDS. The word retro refers to the possession of the enzyme reverse transcriptase, which transcribes RNA into DNA during the process of the viral nucleic acid synthesis. The virus is produced from a proviral DNA in infected cells. *(Joklik et al, pp 878–879)*

459. **(C)** The ability of certain viruses, such as influenza, mumps, and parainfluenza viruses, to agglutinate red blood cells is used to diagnose these viruses. In general, chicken—or human type O red blood cells—are employed for the identification of influenza, and other viruses. Red blood cells have receptors for the surface component of the influenza virus called hemagglutinin. This hemagglutinin is a glycoprotein. In a hemagglutination assay, a fixed number of red blood cells is mixed with increasing dilutions of the influenza virus. Then, following incubation at 4°C for 2 hours, the tubes containing the red blood cells and the virus are examined for hemagglutination. Unagglutinated cells form a dark bottom (virus dilutions 1:160; 1:320). Cells agglutinated by the virus

form a lattice that covers the entire bottom of the test tube (virus dilutions 1:20; 1:40; 1:80). The hemagglutination titer of the virus is the highest dilation of virus that forms a lattice. In this case, the hemagglutination titer is 1:80. *(Joklik et al, pp 746,766)*

460. **(C)** The site of action of erythromycin (as macrolide antibiotic) is the 50 s portion of the bacterial ribosome, while the aminoglycosides kanamycin, amikacin, gentamicin, and streptomycin act on the 30 s portion of the bacterial ribosome. Erythromycin inhibits the release of the charged tRNA bound to the donor site of the ribosome following peptide bond formation. This results in a blockage of *transfer* peptidyl-tRNA from the acceptor site back to the donor site of the ribosome. Erythromycin has an antibacterial spectrum similar to that of penicillin, but individuals allergic to penicillin are not allergic to erythromycin. It is bacteriostatic, and it is the drug of choice for *Legionella pneumophila, Coempylateaseter jejune,* and *Mycoplasma pneumoniae* infections. Streptomycin (SM) and other aminoglycoside antibiotics (neomycin, kanamycin, gentamicin, tobramycin, and amikacin) have a selectivity for gram-negative and acid-fast bacteria. The primary effect of aminoglycosides is on protein synthesis by permitting formation of an initiation complex, but blocking its further activity. As a result, the ribosomes drop off and there is an accumulation of monosomes. At higher concentration of SM, there is interference with the functioning of the mRNA so that there is some misreading of the code and a resulting insertion of the "wrong" amino acid (loss of fidelity). mRNA binds to the 30 s particle. *(Joklik et al, pp 169–175)*

461. **(C)** Plasmids are extrachromosomal double-stranded DNA circles that exist in bacterial cytoplasm independently of the host chromosome. They are of tremendous importance to medicine because they play a major role in the development of antibiotic-resistant bacterial strains. Plasmids replicate independently in the bacterial cytoplasm. Occasionally, plasmids will integrate into the bacterial chromosome. Usually, integration is a rare event. These plasmids that can replicate either autonomously in the cell cytoplasm, or as an integral part of the bacterial chromosome, are called *episomes*. Transposons are genetic elements that are highly mobile and that can be transposed from one piece of DNA to another at high frequency. Unlike plasmids, they do not contain genetic information for their synthesis. Competence factor is a special set of proteins required for bacterial transformation. Hfr refers to high frequency recombination donors from which chromosomal DNA is transferred to the donor cells. *(Jawetz et al, pp 85–89)*

462. **(D)** Since there are memory lymphocytes primed by a previous tetanus toxoid infection, booster immunization with tetanus toxoid will lead to rapid production of adequate levels of protective antibody. This is the routine procedure followed by physicians for patients with trauma who have been vaccinated against tetanus and received booster immunization for the last 5–7 years. The antibody titer to tetanus toxoid remains at protective levels for 5–10 years. Aminoglycosides will not be effective against the spores or vegetative cells of *Clostridium tetani.* Tetanus immune globulin is administered to individuals who already exhibit the symptoms of tetanus in an effort to neutralize tetanus toxin that has not yet been bound to nervous tissue. *(Joklik et al, pp 646–648)*

463. **(E)** Duplication of the eukaryotic chromosomes involves mitosis during which the chromosomes undergo a number of phases known as prophase, metaphase, anaphase, and telophase. However, replication of the bacterial chromosome does not involve mitosis. Therefore, in this respect bacteria differ from eukaryotic cells. DNA replication occurs continuously throughout the growth of the bacterial cell, and completion of a round of chromosome replication is required for cell division. The replication of the bacterial chromosome is semiconservative. That is, each one of the two strands that constitute the bacterial chromosome acts as a template for the synthesis of a complimentary DNA strand. Synthesis of the DNA strands occurs in both directions. Thus, it is bi-directional. Replication begins at a specific site called the origin, located in the cytoplasmic membrane. Protein synthesis is required for the completion of DNA bacterial replication. *(Joklik et al, pp 66–68)*

464. **(A)** The antiviral drug used currently against the immunodeficiency virus is AZT, or 3-azido-3-deoxythymidine (azidothymidine). Its structure is shown in this question. The structures of dideoxyinosine, idoxuridine, acyclovir, and enviroxine, which inhibit poliovirus replication, herpes virus thymidine kinase, herpes virus encoded DNA polymerase, and rhinoviruses, respectively, follow. *(Jawetz et al, pp 398–400)*

Acyclovir (acycloguanosine)

Enviroxime

Idoxuridine

Dideoxyinosine (ddl)

to phagocytosis, inside the phagocytic cell they are as readily destroyed as nonpiliated cells. *(Joklik et al, pp 450–456)*

467. **(E)** Immunosuppression, whether it is genetically acquired (as in the case of Bruton's agammaglobulinemia) or is caused by such diseases as cancer or autoimmunity or is the result of some of the therapeutic modalities employed today, will definitely predispose an individual to infections by various microbes. Indigenous flora will become opportunistic pathogens. Latent infections, such as those caused by the Herpesviridae, will exacerbate, and infections that would be mild or even subclinical in a normal individual will become life threatening. The majority of adult humans carry the agents listed in the question either as a latent infection or as normally occurring flora. The best example of nonpathogenic organism is *Saccharomyces cerevisiae*. *(Joklik et al, pp 333,399,935,1140)*

468. **(A)** Although there are relatively few effective antifungal drugs, in contrast to innumerable antibiotics that have been developed as antibacterial therapeutic agents (chloramphenicol, methicillin, streptomycin, penicillin), prognosis of many fungal diseases is greatly improved when a correct, specific diagnosis has been made and a proper therapeutic regimen can be instituted. Ketoconazole is a useful antifungal agent, which is clinically active against dermatophytes, dimorphic fungi, and yeasts. Thus, ketoconazole is used for the treatment of chronic mucocutaneous candidiasis, superficial candidiasis, dermatophytosis, systemic mycoses, and especially paracoccidioidomycosis. Ketoconazole interferes with the synthesis of ergosterol, which is a component of the fungal cytoplasmic membrane. *(Joklik et al, pp 165–166)*

469. **(D)** Immunity to tuberculosis requires such key players as activated macrophages and T lymphocytes, which had a previous interaction with the antigens of *Mycobacterium tuberculosis*, or related mycobacteria that are classified as facultative intracellular parasites. Activation of macrophages occurs via lymphokinins released by immunocompetent T lymphocytes. Now the macrophages, within which the causative agent of tuberculosis was able to multiply, have acquired the ability to suppress the growth of *M. tuberculosis*. Tuberculosis represents the best example of cell-mediated immunity in which activated macrophages play a key role. Diphtheria, pneumococcal pneumonia, furunculosis, and botulism are caused by extracellular parasites for which activated macrophages do not play a key role for their destruction. For these, extracellular parasites, normal macrophages, and/or specific antibody to their main virulence factor(s) will suffice. *(Joklik et al, pp 506–508)*

465. **(A)** Some soil microorganisms, such as members of the genes *Azotobacter, rhizobium,* and *clostridium,* can fix atmospheric nitrogen (N_2) and convert it to NH_4, which then can be assimilated into amino acids, purines, pyrimidines, and other nitrogen-containing compounds by plants, some bacteria, and other cells. The conversion of atmospheric nitrogen to NH_4 is catalyzed by an enzyme complex known as nitrogenase. Bacteria that can utilize CO_2 as their sole carbon, such as species of *Nitrobacter, Nitrosomonas,* etc., are called autotrophic bacteria, and nitrogen fixation is not a feature of these microorganisms. *(Joklik et al, p 54)*

466. **(D)** The pili of *N. gonorrhoeae* confer on the cells an enhanced ability to adhere to each other and to host cells. This has been demonstrated in vitro, where piliated organisms of colony types 1 and 2 adhere to cultured human cells better than do nonpiliated organisms of colony type 4. The pili are composed of proteins; therefore, they do not have endotoxin activity. Secretory IgA can be detected early in the urethral secretions of infected males. Thus, pili do not inhibit IgA secretion. Although the piliated strains are relatively resistant

470. **(A)** The genome of reoviruses is segmented double stranded. It has a cubic symmetry and it is resistant to ether. Rotaviruses are members of the reoviruses. They have a wheel-shaped morphology and are the causative agents of infantile gastroenteritis. Papovaviruses are ether-resistant, circular double-stranded DNA viruses. They cause human warts and they can be tumorigenic. Influenza viruses are members of the orthomyxoviruses, containing a segmented, single-stranded RNA genome. Orthomyxoviruses have hemagglutinin, or neuraminidase, on their surface, and they are sensitive to ether. The genome of arenaviruses is segmented, single stranded. The Lasa fever virus is a member of the arenaviruses, which are prominent in tropical America. Lasa fever is characterized by ulcers, skin rashes, higher fever, hemorrhages, pneumonia, and kidney and heart lesions. The mortality rate ranges between 36–67%. Rhabdoviruses have a single stranded, nonsegmented RNA genome. The rabies virus is an example of a rhabdovirus. It has a bullet-shaped morphology, and it is ether sensitive. *(Jawetz et al, pp 368–370)*

471. **(E)** Lymphocytes existing in fetal liver, or bone marrow, will be rich in cell surface TdT. This transferase is an indicator of a rather primitive cell state and is found only in very young cells that have not undergone extensive membrane differentiation or developed cell receptors. Sheep cell rosetting factors, subpopulation determinants, and cytotoxic potential appear after thymic migration. An abundance of idiotype determinants will appear after specific antigen stimulation and an appearance of the final heavy class chain on the cell surface. *(Joklik et al, pp 208,221,235,250–253)*

472. **(D)** Q (query) fever is a zoonosis caused by *Coxiella burnetii*. It is a respiratory disease that may be severe enough to develop into interstitial pneumonia. The microorganism is a natural parasite of cattle and sheep, and humans are incidental hosts, being infected by inhalation of infected excreta or contact with animal tissues. *C. burnetii* is spread from animal to animal by ticks and remains as an inapparent infection in the mammalian host until parturition. The organisms multiply readily in the placenta and other birth tissues and also are found in the urine and stool. These wastes contaminate the soil and serve as the source of infection for humans. *(Joklik et al, pp 713–714)*

473. **(C)** *Sporothix schenckii* is found on thorns, and it is introduced into the skin of extremities through trauma. A regional lesion begins as a pustule, abscess, or ulcer, and then nodules and abscesses are formed along the lymphatics. The history and the symptoms described in this patient are consonant with a diagnosis of sporotrichosis. *Trichophyton rubrum* is the cause of dermatophytosis (ringworm) of skin, scalp, and especially nails. The nails thicken and are discolored. *Aspergillus fumigatus* and *Candida albicans* are associated with deep opportunistic infections in immunocompromised patients such as AIDS patients. Aspergillosis is basically a pulmonary infection. Candidiasis can be associated with pathological conditions of the mucous membranes of the respiratory, genital, and gastrointestinal tract, where it is found as a normal inhabitant. *Cryptococcus neoformans* is the cause of meningitis. *(Jawetz et al, pp 310–327)*

474. **(E)** The genome of hepatitis B virus is composed of a circular, double-stranded DNA genome. It has a negative strand of 3200 nucleotides and another positive, incomplete strand of 1700–2600 nucleotides. Hepatitis A virus, the cause of infectious hepatitis, has a linear single-stranded RNA genome, and as such it is a member of the enteroviruses. Papilloma and polyomaviruses belong to the family of Papoviridae, which are viruses without envelopes and have a double-stranded, circular DNA genome. Both DNA circular strands are complete and thus differ from the genome of hepatitis B virus that has 2 incomplete circular DNA strands. J.C. virus is a member of the polyomaviruses. Epstein-Barr virus (EBV) is a member of the herpes viruses and as such has a double-stranded, linear DNA genome. EBV has been associated with infectious mononucleosis, Burkitt's lymphoma, and nasopharyngeal carcinoma. *(Joklik et al, pp 803,810–811,874,877,975,980)*

475. **(D)** The most appropriate laboratory diagnostic procedure for cases of suspected tinea corporis is digestion of tissue biopsies with 10–20% KOH and a search for hyaline, branched septate hyphae on squamous epithelial cells. A 10–20% potassium hydroxide solution dissolves the tissue without destroying the fungal cytology, thus allowing easy visualization of the fungal cells. Silver staining is used for the detection of spirochetes. Acid-fast stain is employed for the identification of mycobacteria. Culture of the vesicular fluid on agar does not permit growth of the fungal cells. Fungi are grown on Sabouraud's nutrient agar, which contains peptones, carbohydrates, vitamins, minerals, and water, and it has a pH of 5.3, which is optimal for fungal growth. Serology for *Blastomyces dermatitides* is inappropriate, because *Trichophyton rubrum* is the causative agent of tinea corporis. Furthermore, serology is of marginal value for the diagnosis of tinea corporis. *(Joklik et al, p 1130)*

476. **(D)** The cause of antigenic drift of influenza viruses is accumulated point mutations in the hemagglutinin gene. The genome of the influenza virus is composed of segmented, simple-stranded RNA. Influenza virus has a lipid envelope where the important antigens of influenza virus are localized. The virus-encoded surface glycoproteins hemagglutinin and neuraminidase undergo frequent variation independent of each other. Minor antigenic alterations are called *antigenic drift,* while major antigenic variations are termed *antigenic shift.* Antigenic drifts can be diagnosed by amino acid changes in the hemagglutinin glycoprotein molecule, and are the results of the accumulations of point mutations in the hemagglutinin gene. Antigenic shifts are due to reassortment of the 8 RNA segments of the viral genome. This occurs when persons are infected with two influenza viruses, i.e., a human influenza virus to which the person has partial immunity and an animal influenza virus possessing different hemagglutinins and neuraminidases. Now, the proteins surrounding the RNA influenza virus genome (capsids) may be encoded by the genomes of the human and animal viruses (*phenotypic mixing*) or specified entirely by the animal influenza virus genome (*phenotypic masking*). This situation can be detected by antigenic analysis. *(Joklik et al, pp 825,844–846,993–998)*

477. **(E)** The history of the patient described in the question would require careful consideration of all of the diseases listed, and the serology would not serve to rule out any. In the acute phase of the illness, an elevation of antibodies specific for the causative agent might not occur. Usually the rise in antibody levels does not occur until the second or third week of the infection, thus the significance of paired (acute and convalescent) serum samples, which allow the observation of an increase in the antibody specific for the causative agent of the infection. Identifying the cause of most bacterial infections is ideally accomplished by culture of the organism. Serology is used to confirm these identifications and is used also when the agent is slow growing or very expensive to culture or when the agent cannot be grown at all (as in the case of syphilis). *(Joklik et al, pp 561–562,596–597,611–613,705–707)*

478. **(D)** Creutzfeldt-Jacob disease is a degenerative central nervous human disease. The etiological agent does not seem to be a conventional virus, but infectivity is related to a proteinaceous macromolecule that appears to be devoid of any nucleic acid. This macromolecule is resistant to formaldehyde. It is inactivated by autoclaving, iodine disinfectants, ether, acetone, 6 M urea, 10% sodium dodecyl sulfate, or 0.5% sodium hypochlorite. Subacute sclerotizing panencephalitis is currently believed to be caused by measles virus, or a defective variant of the measles virus (rubeola virus). Distemper is a canine viral infection. It is caused by an RNA virus that is a member of the paramyxoviridal family. Progressive multifocal leukoencephalopathy has been associated with the J.C. virus, which is a member of the polyomaviruses. These viruses have a double-stranded, circular DNA genome. Dengue fever is caused by an arbovirus. Arboviruses have a RNA genome. Dengue fever is transmitted by a mosquito bite, and it is prevalent in tropical areas. It can be prevented by vaccination. *(Joklik et al, pp 778,874, 1014–1015,1019–1025,1066)*

479. **(E)** Plasmid encoded genes specify a variety of functions that include multiple drug resistance, resistance to heavy metals, and sex pilus formation (F plasmids). Bacteriocinogens are a group of plasmids that specify the production of the bactericidal proteins known as bacteriocins. The heat-labile and heat-stable enterotoxins of *E. coli* are plasmid encoded. The gene for exfoliative toxin, an exotoxin responsible for the staphylococcal scalded skin syndrome, is also located on a plasmid. Plasmids also contain genes responsible for the production of proteases (of *Streptococcus lactis*), resistance to phages (*E. coli*), metabolism of sugars and hydrocarbons, exotoxin of *Clostridium botulinum*, and tumorigenesis in plants. *(Joklik et al, pp 145–149,404–409,546)*

480. **(C)** Burkitt's lymphoma is associated with Epstein-Barr virus (EBV), which is a member of the herpes viruses. In this herpetic virus lymphoma, under the influence of EBV, an oncogene called c-myc, that is usually located on the 8th chromosome of B lymphocytes, is translocated to chromosome 14 of the B lymphocytes at the region of immunoglobulin heavy chain genes. This translocation places the c-myc gene side by side to an active promoter, and high levels of c-myc RNA are formed. The oncogenes, or transforming genes v-abl and v-fms, have been associated with the Abelson murine leukemia virus. They appear to be involved in the synthesis of proteins p160 and gp 180. The v-ras oncogene has been linked to Harvey murine sarcoma virus that causes sarcoma and leukemia in rats. The v-ras oncogene is involved in the production of a protein known as p21. The v-src oncogene has been connected with the Rous sarcoma virus, which is the etiological agent of chicken sarcoma. The product of the v-src oncogene appears to be a protein known as pp 60. *(Joklik et al, pp 886–891)*

481. **(E)** In contrast to rheoviruses, picornaviruses, poxviruses, and paramyxoviruses, the genomes of which replicate in the cytoplasm of the host cells, the genome of herpes viruses is replicated in the nucleus of the host cell. The first genes expressed are the alpha genes, which encode for phosphoproteins that act as activators of the next set of genes called beta genes. Expression of the beta 1 and 2 genes results in the synthesis of a DNA-binding protein, a DNA polymerase, a deoxypyrimidine kinase, and a moiety of a ribonucleotide reductase. The formation of these enzymes leads to the synthesis of visual DNA. Following initiation of the synthesis of the viral DNA, another set of genes called gamma genes is activated, giving rise to the formation of more than 50 viral proteins. *(Joklik et al, pp 804–805)*

482. **(D)** The best way to detect congenital syphilis is by the use of fluorescent-treponema-antibody-absorption-IgM (FTA-ABA IgM). All newborn infants of mothers with reactive VDRL, or reactive FTA-ABS tests, will themselves have reactive tests, whether or not they have actually acquired syphilis, because of the passive placental transfer of maternal immunoglobulins. However, if IgM antisyphilitic antibody is present in the infant's serum, it will reflect fetal antibody production in response to intrauterine infection (congenital syphilis) because maternal IgM antibody does not penetrate a healthy placenta. *(Joklik et al, pp 664–665)*

483. **(E)** A positive PPD skin test indicates that the individual has experienced mycobacterial infection at some time. It does not necessarily indicate current disease or give any information on the health status of the individual. Conversion to negative does not occur naturally and, if it occurs, has grave significance. Conversions occur in the terminal stages of tuberculosis and in certain immunodeficiency states (e.g., AIDS). *(Joklik et al, pp 502–508)*

484. **(D)** Amantadine (generic name) or symmetral (trade name) inhibit an early event in the multiplication cycle of influenza virus as well as arenaviruses. It blocks the uncoating process. Mutations in the M protein genes result in the development of drug-resistant mutants. The drug is not used extensively in the United States because it seems impractical to control this type of infectious disease that is not ordinarily fatal. To protect individuals at high risk, and in those when the infection is of potential danger, there is a choice between this drug and the influenza vaccine. In most cases, the vaccine would seem to be preferred. *(Joklik et al, pp 996–997)*

485. **(E)** The immunologic basis of graft rejection was proved by the classic experiments, which showed that accelerated destruction of second grafts from the original donor could be reproduced by infusion of B and T cells from a graft recipient into a naive animal before transplantation. It is logical, then, to expect that destruction of the effector B and T cells would suppress graft rejection. Irradiation, antilymphocyte globulin, and steroids all have been shown to cause lymphoid cell destruction when they were administered in appropriate doses. Cyclosporine is thought to inhibit interleukin 2, which drives antigen-activated cells into proliferation. *(Joklik et al, pp 282–283)*

486. **(C)** Adenoviruses do not have an envelope. Their linear, double-stranded DNA is enclosed within a capsid with icosahedral symmetry. Spikes project from each of the 12 vertices. The viral DNA contains a virus-encoded protein that is covalently crosslinked to each 5′ end of the linear adenovirus genome. Herpes viruses, and varicella-zoster virus, belong to the same family of herpesviridae and have a linear, double-stranded DNA genome, in which the complementary strands are not covalently crosslinked at the termini of the genome. SV40 virus is a member of the polyoma group of viruses which possesses a circular, double-stranded DNA genome. Finally, the genome of the vaccinia virus is linear, double-stranded DNA with inverted terminal repeats. *(Jawetz et al, pp 408,418,427,441,562)*

487. **(E)** Immune complexes are involved in the pathogenesis of all of the diseases listed in the question. They contribute to tissue damage by activating complement and attracting neutrophils that, through a process of exocytosis, release lysosomal enzymes into the microenvironment. Poststreptococcal nephritis is a nonsuppurative sequela of infection by a few M types of group streptococci. The Arthus reaction is a laboratory phenomenon that is usually evoked in the skin of an immune rabbit by the intradermal injection of antigen. Lupus glomerulonephritis is one of the most significant complications of this autoimmune disease and occurs as a result of DNA/antiDNA antibody complexes (and others) being deposited on the glomerular basement membrane. Serum sickness occurs in humans after the injection of foreign materials. Any foreign substance against which the host can produce antibody can cause this disease, although horse serum historically was the culprit. The immune complexes in serum sickness may localize in the vascular bed, producing vasculitis, or may cause arthritis or glomerulonephritis. *(Joklik et al, pp 321–322)*

488. **(E)** To be useful as a cloning vector, a plasmid should possess several properties. It should code for one or more selectable markers (such as antibiotic resistance) to allow identification of transformants and to allow maintenance of the plasmid in a bacterial population. Also, it should contain single sites for restriction enzymes in regions of the plasmid that are not essential for replication. Single sites for restriction enzymes allow for insertion of foreign DNA molecules that have been cleaved with the restriction enzymes. Autonomous replication is necessary and allows a high copy number of plasmids to be obtained. With high copy numbers, large amounts of a specific segment of foreign DNA can be obtained readily in pure form. *(Jawetz et al, pp 95–104)*

489. **(E)** Legionellosis, or legionnaire's disease, was first detected in 1976 when an outbreak of deadly pneumonia occurred in over 200 persons attending an American Legion convention. Epidemiologic investigations showed that the disease was caused by a gram-negative rod that was named *L. pneumophila*. The organism was spread from water reservoirs, contaminated air-conditioning units, nebulizers filled with water, or evaporative condensers. The organism can survive for over a year in tap water at room temperature (23 to 25°C). *L. pneumophila* is difficult to stain with the Gram stain or other common bacterial stains. It will stain faintly gram-negative when the safranin is left on for an extended period. The organism can be demonstrated by the direct fluorescent antibody procedure or by the silver impregnation method. *(Joklik et al, pp 694–697)*

490. **(E)** The physical examination supports a provisional diagnosis of streptococcal pharyngitis. This is a common infection caused by Group A, beta hemolytic streptococci, which are usually susceptible to penicillin and bacitracin. Laboratory diagnosis of Group A streptococcal pharyngitis is based on blood agar cultures, bacitracin sensitivity tests, and various serologic assays. *(Joklik et al, pp 418–424)*

491–492. **(491-B, 492-D)** A few parasitic diseases are acquired by ingestion of the eggs of organisms, such as *Enterobius vermicularis, Ascaris lumbricoides, Toxocara canis,* and *Trichuris trichiura.* Cysts are the infective form of *Entamoeba, Toxoplasma,* and *Giardia.* Ingestion of larvae is the source of *Trichinella* and *Taenia* infestations. Larval penetration of skin is the mode of transmission for hookworms, *Strongyloides,* and *Schistosoma.* Larval inoculation by vector insects occurs in onchocercal and wuchererial infections. Although both organisms have an intestinal phase in their life cycle in humans, major pathology involves tissues other than the gut. In addition to the primary abscesses affecting the large intestine of patients with *E. histolytica* infection, secondary abscess formation may occur in the liver or, rarely, in other organs. *S. mansoni* (and *Schistosoma japonicum* as well) causes granulomatous reactions in the host to the eggs deposited in in-

testinal venules or to those trapped in the liver or other organs. *(Joklik et al, pp 1164,1170,1183,1189, 1192,1209)*

493–495. **(493-E, 494-C, 495-B)** The antibody molecule is composed of two identical light chains and two identical heavy chains. The light chains are either κ or λ chains and have two domains, a constant domain (represented by the straight line in the figure that accompanies the question) and a variable domain (represented by the wavy line). The heavy chains carry the determinant group responsible for the immunoglobulin class of the molecule and are either α, γ, μ, σ, or ε chains. They have either four or five domains, only one of which is variable (represented by the wavy line). The portion of the molecule marked **A** is called the Fd fragment; this is the heavy-chain portion of the fragment antigen binding (Fab) fragment, which results from mild proteolysis of the molecule. Another fragment of the pepsin digestion of the molecule is the fragment crystallizable (Fc) fragment, marked by the **D** in the diagram. It is in this area of the molecule where most of the carbohydrate is located. Various biologic properties are controlled by this area as well. For example, complement is bound in this portion, and the ability of the IgE molecule to fix to mast cells is controlled here. *(Joklik et al, pp 223–230)*

496–498. **(496-C, 497-B, 498-A)** When an antigen is injected into an animal, it first undergoes an equilibration (choice **A** in the question) in which the concentration in the intravascular compartment is equalized with that outside this compartment (if the material can readily escape through the vascular endothelium), and any aggregated material is rapidly removed by the reticuloendothelial system. The next phase **(B)** is the phase of normal metabolic decay that reflects the molecule's half-life intravascularly. This will vary in slope depending on the half-life of the molecule in question. If the substance is antigenic, the host will respond immunologically to it and a phase of immune elimination, or clearance **(C)**, will ensue. It is during this period of rapid removal of the antigen in the form of antigen-antibody complexes that tissue damage can occur (such as that seen in serum sickness). If the host has been exposed to the antigen before, the metabolic clearance (or decay) phase will be very short, since there either are already circulating antibodies present to opsonize the antigen, or the anamnestic response will occur, in which event new antibodies will be produced very rapidly. *(Joklik et al, pp 247–249)*

499–500. **(499-A, 500-C)** Pili are hair-like proteinaceous appendages found on some bacteria. Pili are of two kinds. The thin, abundant, short ones (ordinary pili) are responsible for the adherence of bacteria to host cells. The few, long pili, known as sex pili, play a role in the transfer of genetic information from one bacterial cell to the other during the process of bacterial conjugation. The sex pili appear to be responsible for the attachment of DNA donor and recipient cells in bacterial conjugation. Members of the genus *Bacillus* and *Clostridium* produce spores. These are considered resting cells that are resistant to dryness, heat, and chemical agents. When spores are returned to an appropriate growth environment, they germinate to produce a vegetative cell. Part of their heat resistance has been attributed to a unique chemical known as calcium dipicolinate. *(Jawetz et al, pp 25–28)*

501–503. **(501-B, 502-A, 503-D)** Conjugation is the contact-dependent transfer of DNA from one bacterial cell to another. Auxotrophic mutants are those that differ from the wild-type organism in having one or more additional nutritional requirements. In the case presented in the question, one organism requires exogenous tryptophan, lysine, and histidine (Try⁻ Lys⁻ His⁻) and is able to synthesize its own proline, pantothenic acid, and biotin (Pro⁺ Pan⁺ Bio⁺). The second organism in the pair has the opposite genetic capabilities (i.e., it is Try⁺ Lys⁺ His⁺ Pro⁻ Pan⁻ Bio⁻). Conjugation that resulted in complete restitution of biosynthetic capabilities would produce an organism (Try⁺ Lys⁺ His⁺ Pro⁺ Pan⁺ Bio⁺) that could grow on minimal medium devoid of any of these nutrients. Colony 6 in the question is such an organism. Colony 1 still needs tryptophan and lysine for growth, as it was only able to grow on a plate supplemented with these two amino acids; its genotype then is Try⁻ Lys⁻. Colonies 2 and 4 both need tryptophan only; they are Try⁻. Colony 3 is Bio⁻, 5 is Pan⁻ Bio⁻, and colony 7 needs something in the complete medium that has not been added to the plates used in this experiment. *(Joklik et al, pp 139–141)*

504. **(D)** Autoantibody reactions can develop in individuals who have formed antibodies to their own modified cellular components that the immunological system, due to modification of cell molecules, can no longer recognize as part of itself. Thus, autoantibody to acetylcholine receptors of neuromuscular junctions is now considered the basis of myasthenia gravis. Certain individuals with Graves' disease develop autoantibodies to thyroid stimulating hormone (TSH) receptors. When these autoantibodies bind to TSH receptors, they resemble biologically-active TSH and induce the thyroid gland to synthesize thyroxine. Thrombocytopenia has been attributed to the development of autoantibodies to the cell surface receptors of the thrombocytes and the subsequent destruction of thrombocytes. The presence of autoantibodies to DNA

has been associated with the development of systemic lupus erythematosus. *(Joklik et al, pp 320–321)*

505. **(E)** Rheumatoid arthritis is an autoimmune disease. Autoimmune diseases involve the production of antibodies to an individual's own components. Thus, these antibodies are called autoantibodies. Normally, an individual does not produce antibodies to his own components. However, when his antigenic components become altered to the point that the immunological system can no longer recognize a component as being part of itself, it responds with the development of autoantibodies that can cause damage to this individual. Rheumatoid arthritis has been associated with the production of autoantibodies to immunoglobulin G (rheumatoid factor). It has been reported that there are over 100 diseases that have associated with a given human lymphocyte antigen (HLA) allele. For example, rheumatoid arthritis has been connected with possession of the HLA-DR4 allele, while Graves' disease, myasthenia gravis, and systemic lupus erythematosus have all been associated with the HLA-DR3 allele. *(Joklik et al, pp 281,320–321)*

506–508. **(506-G, 507-F, 508-B)** "Shingles" or herpes zoster is a recurrence of chickenpox caused by the varicella-zoster virus, which is a medium-sized, square-like, enveloped virus containing double-stranded DNA genome. The disease is characterized by inflammation of the dorsal root ganglion, neuralgic pain, and crops of clustered vesicles located along the affected nerves. Adenoviruses cause such diseases as pharyngitis, conjunctivitis, pneumonia, hemorrhagic cystitis, and gastroenteritis. Adenovirus is a nonenveloped, cubical virus with a double-stranded genome. Rhabdovirus is a bullet-shaped, enveloped virus, which contains a single-stranded genome. An example of a rhabovirus is the rabies virus. Measles, or rubeola virus, is an enveloped, round, single-stranded RNA virus. Measles is characterized by the development of maculapapules that coalesce to form blotches, becoming brownish in 5–10 days. There is also sneezing, coughing, Koplik spot formation, and lymphopenia. Mumps virus, like the measles virus, is a member of the paramyxoviridae family, which is composed mostly of spherical, enveloped viruses that are single stranded: linear, nonsegmented RNA genomes. Mumps is characterized by swelling of the parotid glands. Significant complications include orchitis and aseptic meningitis. J.C. virus is a member of the polyoma viruses that has been implicated in progressive multifocal leucoencephalopathy. It is a spherical, nonenveloped virus that belongs to the family of papoviridae, the members of which possess a double-stranded, circular DNA genome. Bunyavirus is a spherical, enveloped virus. It is transmitted by arthropods, *insects* and can cause encephalitis. Cytomegalovirus and molluscum contagiosum viruses are brick-shaped, enveloped viruses. Cytomegalovirus has been associated with microcephaly, seizures, deafness, jaundice, and purpura in 20% of infants infected during pregnancy. Molluscum contagiosum virus causes small, pink, wartlike, benign skin tumors. *(Levinson and Jawetz, pp 158,160,163,164,168–170,173, 187)*

BIBLIOGRAPHY

Joklik WK, Willett HP, Amos DB, Wilfert CM. *Zinsser Microbiology*. 20th ed. Norwalk, Conn: Appleton & Lange; 1992

Jawetz E, Melnick JL, Adelberg EA, et al. *Review of Medical Microbiology*. 19th ed. Norwalk, Conn: Appleton & Lange; 1991

Levinson WE, Jawetz E. *Medical Microbiology and Immunology*. 2nd ed. Norwalk, Conn: Appleton & Lange; 1992

Subspecialty List: Microbiology

Question Number and Subspecialty

382. Antigen-antibody reaction
383. Pathogenic bacteriology
384. Virology
385. Virology
386. Microbial genetics
387. Pathogenic bacteriology
388. Virology
389. Cellular immunology
390. Antigen-antibody reactions
391. Microbial genetics
392. Microbial genetics
393. Microbial genetics
394. Virology
395. Pathogenic bacteriology
396. Pathogenic bacteriology
397. Microbial genetics
398. Microbial physiology
399. Microbial physiology
400. Microbial physiology
401. Mycology
402. Virology
403. Pathogenic bacteriology
404. Antibody structure
405. Pathogenic bacteriology
406. Microbial genetics
407. Cellular immunology
408. Cellular immunology
409. Virology
410. Microbial genetics
411. Immune deficiency disease
412. Virology
413. Autoimmune disease
414. Immune deficiency disease
415. Microbial physiology
416. Microbial genetics
417. Virology
418. Antigen-antibody reaction
419. Microbial genetics
420. Parasitology
421. Pathogenic bacteriology
422. Virology
423. Antigen-antibody reaction
424. Parasitology
425. Antigenicity
426. Pathogenic bacteriology
427. Serology
428. Pathogenic bacteriology
429. Mycology
430. Virology
431. Mycology
432. Pathogenic bacteriology
433. Pathogenic bacteriology
434. Mycology
435. Parasitology
436. Pathogenic bacteriology
437. Microbial genetics
438. Pathogenic bacteriology
439. Pathogenic bacteriology
440. Pathogenic bacteriology; Oral microbiology
441. Cellular immunity
442. Cellular immunity
443. Pathogenic bacteriology
444. Pathogenic bacteriology
445. Pathogenic bacteriology
446. Pathogenic bacteriology
447. Pathogenic bacteriology
448. Immunology
449. Parasitology
450. Microbial physiology
451. Virology
452. Microbial genetics
453. Microbial physiology
454. Immunology
455. Immunology
456. Physiology
457. Microbial genetics
458. Virology
459. Virology
460. Microbial physiology
461. Microbial physiology
462. Pathogenic bacteriology
463. Microbial genetics
464. Virology
465. Microbial physiology
466. Pathogenic bacteriology
467. Acquired immunity
468. Mycology
469. Cellular immunity
470. Virology
471. Cellular immunity

472. Pathogenic bacteriology
473. Mycology
474. Virology
475. Mycology
476. Virology
477. Pathogenic bacteriology
478. Virology
479. Microbial genetics
480. Virology
481. Virology
482. Pathogenic bacteriology
483. Pathogenic bacteriology
484. Virology
485. Cellular immunology
486. Virology
487. Allergy
488. Microbial genetics
489. Pathogenic bacteriology
490. Pathogenic bacteriology

491. Parasitology
492. Parasitology
493. Antibody structure
494. Antibody structure
495. Antibody structure
496. Immune response
497. Immune response
498. Immune response
499. Microbial physiology
500. Microbial physiology
501. Microbial genetics
502. Microbial genetics
503. Microbial genetics
504. Autoimmunity
505. Autoimmunity
506. Virology
507. Virology
508. Virology

CHAPTER 5

Pathology
Questions

DIRECTIONS (Questions 509 through 572): Each of the numbered items or incomplete statements in this section is followed by answers or by completions of the statement. Select the ONE lettered answer or completion that is BEST in each case.

509. Which of the following chronic pulmonary conditions is associated with α_1-antitrypsin deficiency?

(A) Goodpasture's syndrome
(B) panlobular emphysema
(C) bronchiectasis
(D) Hamman-Rich syndrome
(E) bronchitis

510. The major pathologic change found in the hearts of persons with hypertensive heart disease is

(A) right ventricular dilatation
(B) right ventricular hyperplasia
(C) right ventricular hypertrophy
(D) left ventricular dilatation
(E) left ventricular hypertrophy

511. "Bronze diabetes" is a term used to describe

(A) melanoma
(B) hemosiderosis
(C) diabetes mellitus
(D) kwashiorkor
(E) hemochromatosis

512. The inflammatory process depicted in the illustration below shows a preponderance of which of the following cell types?

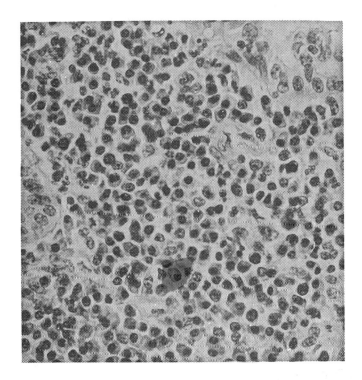

(A) polymorphonuclear leukocytes
(B) plasma cells
(C) eosinophil leukocytes
(D) macrophages
(E) giant cells

513. All of the following statements are true about primary biliary cirrhosis EXCEPT that

(A) it is believed to be an autoimmune disorder
(B) it most commonly occurs in females
(C) it is also called Wilson's disease
(D) it is characterized by destruction of the intrahepatic bile ducts
(E) it is commonly associated with anti-mitochondrial antibodies

514. Which of the five major classes of immunoglobulins has the highest mean serum concentration in humans?

(A) IgA
(B) IgD
(C) IgE
(D) IgG
(E) IgM

515. All of the following statements are true about gout EXCEPT that

(A) it is caused by elevated uric acid levels
(B) affected patients suffer transient attacks of acute arthritis
(C) multiple joints are typically affected
(D) tophi are the characteristic lesions
(E) precipitated urate crystals damage lysosomal membranes

516. Metaplasia is defined as

(A) an increase in the size of cells
(B) an increase in the number of cells
(C) irregular, atypical proliferative changes in epithelial or mesenchymal cells
(D) replacement of one type of adult cell by another type of adult cell
(E) loss of cell substance producing shrinkage of cell size

517. Niacin deficiency is associated with

(A) night blindness
(B) a bleeding diathesis
(C) altered formation of connective tissues
(D) neuromuscular and cardiac problems and edema
(E) dermatitis, diarrhea, and dementia

518. Adult polycystic disease of the kidneys is characterized by the following EXCEPT

(A) autosomal dominant inheritance
(B) autosomal recessive inheritance
(C) associated with polycystic change in the liver in some cases
(D) associated with polycystic change in the pancreas in some cases
(E) associated with berry aneurysm of the circle of Willis in some cases

519. Which statement is false about vitamin C?

(A) water-soluble vitamin
(B) necessary for synthesis of clotting factors
(C) lack causes bleeding in joints and gums
(D) deficiency state is termed scurvy
(E) necessary for synthesis of normal collagen

520. An elevation in the serum of which substance would be an unexpected finding in chronic liver disease?

(A) alanine aminotransferase
(B) aspartate aminotransferase
(C) albumin
(D) gamma globulin
(E) lactate dehydrogenase

521. The type of inflammatory change depicted in the illustration below is seen characteristically in all of the following EXCEPT

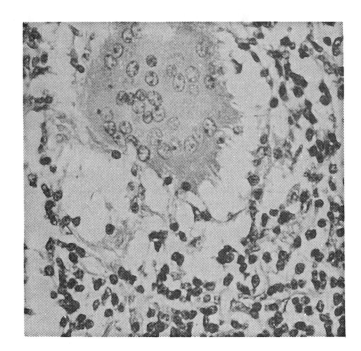

(A) Crohn's disease
(B) sarcoidosis
(C) ulcerative colitis
(D) temporal arteritis
(E) tuberculosis

522. Patients with Sjögren's syndrome show an increased risk for the development of

(A) pleomorphic adenoma
(B) melanoma
(C) lymphoma
(D) esophageal carcinoma
(E) leukemia

523. The human embryo or fetus is most susceptible to malformation caused by environmental factors during

(A) days 1 to 15
(B) days 15 to 60
(C) the second trimester
(D) the third trimester
(E) delivery

524. The Philadelphia chromosome is most often associated with which disease?

(A) follicular lymphoma
(B) Burkitt's lymphoma
(C) Down's syndrome
(D) acute lymphoblastic leukemia
(E) chronic myelogenous leukemia

525. The constellation of abnormalities seen in DiGeorge's syndrome includes

(A) an immune defect that improves with age
(B) a deficiency of B lymphocytes
(C) a decrease in serum immunoglobulin levels
(D) developmental failure of the second and third pharyngeal pouches
(E) an autosomal recessive genetic defect

526. Diverticulosis occurs most frequently in the

(A) cecum
(B) ascending colon
(C) transverse colon
(D) descending colon
(E) sigmoid colon

527. Which of the following disease states characteristically produces the nephrotic syndrome?

(A) interstitial nephritis
(B) membranous glomerulonephritis
(C) unilateral hydronephrosis
(D) acute crescentic glomerulonephritis
(E) polycystic disease of the kidneys

528. Which condition would not occur as a tumorous lesion in the duodenum?

(A) ulcer
(B) celiac sprue
(C) ectopic pancreas
(D) Brunner gland adenoma or hamartoma
(E) leiomyoma

529. The histologic changes seen in the connective tissue from the joint space of the great toe shown in the photomicrograph below are pathognomonic for

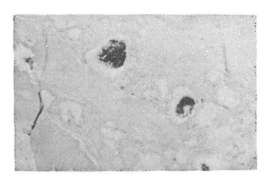

(A) rheumatoid arthritis
(B) suppurative arthritis
(C) gout
(D) osteoarthritis
(E) ankylosing spondylitis

530. Which of the following options is LEAST appropriate regarding the lesion depicted in the photomicrograph below?

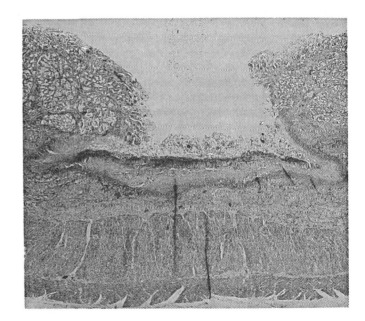

(A) focal loss of epithelial continuity
(B) associated with increased acid and pepsin secretion
(C) may be complicated by hemorrhage
(D) a malignant neoplasm
(E) may be complicated by perforation of the organ

531. Common findings in myelofibrosis with myeloid metaplasia include all of the following EXCEPT

   (A) fibrosis in the bone marrow
   (B) enlarged spleen
   (C) extramedullary hematopoiesis
   (D) teardrop-shaped erythrocytes
   (E) usually a neonatal disorder

532. Which of the following tumors is LEAST characteristically seen in early childhood?

   (A) neuroblastoma
   (B) retinoblastoma
   (C) medulloblastoma
   (D) astrocytoma
   (E) meningioma

533. All of the following are characteristic of neuroblastoma EXCEPT that it

   (A) is rare in childhood
   (B) may arise in the adrenal medulla
   (C) may arise in the posterior mediastinum
   (D) secretes catecholamines
   (E) shows a rosette pattern

534. Which of the following neoplasms is benign?

   (A) adenocarcinoma
   (B) cystadenoma
   (C) fibrosarcoma
   (D) lymphocytic leukemia
   (E) melanoma

535. Which characteristic best determines the genotype of an organism?

   (A) number of microvilli
   (B) DNA structure
   (C) pinocytosis
   (D) lysosomal content
   (E) rate of metabolism

536. All of the following statements are true about the relationship of leukocytes to the sequence of events occurring in acute inflammation EXCEPT that

   (A) in response to the inflammation, neutrophils tend to marginate or pavement along the blood vessel walls
   (B) endothelial cell contractions allow neutrophils to emigrate from the blood vessels through intercellular gaps
   (C) WBCs may stick to endothelial cells by undergoing surface changes and by the formation of pseudopods

   (D) neutrophils arrive at the site of the inflammation in response to bacterial chemotactic products
   (E) C3 and C5 complement compounds are important factors in the chemotaxis of neutrophils

537. The characteristic inflammatory cell seen in the tissues in response to infection by *Salmonella typhi* is the

   (A) polymorphonuclear leukocyte
   (B) eosinophil leukocyte
   (C) monocyte
   (D) multinucleate giant cell
   (E) plasma cell

538. All of the following are true about a fibrinous exudate EXCEPT that it

   (A) induces connective tissue organization
   (B) is associated with pneumococcal pneumonia
   (C) has a low protein content
   (D) is seen in bread-and-butter pericarditis
   (E) has fibrin precipitates

539. Renal cell carcinoma is characterized by all of the following EXCEPT that

   (A) it may reach a large size before hematuria occurs
   (B) it is usually seen in infants or in early childhood
   (C) it invades the renal capsule and perirenal fat
   (D) it invades the renal vein frequently
   (E) frequent metastases include those to bone and lung

540. Identify the false statement about breast cancer.

   (A) incidence in United States is higher than in Japan
   (B) increased incidence with early menarche
   (C) increased incidence with family history of breast cancer
   (D) increased incidence with high fat diet or late menopause
   (E) decreased incidence with atypical mammary hyperplasia

541. A rectal biopsy is the usual approach to the morphologic documentation of Hirschsprung's disease. Which of the following findings is considered diagnostic of Hirschsprung's disease on histologic examination of the rectal biopsy specimen?

   (A) hypertrophy of the muscle coat of the wall of the rectum

(B) atrophy of the mucosal lining of the wall of the rectum

(C) absence of the nerve fibers that innervate the wall of the rectum

(D) absence of parasympathetic ganglion cells in the submucosal and myenteric plexus

(E) presence of multiple small polyps along the mucosal surface of the rectal wall

542. The most common cause of neonatal cholestasis is

(A) intrahepatic biliary atresia

(B) extrahepatic biliary atresia (EBA)

(C) choledochal cyst

(D) primary biliary cirrhosis

(E) Budd-Chiari syndrome

543. Adult respiratory distress syndrome is characterized by all of the following EXCEPT

(A) hyaline membrane formation

(B) proliferation of type I pneumonocytes

(C) intra-alveolar fibrosis

(D) heavy, meaty lungs

(E) unresponsiveness to oxygen therapy

544. Red hepatization is a pathologic term characterizing

(A) fibroblast proliferation

(B) WBCs, RBCs, and fibrin filling the alveolar spaces

(C) hyaline membrane formation

(D) congestion of the hepatic sinusoids

(E) hemorrhage and abscess formation

545. Chronic granulomatous disease includes all of the following EXCEPT that

(A) there is poor bacterial killing by neutrophils

(B) it usually afflicts males

(C) there are symptoms of pneumonia, lymphadenitis, or splenomegaly

(D) it is usually manifest in the first 2 yrs of life

(E) there is increased nitroblue tetrazolium (NBT) reduction

546. Which of the following is NOT a characteristic feature or complication of syphilis and its effects on the heart and great vessels?

(A) endarteritis obliterans and perivascular plasma cell infiltration of the vasa vasorum of the aortic arch

(B) dissecting aneurysm of the aorta

(C) stellate fibrosis and loss of elastic tissue in the media

(D) saccular aneurysm of the ascending thoracic aorta

(E) narrowing of the coronary ostia

547. The vegetation characteristically seen in acute rheumatic carditis most commonly occurs in

(A) the aortic sinuses of Valsalva

(B) the line of closure (free margins) of mitral valve

(C) the insertion of the chordae tendinae

(D) the mitral valve annulus

(E) just lateral to the coronary artery ostia

548. Edema is caused by all of the following mechanisms EXCEPT

(A) increased vascular permeability

(B) obstruction to lymphatic flow

(C) sodium retention

(D) increased plasma proteins

(E) increased capillary blood pressure

549. All of the following statements are true about radiation-induced carcinogenesis EXCEPT that

(A) the amount of damage is related to the dose of radiation

(B) RNA is the major cell target for radiation injury

(C) cells can repair radiation-induced cell damage

(D) past history of therapeutic radiation has been implicated in carcinogenesis

(E) occupational exposure to radiation is a well-documented cause of cancer

550. The teratogenic effect of high-dose radiation to the fetus in utero may produce all of the following abnormalities EXCEPT

(A) microcephaly

(B) mental retardation

(C) skeletal malformation

(D) mutation in fetal germ cells

(E) masculinization of the female fetus

551. All of the following statements concerning skin melanocytes and the response of skin melanocytes to ultraviolet (UV) light are true EXCEPT that

(A) in whites, an increase in the size and functional activity of melanocytes can be seen after a single exposure to UV light

(B) in whites, repeated UV light exposure produces an increase in the concentration of melanocytes

(C) melanocytes may undergo mitosis when exposed repeatedly to UV light

(D) blacks have a higher concentration of melanocytes for any given area of skin than do whites

(E) the skin of blacks has larger melanocytes with more dendritic processes than does the skin of whites

552. All of the following statements concerning Duchenne muscular dystrophy are true EXCEPT that

(A) pseudohypertrophy of the calf is the result of regeneration of the muscle

(B) it is the most common type of muscular dystrophy

(C) it occurs as symmetrical involvement of the pelvic girdle muscles

(D) Becker's muscular dystrophy is a more benign form of the disease

(E) elevated serum creatine phosphokinase (CPK) levels may be helpful in detecting the carrier state

553. Prenatal exposure to diethylstilbestrol (DES) has been linked to the development of

(A) granulosa cell tumor of the ovary

(B) squamous cell carcinoma of the endometrium

(C) clear cell carcinoma of the vagina

(D) carcinoma in situ of the cervix

(E) adenomatous hyperplasia of the endometrium

554. The bone marrow biopsy specimen shown below is diagnostic of

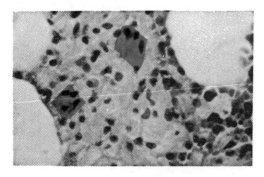

(A) amyloidosis

(B) acute myelocytic leukemia

(C) chondrosarcoma

(D) Gaucher's disease

(E) Pompe's disease

555. Which of the following is the most correct statement concerning acquired immunodeficiency syndrome (AIDS)?

(A) The disease is most prevalent in the United States in homosexual males.

(B) The disease is most frequent in Central Africa in homosexual males.

(C) The disease is most frequent in Central Africa in intravenous drug users.

(D) The disease is most frequent in Scandinavia in prostitutes.

(E) The disease is most frequent in the United States in hemophiliacs.

556. Which of the following statements concerning carcinoma of the uterine cervix is FALSE?

(A) The majority of tumors are squamous cell in type.

(B) The 5-yr survival in treated stage I is 90 percent.

(C) The 5-yr survival in stage IV is 10 percent.

(D) The disease is rare in black Africans.

(E) There is often a recognizable preinvasive stage.

557. Which of the following statements concerning *Schistosoma mansoni* infestation is FALSE?

(A) The eggs are usually shed in the feces.

(B) Liver fibrosis may be a long-term complication.

(C) One of the phases in the life cycle includes the fresh water snail.

(D) The initial phase of infection in humans is from water contact with the skin.

(E) It is a frequent cause of hematuria.

558. An expected finding in an anaphylactic reaction, or type I immunologic response, would be

(A) reaction to an antigen on first exposure to the antigen

(B) an interaction of antibody with the eosinophilic leukocyte

(C) release of vasoactive amines

(D) IgA antibody as the mediator of response

(E) tuberculin type giant cells

559. Malignant neoplasms differ from benign neoplasms by showing all of the following features EXCEPT

(A) metastases to distant viscera

(B) encapsulation

(C) blood vessel invasion

(D) rapid, erratic growth

(E) disorganized cell architecture

560. Hyponatremia secondary to the inappropriate secretion of ADH is seen most often in association with which type of lung tumor?

(A) squamous cell carcinoma

(B) adenocarcinoma

(C) large cell carcinoma

(D) oat cell carcinoma

(E) bronchioalveolar carcinoma

561. The major scavenger cell involved in the inflammatory response is the

(A) neutrophil

(B) lymphocyte

(C) plasma cell

(D) eosinophil

(E) macrophage

562. Liquefaction necrosis is the characteristic result of infarcts in the

(A) brain

(B) heart

(C) kidney

(D) spleen

(E) small intestine

563. Which is least likely to produce an intravascular thrombus?

(A) damage to endothelium

(B) hypercoagulable states

(C) warfarin therapy

(D) stasis of blood

(E) hyperviscosity syndromes

564. A child has a vesicular skin rash. His immunization history is not available. The Tzanck test smear shown in the photomicrograph below supports the preliminary diagnosis of

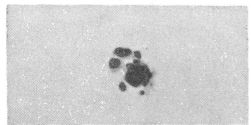

(A) measles

(B) Rocky Mountain spotted fever

(C) German measles

(D) chickenpox

(E) none of the above

Questions 565 and 566

A 60-yr-old man is suffering from the nephrotic syndrome and microscopic hematuria. A renal biopsy is performed.

565. The electron micrograph (EM) of the glomerular lesions, shown below, demonstrates

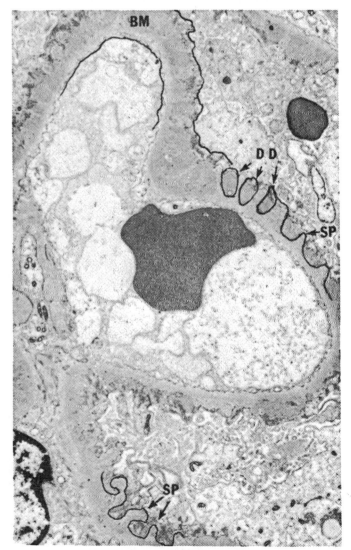

(A) acute or postinfection glomerulonephritis (AGN)

(B) membrane glomerulonephritis (MGN)

(C) minimal change disease (MCD)

(D) membranoproliferative glomerulonephritis (MPGN)

(E) focal glomerulonephritis (FGN)

566. Immunofluorescence (IF) studies performed on the biopsy specimen reveal granular staining with IgG and complement antibodies. This patient's renal disease is most likely

(A) postinfectious glomerulonephritis

(B) secondary to diabetes mellitus

(C) idiopathic

(D) IgA nephropathy (Berger's disease)

(E) a manifestation of Goodpasture's syndrome

567. A photomicrograph of immunohistochemical stain of a lesion in the region of the pituitary gland of a 50-yr-old woman with Cushing's syndrome is shown below. The lesion is most likely

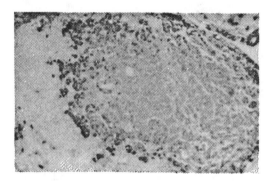

(A) a pituitary granuloma

(B) a parapituitary glioma

(C) a craniopharyngioma

(D) an adrenocortical carcinoma

(E) a pituitary adenoma

568. Auer rods are most characteristic of

(A) chronic lymphocytic leukemia (CLL)

(B) acute lymphoblastic leukemia (ALL)

(C) chronic myelocytic leukemia (CML)

(D) acute myeloblastic leukemia (AML)

(E) erythroleukemia (DiGuglielmo's syndrome)

569. A neoplastic disease of T cell lymphocytes is

(A) multiple myeloma

(B) macroglobulinemia

(C) chronic myelocytic leukemia (CML)

(D) acute myeloblastic leukemia (AML)

(E) mycosis fungoides

570. All of the following statements characterize chronic lymphocytic leukemia (CLL) EXCEPT that

(A) it is a malignancy of elderly persons

(B) patients may be asymptomatic at diagnosis

(C) patients may exhibit hepatosplenomegaly

(D) patients often have a history of fever

(E) the peripheral blood smear alone may be diagnostic

571. Hypochromic microcytic anemia is classically caused by

(A) recent blood loss

(B) vitamin B_{12} deficiency

(C) iron deficiency

(D) folic acid deficiency

(E) accelerated erythropoiesis

572. The lactate dehydrogenase (LDH) isoenzyme pattern shown below is diagnostic of

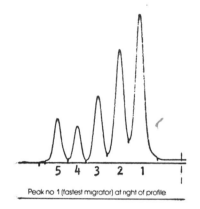

Peak no 1 (fastest migrator) at right of profile

(A) pulmonary embolism

(B) hepatitis

(C) meningitis

(D) myocardial infarction

(E) skeletal muscle trauma

DIRECTIONS (Questions 573 through 635): Each set of matching questions in this section consists of a list of up to ten lettered options followed by several numbered items. For each item, select the ONE lettered option that is most closely associated with it. *Each lettered heading may be selected once, more than once, or not at all.*

Questions 573 through 575

For each description below, choose the compound with which it is usually associated.

(A) histamine

(B) bradykinin

(C) C567

(D) prostaglandin E

(E) neutral proteases

573. Vasodilatory product of Hageman factor with no chemotactic action

574. Important in early increases in vascular permeability

575. Lysosomal product important in extracellular degradation

Questions 576 through 578

(A) synaptophysin
(B) actin
(C) cytokeratin
(D) desmin
(E) glial fibrillary acid protein

576. Intermediate filament most likely to be found in malignant epithelial tumors

577. Intermediate filament most likely to be found in smooth muscle tumors

578. Intermediate filament most likely to be found in glial cell tumors

Questions 579 through 581

For each infectious agent listed below, select the disease for which it is responsible.

(A) tularomia
(B) lymphogranuloma venereum
(C) pertussis
(D) plague
(E) Rocky Mountain spotted fever

579. *Rickettsia rickettsi*

580. *Chlamydia trachomatis*

581. *Yersinia pestis*

Questions 582 through 584

For each organism listed below, select the microscopic or anatomic finding with which it is associated.

(A) relatively intact colonic mucosa
(B) ulceration of esophageal mucosa
(C) necrotizing interstitial pneumonia
(D) ulceration of colonic mucosa
(E) diffuse reticuloendothelial hyperplasia

582. *Salmonella* species

583. *Shigella* species

584. *Vibrio cholerae*

Questions 585 through 587

(A) Addison's disease
(B) Hashimoto's disease
(C) Cushing's syndrome
(D) de Quervain's thyroiditis
(E) Cori's disease

585. Autoimmune thyroid disorder

586. Chronic adrenocortical insufficiency

587. Hereditary disorder of glycogen metabolism

Questions 588 through 590

(A) squamous cell carcinoma of the uterine cervix
(B) adenocarcinoma of the endometrium
(C) malignant teratoma of the ovary
(D) sarcomas of the fallopian tube
(E) clear cell carcinoma and adenosis of the vagina

588. In utero exposure to diethylstilbestrol

589. Highest incidence associated with multiple sexual partners, viral infections, and preceding dysplasia

590. Highest incidence associated with nulliparity, diabetes, and obesity

Questions 591 through 593

(A) ventricular septal defect
(B) tricuspid atresia
(C) tetralogy of Fallot
(D) patent ductus arteriosus
(E) truncus arteriosus

591. Failure to close intrauterine vascular channel between pulmonary artery and aorta

592. Most common congenital heart anomaly

593. Developmental failure of aorta and pulmonary artery to separate

Questions 594 through 596

(A) beryllium granulomatosis
(B) stannosis
(C) byssinosis
(D) silicosis
(E) asbestosis

594. Asthma-like disorder caused by inhaled cotton fibers

595. Increased risk of malignant mesothelioma

596. Associated with tin oxide inhalation

Questions 597 through 599

    (A) Goodpasture's syndrome
    (B) Chagas's disease
    (C) Dubin-Johnson syndrome
    (D) Peutz-Jeghers syndrome
    (E) Kawasaki's disease

597. Myocarditis caused by protozoan organism

598. Familial disease with intermittent jaundice and black pigmentation of the liver

599. Diffuse pulmonary hemorrhages and rapidly progressive glomerulonephritis

Questions 600 through 602

    (A) autosomal dominant inheritance
    (B) autosomal recessive inheritance
    (C) X-linked recessive inheritance
    (D) X-linked dominant inheritance
    (E) non-hereditary disorder

600. Hemophilia A

601. Achondroplasia

602. Alkaptonuria (ochronosis)

Questions 603 through 605

    (A) *Streptococcus viridans*
    (B) *Klebsiella pneumoniae*
    (C) *Pneumocystis carinii*
    (D) tricuspid valve
    (E) aortic valve

603. Which cardiac valve is most likely to be affected by the chronic form of this disorder?

604. Which organism is most commonly cultured from the chronic form of this disorder?

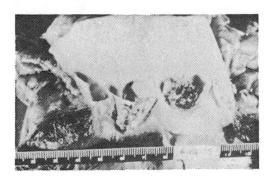

605. Which cardiac valve with this disorder is most likely to give rise to embolic infarcts of the kidney?

Questions 606 through 608

    (A) Sipple syndrome
    (B) Stein-Leventhal syndrome
    (C) Wermer syndrome
    (D) Zollinger-Ellison syndrome
    (E) MEN I

606. Peptic ulcer disease, gastric hypersecretion, and ectopic gastin production

607. Medullary thyroid carcinoma, parathyroid neoplasms, and pheochromocytoma

608. Polycystic ovaries, obesity, oligomenorrhea, and hirsutism

Questions 609 through 611

    (A) pemphigus
    (B) mycosis fungoides
    (C) actinic keratosis
    (D) ichthyoses
    (E) dermatitis herpetiformis

609. Cutaneous T cell lymphoma

610. Immunologically mediated dysadhesion between keratinocytes

611. Hereditary disorder with marked hypertrophy of stratum corneum

Questions 612 through 614

    (A) thalassemia
    (B) myelophthisic anemia
    (C) sideroblastic anemia
    (D) hereditary elliptocytosis
    (E) pernicious anemia

612. Pancytopenia due to cobalamin deficiency

613. Usually seen with carcinomatous metastases to the bone

614. Hereditary disease of discordant globin chain synthesis

Questions 615 through 617

(A) acetaminophen overdose
(B) methyl alcohol poisoning
(C) carbon monoxide poisoning
(D) chronic lead poisoning
(E) cocaine overdose

615. Toxic metabolite causes massive hepatic necrosis

616. Systemic asphyxiant

617. Toxic metabolites formaldehyde and formic acid can cause blindness and neuronal damage

Questions 618 through 620

(A) hypertrophy
(B) hyperplasia
(C) atrophy
(D) metaplasia
(E) dysplasia

618. A reversible change in which one adult cell type is replaced by another adult type

619. Shrinkage in cell size by loss of substance

620. Atypical cellular development that may be precancerous

Questions 621 through 626

(A) Down's syndrome
(B) Edwards' syndrome
(C) Patau's syndrome
(D) Cat-cry syndrome
(E) Klinefelter's syndrome
(F) Turner's syndrome
(G) Double Y males
(H) Normal male karyotype
(I) Normal female karyotype
(J) Multi-X female

621. On physical examination 17-year-old male is noted to have only minimal secondary sexual development, gynecomastia, and an eunuchoid, tall habitus. His chromosome analysis is reported as 47,XXY.

622. An amniocentesis is performed on a 16-week fetus because of advanced maternal age. The chromosome analysis is reported as 46,XX.

623. A mentally retarded female adolescent with a history of congenital cardiac disease has a chromosome analysis reported as 47,XX,+21.

624. An autopsy is done on a 53-year-old woman who was killed in an accident. She had been in apparent good health. The chromosome analysis is reported as 47,XXX.

625. A 17-year-old short-statured girl is found to have streak gonads. Her karyotype is reported as 45,X.

626. An infant dies shortly after birth. At autopsy the occiput is prominent, there are multiple renal and intestinal defects, and there is micrognathia. A chromosome analysis is reported as 47,XX,+18.

Questions 627 through 630

(A) sarcoidosis
(B) tuberculosis
(C) histoplasmosis
(D) coccidiomycosis
(E) amyloidosis
(F) bacterial pneumonia
(G) mesothelioma
(H) carcinoma
(I) fibrosing alveolitis
(J) silicosis

627. A right lower lobectomy specimen contains a solitary 1.2 cm diameter solid nodule. The center of the nodule is fibrous. The periphery has granulomatous inflammation. With special stains, multiple 2 to 5 μm budding yeasts are evident within the nodule. Acid fast stains are negative.

628. A left upper lobectomy specimen is received containing a 4.6 cm nodule with central cystic degeneration. Microscopically, the nodule is composed of anaplastic squamous cells. Similar abnormal cells are seen in a concomitant biopsy of a hilar lymph node.

629. After a long history of multiple myeloma, a 67-year-old male is noted to have abundant acellular eosinophilic deposits around the pulmonary microvasculature at autopsy. A congo red special stain demonstrates apple green birefringence.

630. A large, pleural-based lesion is found on chest X-ray of an asbestos worker. Electron microscopy of the biopsy shows abundant long microvilli.

Questions 631 through 635

    (A) renal cell carcinoma

    (B) diabetic kidney

    (C) renal papillary necrosis

    (D) glomerulonephritis

    (E) endometriosis

    (F) transitional cell carcinoma

    (G) seminoma

    (H) teratoma

    (I) prostatic carcinoma

    (J) condyloma acuminatum

631. A sexually active 24-year-old male has recently developed multiple 0.2 to 0.6 cm normally pigmented papillary tumors at his penile meatus. Histologic examination reveals perinuclear vacuoles, papillomatosis, and positive immunoperoxidase stains for human papilloma virus.

632. The left kidney is surgically removed and found to contain a 6.3 cm diameter solitary solid nodule with a variegated red, white, and yellow hue. The nodule grows into the renal vein. Histologically, the nodule is composed of anaplastic cells with clear cytoplasm and focal abortive gland formation.

633. A 34-year-old female is found to have intermittent hematuria. A bladder biopsy demonstrates a focus of benign endometrial glands and stroma with associated hemorrhage.

634. A 77-year-old male has bone pain and a markedly elevated prostatic specific antigen. A prostate biopsy demonstrates anaplastic glands in a fibrous stroma and in perineural spaces.

635. A 7-year-old female suddenly experiences hematuria and hypertension two weeks after a streptococcal throat infection.

Answers and Explanations

509. **(B)** Panlobular emphysema is a diffuse loss of alveolar septa throughout the lung, extending from the hilum to the periphery. In 1963, an association was shown between patients with a hereditary deficiency of α_1-antitrypsin and patients with severe panlobular emphysema. These patients have bilateral emphysema, primarily basilar, which occurs in both sexes and at an earlier age than do other forms of chronic obstructive pulmonary diseases. This disease has an autosomal recessive inheritance pattern. Heterozygous individuals with the α_1-antitrypsin deficiency gene also may show an increased risk of developing emphysematous changes in their lungs, especially with environmental and smoking insults. Homozygous patients with α_1-antitrypsin deficiency account for fewer than 10 percent of all patients with emphysema. *(Cotran, pp 766–772)*

510. **(E)** Hypertensive heart disease is a common form of heart disease in the elderly population, affecting men more often than women and blacks more often than whites. The majority of cases are of idiopathic origin, but some cases are secondary to renal, cerebral, endocrine, or cardiovascular disease. Because of the increased resistance to blood flow, the most significant pathologic change is left ventricular hypertrophy with increasing size of the myocardial cells. There is no actual increase in cell number (hyperplasia). There is thickening of the left ventricular muscle wall concentrically, with narrowing of the chamber size. Endocardial fibrous thickening also may occur. The left ventricular wall thickness is increased as much as 2 cm, and the heart weight may be doubled. With long-standing hypertrophic heart disease, there is gradual dilatation and hypertrophy of the right ventricle and dilatation of the right and left atria. Enlargement of the myocardial cells, an increased number of nuclei per cell (boxcar nuclei), degenerative changes, and fibrosis may be seen microscopically. *(Rubin and Farber, pp 477–481)*

511. **(E)** Hemochromatosis, or bronze diabetes, is an inherited disease characterized by cirrhosis, diabetes, and increased skin pigmentation. Affected persons are usually middle-aged or elderly, often male, and have elevated serum iron levels, high saturation of total iron-binding capacity, elevated serum ferritin levels, and increased urinary iron excretion. Sufferers are thought to have a defect in mucosal iron absorption in the gastrointestinal tract, resulting in increased iron absorption with iron overload. The excess iron accumulated is stored in parenchymal organs, especially in the liver, pancreas, endocrine glands, myocardium, and skin. Iron is not stored to any great extent in the reticuloendothelial system, as is the case of hemosiderosis with iron overload secondary to increased intake or release. In patients with hemochromatosis, the excess iron deposits in organs cause parenchymal destruction and fibrosis. This is manifested as cirrhosis and hepatic failure and diabetes due to islet cell destruction in the pancreas. Sufferers also have an increased risk of developing hepatomas. Hyperpigmentation results from increased melanin production in the epidermis and not from increased iron pigment in the dermis, as was previously thought. Affected patients have diabetes, hepatomegaly, and endocrine abnormalities, such as impotence or adrenal dysfunction. Treatment is aimed at reducing the iron load by phlebotomy or the use of iron chelators. *(Cotran, pp 950–953)*

512. **(B)** The photomicrograph shows tissue in which there are sheets of plasma cells with eccentric nuclei and ample cytoplasm, typical of these cells. The recognition of plasma cells implies either that the disorder is one in which there may have been a transient acute inflammatory change that has now subsided or the disease has not yet gone into a more long-term, or chronic, phase. It is of some interest that plasma cells, although associated with such subacute inflammations, are not always seen and sometimes can be seen characteristically in certain settings. Plasma cells, for instance, are seen very frequently in these large numbers, being the predominant cell in the primary chancre of syphilis and maybe, as in the illustration, the predominant cell in chronic salpingitis. It is still not entirely clear why plasma cells that secrete immunoglobulin should be in the tissues in such large numbers in certain types of inflammation. *(Rubin and Farber, pp 59–62)*

513. **(C)** Primary biliary cirrhosis is a chronic liver disorder occurring in middle-aged women. Autoimmune destruction of intrahepatic bile ducts is the characteristic pathologic finding early in the disorder, with cirrhosis following later in those individuals with progressive disease. Anti-mitochondrial antibodies are found in about 90% of patients with primary biliary cirrhosis. Wilson's disease, also termed hepatolenticular degeneration, is a hereditary disorder of copper metabolism that adversely affects both the liver and the brain. *(Rubin and Farber, pp 760–764)*

514. **(D)** Five major classes of immunoglobulins are identified in humans on the basis of the characteristics of their heavy-chain constituents. Of the five, IgG is the major immunoglobulin in humans. It has the highest mean immunoglobulin serum concentration, 1200 mg/100 ml, and accounts for approximately 75 percent of the body's total γ-globulin pool. The remaining four major immunoglobulin classes have mean serum concentrations as follows: IgA, 250 mg/100 ml; IgM, 120 mg/100 ml; IgD, 3 mg/100 ml; and IgE, 0.03 mg/100 ml. *(Kissane, p 489)*

515. **(C)** Gout is a disease caused by elevated uric acid levels. It may be idiopathic or secondary to enzyme defects causing overproduction of uric acid. Patients with secondary gout may also have hyperuricemia due to increased production from cell breakdown or decreased excretion. The uric acid tends to build up in joint fluids and precipitate out. Initially, affected patients suffer transient attacks of acute arthritis because of an acute inflammatory reaction to the precipitated urate crystals. One or two joints are typically affected, most commonly the great toe and ankle joints. The precipitated urate crystals are taken up by macrophages and neutrophils in phagosomes. These crystals then damage the lysosomal membranes, causing release of the inflammatory mediators, enzymes, and cell debris, which stimulate the arthritis. The tophus is the characteristic lesion of gout and is caused by the inflammatory reaction. It is a urate deposit composed of chronic inflammatory cells, macrophages, and foreign body giant cells. These tophi are found in the external ear, around the knee joints, in connective tissue, and in the medullary pyramids of the kidney. Treatment is directed toward lowering the concentration of serum uric acid and inhibiting its synthesis. *(Cotran, pp 1355–1360)*

516. **(D)** A number of cell alterations can be produced or identified as a response to a variety of changes or stresses in the cell's environment. Hypertrophy refers to an increase in the size of cells—for example, myocardial fiber hypertrophy in response to increased demands in the setting of hypertension. Hyperplasia refers to an increase in the number of cells—for example, the increase in breast glandular epithelium in females at the time of puberty. Dysplasia refers to irregular, atypical proliferative changes of epithelial or mesenchymal cells in response to chronic inflammation or irritations—as is often seen, for example, in the uterine cervix. Atrophy is the loss of cell substance, producing a shrinkage in cell size—striated muscle response to disuse is an example. Metaplasia refers to the replacement of one type of adult cell, epithelial or mesenchymal, by another type of adult cell. The replacement of the normal type of adult ciliated columnar epithelium of the bronchial mucosa by the adult type of squamous epithelium in response to chronic irritation due to cigarette smoking is such an example. *(Cotran, pp 30–35)*

517. **(E)** A wide variety of afflictions may be caused by vitamin deficiencies. Niacin deficiency, also known as pellagra, is associated with dermatitis, diarrhea, and dementia. Night blindness (nyctalopia), with or without keratomalacia, and papular dermatitis suggest vitamin A deficiency. Vitamin K deficiency may manifest itself as a bleeding diathesis due to the role of vitamin K in the formation of prothrombin and clotting factors VII, IX, and X. Scurvy, or vitamin C deficiency, results in the altered formation of connective tissues, such as collagen, osteoid, dentin, and intercellular cement substance. Vitamin B deficiency, or beriberi, occurs in three ways that generally overlap to some extent in any given patient. Neuromuscular signs and symptoms alone are known as "dry beriberi" but in association with edema are known as "wet beriberi." Heart failure, generally high-output failure, accounts for so-called cardiac beriberi. *(Cotran, pp 438–459)*

518. **(B)** Adult polycystic disease of the kidneys is inherited by an autosomal dominant mechanism with almost complete penetrance. It is associated in a number of cases with polycystic change in the liver and to a lesser degree with polycystic change in the pancreas. Approximately 20 percent of patients with polycystic disease of the kidneys may have berry aneurysms in the circle of Willis, and sometimes it is rupture of these aneurysms that brings to attention the polycystic disease in general. There are some forms of childhood cystic disease of the kidneys that are autosomal recessive, but this is not true of adult polycystic disease. *(Rubin and Farber, pp 838–840)*

519. **(B)** Vitamin C, ascorbic acid, is a water-soluble vitamin widely distributed in nature. Citrus fruits and fresh vegetables are particularly rich sources of the vitamin. Vitamin C plays a pivotal role in collagen synthesis through hydroxylation of proline and lysine residues. Hypovitaminosis C leads not only to a bleeding diathesis but also to poor wound healing, loose teeth, and in children, abnormalities of bone development. Subperiosteal hemorrhage and joint hemorrhage are particularly characteristic in scorbutic infants. Although bleeding is a significant component of hypovitaminosis C, the clotting factors themselves usually are normal in structure, function, and quantity. *(Cotran, pp 456–459)*

520. **(C)** Hepatocytes synthesize a diverse population of proteins, including albumin, blood clotting factors, and enzymes (lactate dehydrogenase, aminotransferases, glutamate dehydrogenase, ornithine carbamyl transferase, and isocitrate dehydrogenase). In chronic liver disease, albumin production is reduced, leading to a drop in serum albumin levels. Elevated albumin levels in chronic liver disease would be truly exceptional. Increased serum levels of hepatic enzymes (alanine aminotransferase, aspartate aminotransferase, and lactate dehydrogenase) are seen with chronic liver disorders as damaged or dying hepatocytes release these enzymes into the serum. Gamma globulin levels are increased in all chronic disease states, particularly in chronic liver diseases. *(Rubin and Farber, pp 726–727)*

521. **(C)** In the photomicrograph, there is clearly a multinucleated giant cell surrounded by some monocytes and lymphocytes. This is the typical picture of a granulomatous form of inflammation without, in this illustration, any evidence of caseation. This is seen in such diseases as Crohn's disease, sarcoidosis, temporal arteritis, and some stages of tuberculosis. Ulcerative colitis is an inflammatory condition that may be acute or subacute and occurs predominantly in the colonic mucosa but does not extend into the submucosa and does not produce the granulomatous change seen in Crohn's disease or in the other granulomatous diseases mentioned. Tuberculosis is the only form of such granulomas that produces the breakdown characteristic of caseation, although this is not always seen, particularly in the early stages of the disease. *(Cotran, pp 65–68)*

522. **(C)** The constellation of dry eyes (keratoconjunctivitis sicca or xerophthalmia), dry mouth (xerostomia), and chronic arthritis constitutes the clinicopathologic entity known as Sjögren's syndrome. In the absence of arthritis, the symptoms are referred to as the sicca syndrome. Sjögren's syndrome primarily affects middle-aged women, either alone or in combination with other connective tissue disorders. About 50 percent of patients have rheumatoid arthritis. Large numbers of autoantibodies are seen in the serum of patients with Sjögren's syndrome. Symptoms are, in part, the result of the infiltration of salivary and lacrimal glands by lymphocytes, both B and T cell types. Over time, atrophy, fibrosis, hyalinization, and fatty change ensue. The lymphoid infiltrate may be heavy with the formation of lymphoid follicles with germinal centers and may mimic lymphoma. Of interest, however, is the finding that patients with Sjögren's syndrome show an increased tendency to develop lymphoma and so-called pseudolymphoma. Involvement of the respiratory tract, stomach, and kidneys (tubulointerstitial nephritis) also may occur. *(Kissane, pp 1128–1129)*

523. **(B)** The human embryo is most susceptible to malformations caused by environmental factors during days 15 to 60 of gestation. This time period is referred to as the "organogenetic period." Although environmental factors acting during the first 2 weeks (days 1 to 15) after fertilization may interfere with implantation or the development of the early embryo, rarely do they produce congenital malformations. Instead, these very early disturbances usually result in death or abortion of the blastocyst or early embryo. Exposure to teratogenic agents during the described critical period (days 15 to 60) may lead to death or abortion of the same embryo but usually produces major malformation. *(Cotran, pp 519–523)*

524. **(E)** Ninety percent of individuals with chronic myelogenous leukemia have an acquired Philadelphia chromosome abnormality. The Philadelphia chromosome usually consists of a translocation of a portion of the long arm of chromosome 22 to chromosome 9. The oncogene, c-abelson (c-abl), is present at the breakpoint of chromosome 9 and is usually reciprocally translocated to chromosome 22. *(Rubin and Farber, pp 1069–1071)*

525. **(A)** DiGeorge's syndrome is a deficiency of T lymphocytes due to thymic hypoplasia. Developmental failure of the third and fourth pharyngeal pouches is responsible for total or partial thymic, parathyroid, thyroid, and ultimobranchial pouch abnormalities. These structural anomalies lead to the absence of the cell-mediated T lymphocyte immune response, tetany, and congenital heart and great vessel abnormalities. B lymphocyte and plasma cell populations tend to be normal, as do serum immunoglobulin levels. The syndrome appears to be the result of an intrauterine insult to the fetus sometime before the eighth week of gestation. The syndrome is not genetically determined. As the affected children grow older, T cell function improves so that by age 5 yr, many affected children fail to demonstrate a T cell deficit. Some patients have been treated successfully by transplantation of fetal thymic tissue. *(Cotran, pp 222,1269)*

526. **(E)** Clinically detectable diverticulosis is seen in about 1 in 8 patients beyond 45 yr of age. In autopsy series, this incidence estimate appears to be higher. Diverticulosis occurs in the sigmoid colon in 99 percent of affected individuals. Other segments of the large bowel become involved by diverticulosis as follows: descending colon, 30 percent; transverse colon, 4 percent; entire colon, 16 percent. The sigmoid is the region of the colon exclusively involved in about 41 percent of cases. In underdeveloped and tropical countries and Japan, diverticulosis is rare, apparently partially because of the high-residue diets in these regions of the world. The most consistent abnormality seen in diverticulosis is an abnormality of the muscle wall, leading to herniation of the colonic mucosa and submucosa through the muscularis and eventually into the pericolic adipose tissue. Fecal material may become trapped in the diverticulum, leading to ulceration, inflammation, and rarely perforation. Cecal diverticula differ from those in the other segments of the colon in that they are generally solitary, are not necessarily associated with sigmoid involvement, and classically lack the muscle wall defect. Many reports, however, state that cecal diverticula also lack a muscle wall and thus resemble those seen elsewhere in the large bowel. *(Kissene, p 1155)*

527. **(B)** The nephrotic syndrome is defined as a syndrome in which there are proteinuria, edema, and to a variable degree, hypercholesterolemia. Whatever the cause, the common factor appears to be leakage of protein through the glomerular basement membranes, and the proteinuria is a characteristic finding. In interstitial nephritis, this is a chronic inflammatory change between the renal tubules, and only in a very late stage of disease does it alter glomerular function. There is no proteinuria. Unilateral hydronephrosis may cause complete disruption of the function of one kidney, but the other functions normally. In acute crescentic glomerulonephritis, which usually occurs after a streptococcal infection, there may be hematuria and a rise in blood pressure or even anuria, but proteinuria and edema, in the absence of these other findings so typical of the nephrotic syndrome, are not seen, particularly in the acute phase. Some forms of acute glomerulonephritis may progress to a chronic form that may have some elements of the nephrotic syndrome. Polycystic disease of the kidneys is associated with hypertension and some hematuria but not with the classic nephrotic syndrome. Membranous glomerulonephritis is the most typical form of glomerular disease associated with the nephrotic syndrome, particularly in adults, and can be recognized by both light microscopy and electron microscopy and immunofluorescence. *(Rubin and Farber, pp 841–850)*

528. **(B)** All of the choices, except celiac sprue, usually occur as mass lesions in the duodenum. A mass lesion of the duodenum is a fairly common clinical problem. Ulcers, usually peptic in nature, are the most common cause. Benign tumors, such as ectopic pancreas, Brunner gland adenomas, adenomatous polyps, and lipomas, all occur in the duodenum as tumorous lesions. Malignant tumors of the duodenum are rare and would include adenocarcinomas, carcinoid tumors, and lymphomas. Celiac sprue is an immunologic disease characterized by marked loss of the villi. Females are more often afflicted than males. People with the disease usually have HLA-B8 or D/DR 3 or D/DR 7. Placing the patient on a gluten-free diet will alleviate acute symptoms. Long-term follow-up reveals that celiac sprue patients have an increased risk of developing bowel lymphomas or carcinomas. *(Cotran, pp 860–882)*

529. **(C)** The pathognomonic lesion of gout is the tophus—a collection of crystalline or amorphous urates surrounded by an inflammatory response consisting of macrophages, lymphocytes, fibroblasts, and foreign body giant cells. In the photomicrograph that accompanies the question, the darker stellate deposits denote the center of the tophus. These urate deposits would appear golden brown, in contrast to the pink-staining tissue about them on the actual hematoxylin–eosin (H & E) glass slide. Gout is a systemic disorder of uric acid metabolism resulting in hyperuricemia. Urates precipitate out of the supersaturated blood and deposit in the joints and soft tissues. Rheumatoid arthritis, which includes ankylosing spondylitis, is characterized by a diffuse proliferative synovitis, suppurative arthritis by a prominent neutrophilic inflammation, and osteoarthritis by cartilaginous and subchondral bone changes. Additionally, the various types of arthritis are associated with different causes, symptoms, and extent and distribution of joint involvement. *(Cotran, pp 1355–1360)*

530. **(D)** The photomicrograph shows a typical, chronic peptic ulcer with the loss of epithelial continuity, the ulcer bed with necrotic tissue, and fibrosis between the ulcer bed and the main muscle. These peptic ulcers are associated with increased acid and pepsin secretion, may well be complicated by hemorrhage, since the ulcer erodes major blood vessels in the submucosa and muscularis mucosa, and if the ulcer continues unabated, will perforate through into the peritoneal cavity. Although malignant change may occur at the edge of certain types of gastric peptic ulcers, the illustration shows the ulcer itself, and this is not a neoplastic process at this stage of the disease. Long-standing peptic ulcers that do not heal often produce such malignant transformations, which can be determined by biopsy. *(Rubin and Farber, pp 648–655)*

531. **(E)** Myelofibrosis with myeloid metaplasia is a neoplastic disorder of middle-aged to elderly adults. In the early stages of the disease there is panhyperplasia of bone marrow leukocytes, megakaryocytes, and erythrocytes. Later, the bone marrow becomes fibrotic and extramedullary hematopoiesis occurs. The spleen is almost always enlarged. Teardrop-shaped erythrocytes are a characteristic finding in the peripheral blood. *(Rubin and Farber, pp 1071–1073)*

532. **(E)** The neuroblastoma, retinoblastoma, and medulloblastoma, as the suffix *blastoma* would imply, are primitive tumors ranging from and including the adrenal gland in origin, the retina, and the midline of the brain and characteristically are seen in early childhood. Astrocytomas may occur in all age groups, including childhood, whereas the meningioma is characteristically a neoplasm arising from the dura or its invaginations and is typically seen in a much older population. *(Kissane, pp 573–579)*

533. **(A)** Neuroblastoma is a common tumor of childhood, arising primarily in children younger than 5 yr of age and very rarely in adults. Tumors arising in patients younger than 1 yr old are often benign and regress spontaneously, whereas tumors discovered in older children may be highly malignant. These tumors are from neural crest derivatives and may arise in the adrenal medulla, near the retroperitoneum, in the posterior mediastinum, or along other derivatives of neural crest tissue, such as the sympathetic chains. Grossly, these tumors are large and bulky, and histologically, they are composed of small round cells, often in rosette patterns. Because of the neural crest origin of these tumors, they secrete catecholamines, principally norepinephrine. These secretory products cause the clinical symptoms of diarrhea and flushing. Neuroblastomas may grow rapidly and metastisize widely. *(Cotran, pp 539–540,1418)*

534. **(B)** Benign tumors are designated by adding the suffix *oma* to their primary cell type. However, some malignant neoplasms have retained the *oma* suffix that was used in previous nomenclature schemes. Examples include hepatoma and melanoma, which are accepted names for hepatocellular carcinoma and melanocarcinoma, respectively. An adenoma is a benign epithelial neoplasm composed of glandular tissue. Cystadenomas form benign cystic masses, whereas papillomas form benign fingerlike projections. Sarcomas are malignant tumors arising from mesenchymal tissue. Carcinomas are malignant neoplasms arising from epithelial cells—either endodermal, ectodermal, or mesodermal. A prefix such as *adeno* or *squamous* may further describe the microscopic growth patterns. Melanomas are malignant tumors derived from melanocytes. Leukemias are malignancies derived from hemapoietic cells, and lymphomas are malignant tumors with a lymphoid tissue origin. Teratomas are benign compound tumors derived from more than one germ layer, and teratocarcinoma is the malignant counterpart. *(Cotran, pp 240–243)*

535. **(B)** The genotype (genetic makeup of an organism) is determined by the molecular structure of the DNA contained in its chromosomes. Pinocytosis refers to invaginations of the cell membrane useful in fluid movement. The lysosomal content, number of microvilli, and rate of metabolism of a cell are in part determined by the cell's genotype but do not themselves direct or define the genotype. Rather, they are outward expressions (phenotype) of the DNA structure. *(Kissane, pp 44–45)*

536. **(B)** Leukocytes are important in the first line of defense in acute inflammatory reactions. These WBCs normally are in the blood stream, with a small proportion marginating along the vessel walls. In response to inflammatory stimuli, they line up or marginate along the vessel wall, falling out of the normal flow. RBCs can also stagnate and sludge. These leukocytes become sticky and adhere to the endothelial cells. Normally the WBCs and endothelial cells repel each other, but by intrinsic changes, the WBCs adhere to the endothelial cells in the inflammatory response. Mechanisms for this cell stickiness include changes in the negative charges of the WBC surface coat, pseudopod formation, and the development of divalent cation bridges. The WBCs then emigrate from the blood vessels into the surrounding tissues. They use their pseudopods to crawl into the junctions between the endothelial cells and cause widening of the interendothelial junctions. They cross the basement membranes and escape into the perivascular tissue. This process is one of active mobility and requires considerable flexibility in the leukocytes. Unlike the changes that occur in vascular permeability, there is no contraction of endothelial cells to widen the gap between cells. Also, the emigration of leukocytes is so tight that there is no accompanying vascular leakage. Chemotaxis is the undirectional movement of WBCs toward the inflammatory stimulus.

It is important in attracting leukocytes to the site of injury. The two main chemotactic factors for neutrophils are bacterial products (e.g., proteases) and complement factors. The complement compounds include C3, C5, and C$\overline{567}$, which can be generated both by immunologic reactions and by direct cleavages by bacterial and tissue enzymes. (*Cotran, pp 40–60*)

537. (C) Although most bacteria invoke a polymorphonuclear leukocyte response and produce a characteristic form of inflammation, the organism causing typhoid fever produces a negative chemotaxis toward polymorphs. The cells of first response and those seen most characteristically in either the primary lesions in the Peyer's patches of the intestine or the regional lymph nodes are sheets of monocytes. Eosinophils tend to be attracted toward protozoal and fungal proteins and are not seen particularly in this type of infection. Multinucleated giant cells are characteristically seen in granulomatous disease, and typhoid fever is more in keeping with an acute bacterial infection. Plasma cells have an intermediate function and may be seen in small numbers. (*Kissane, pp 314–317*)

538. (C) A fibrinous exudate is associated with many types of severe inflammation. The fluid that pours into the spaces has a large amount of plasma proteins, fibrinogen, and fibrin precipitates. The inflammatory responses are usually acute and severe, allowing these large protein molecules to escape. It accompanies rheumatic heart diseases, causing bread-and-butter pericarditis, and occurs in pneumococcal pneumonia. Histologically, fibrin strands and eosinophilic proteinaceous material are seen. These fibrinous exudates may stimulate fibroblastic and blood vessel proliferation, with organization of the proteinaceous precipitates and formation of fibrous connective tissue. The exudates also may resolve spontaneously. Serous exudates are fluids with a low protein concentration, arising from either the blood or the mesothelial cell secretions. They are seen early in acute inflammation or with mild injuries. Hemorrhagic exudates are a result of ruptured blood vessels. Suppurative exudates are seen in severe bacterial inflammation with massive neutrophil response and are characteristic of pus or abscess formation. (*Rubin and Farber, p 616*)

539. (B) Renal cell carcinoma is a characteristic tumor arising from renal parenchymal and probably renal tubular cells in adult life. In fact, the majority of cases occur after the age of 50, and it is seen more frequently in males. It invades the renal capsule and perinephric fat and has a marked propensity to invade the renal vein, with extension of the tumor into the vena cava. Although metastases may occur all over the body, bone and lung metastases are seen with a higher frequency. This tumor does not occur in infants or early childhood. The tumor that occurs in early infancy or childhood is the nephroblastoma, or Wilms' tumor, which is an embryonal malignant tumor of the kidney and distinctly different from renal cell carcinoma. (*Rubin and Farber, pp 888–889*)

540. (E) About 1 in 11 women in the United States will have breast cancer in her lifetime. Many western nations (USA, Canada, Australia, western Europe, and New Zealand) have similar, high rates of carcinoma of the breast. Most Asian nations, including Japan, have a much lower incidence of mammary cancer. In one or two generations, Japanese women who emigrate to the United States develop the high rate of breast cancer of native-born American women. Factors other than geography that are associated with an increased rate of breast cancer include menarche at an early age, late age of menopause, a diet high in fat and calories, a family history of breast cancer, and atypical hyperplastic lesions of the breast. (*Kissane, pp 1734–1735*)

541. (D) Hirschsprung's disease (idiopathic megacolon) usually appears soon after birth, with abdominal distention, failure to pass stool, and occasionally, acute intestinal obstruction. The pathogenesis involves abnormal functioning and coordination of the propulsive forces in the distal segment of the large bowel. This motility disorder occurs because of an absence of parasympathetic ganglion cells in the submucosal and myenteric plexus, the diagnostic histologic feature of Hirschsprung's disease. Hypertrophied, disorganized nonmyelinated nerve fibers are often identified in place of ganglion cells. The length of large bowel involved varies. Proximal to the involved segment, however, the colon may be dilated and hypertrophied. The mucosa often appears normal or inflamed. A full-thickness rectal biopsy is the standard procedure employed in diagnosis. Mucosal polyps are not associated with Hirschsprung's disease. (*Cotran, pp 883–884*)

542. (B) Neonatal cholestasis in most cases results from bile duct obstruction, the most common cause (more than 90 percent of cases) of which is EBA. Clinically, EBA may mimic neonatal hepatitis, which is an abnormality of unknown cause and requires a diagnosis by exclusion. α_1-Antitrypsin deficiency, metabolic disorders, and infectious processes must be ruled out before a diagnosis of neonatal hepatitis can be made. Histologically, neonatal hepatitis and EBA may appear similar—in particular, both generally contain giant cells. EBA, however, usually can be identified by evidence of large biliary duct obstruction when examined microscopically. The cause of EBA is still undetermined. Originally, it was thought to represent a congenital anomaly. Some investigators consider it to be an acquired disorder secondary to neonatal hepatitis with cholangitis and sclerosis of large bile ducts, either in utero or in early neonatal life. Overall, few cases can be corrected with standard therapy. The natural history is progression to secondary biliary cirrhosis and death in early childhood. Liver transplantation is a viable alternative therapeutic approach in these patients. Neonatal cholestasis may also, but rarely, be caused by intrahepatic biliary atresia, which is characterized by choledochal cysts and the absence of bile duct elements in the liver. Primary biliary cirrhosis is seen in middle-aged persons, typically females. The Budd-Chiari syndrome describes obstruction of the hepatic veins by a number of varied processes. *(Kissane, pp 1260–1273)*

543. **(B)** Adult respiratory distress syndrome, or shock lung, is a disease characterized by diffuse alveolar wall damage. There is loss of surfactant, with subsequent atelectasis. Both endothelial and epithelial cells are damaged. Type I pneumonocytes are extremely vulnerable to injury and are lost early. Grossly, the lungs are filled with fluid and blood and are heavy, red, and meaty. There is congestion, exudation of pink proteinaceous fluid, and hyaline membrane formation along the alveolar walls. Repair and organization result in proliferation and hyperplasia of type II pneumonocytes and fibroblast proliferation. The alveolar walls become thickened and fibrotic. This syndrome is described in multiple clinical settings, usually when hypotension, sepsis, and oxygen therapy are present. There is severe respiratory failure accompanied by hypoxia unresponsive to oxygen treatment. Physiologically, shock lung is thought to occur secondary to increased permeability of the alveolar capillary walls, with leakage of fluid and subsequent pulmonary edema and atelectasis. *(Rubin and Farber, pp 577–580)*

544. **(B)** Red hepatization is the second stage in the course of bacterial lobar pneumonia. It is histologically described as filling and dilatation of the alveolar spaces with neutrophils, WBCs, fibrin strands, RBCs, and bacteria. There is preservation of the pulmonary architecture, but it is obscured by the massive cellular exudate. This stage of bacterial pneumonia is accompanied by a fibrinous pleuritis. It characteristically develops in untreated, debilitated patients and is caused by a strain of pneumococcus in 90 percent of all cases. *(Cotran, pp 782–783)*

545. **(E)** Chronic granulomatous disease is most often X-linked and associated with a decreased ability

of neutrophils and other phagocytic cells to kill ingested bacteria. As a result, by 2 yr of age, signs of chronic low-grade infections appear, such as lymphadenitis, splenomegaly, pneumonia and sinusitis. The NBT test shows a markedly decreased, not increased, chemical reduction and helps confirm the diagnosis, since lack of NBT reductive capacity correlates with poor bactericidal activity. *(Rubin and Farber, pp 1049–1050)*

546. **(B)** The effect of syphilis on the heart and great vessels is characteristically the result of an endarteritis obliterans of the vasa vasorum of the aortic arch, which produces ischemic change in the media resulting in stellate fibrous replacement of the elastic tissue. Similar changes may occur in the opening of the coronary arteries, giving rise to narrowing of the coronary ostia and possibly producing angina pectoris. The result of the fibrous replacement of the media results in saccular dilatation or aneurysm but does not produce a dissection, since the fibrous tissue makes the media even less likely to split apart. The characteristic appearance of dissection occurs when there is a breakdown of ground substance in the media, which is not a characteristic of syphilis. *(Kissane, pp 766–768)*

547. **(B)** All connective tissue, valves, and muscle of the heart are affected to some degree in rheumatic carditis; hence the term "pancarditis." Certain areas are more selectively involved in a higher proportion of cases. In the early acute phase of rheumatic carditis, the pericardium shows fibrinous pericarditis, and the valve rings, particularly the mitral valve, show thickening and swelling of the free margins, with small fibrinous vegetations on the free margins. The characteristic Aschoff nodules and fibrosis may occur throughout the other mentioned aspects of the heart, but the characteristic vegetation seen in the early phase of the disease is usually confined to the free margins of the mitral valve. It has been thought that, in some instances, if there are no further occurrences of rheumatic fever, these may even resolve. Often, however, with or without recurrence, these fine verrucous vegetations are converted into more dense fibrous tissue, leading to narrowing of the mitral valve. *(Cotran, pp 629–633)*

548. **(D)** Edema is increased volume of extracellular extravascular fluid due to interference with the normal flow of fluids between blood, lymphatics, and tissue. The lymphatic circulation takes up a significant portion of fluid from the interstitial tissues, along with extravascular proteins, and returns it to the blood. If the lymphatic circulation is obstructed, the lymphatic drainage is interrupted. Affected areas have large accumulation of fluid and are edematous. The vascular system

also aids in maintaining fluid volume. The endothelium is the lining of the vessels and serves as a semipermeable membrane for fluids and components, primarily by keeping proteins intraluminally. If the endothelium is damaged, there is increased permeability to proteins, reducing the intraluminal colloidal pressure and causing fluid leakage and edema. Capillary blood pressure (BP), or hydrostatic pressure, is the force in capillaries that drives fluids from the capillaries into the tissues. By increasing the hydrostatic pressure, fluids tend to be forced out of the capillaries into tissues, causing edema. Sodium and water also aid in maintaining fluid balance. Sodium retention causes water retention, leading to an expansion of the extracellular fluid volume both intravascularly and in the tissues with edema. Increased tissue colloid osmotic pressure can be an important factor in causing edema. The protein concentration of plasma also functions in the maintenance of fluid balance. The major protein involved is albumin. By decreasing the plasma protein concentrations, there is a decreased colloid osmotic pressure in the blood, so there is a decreased counterforce to the hydrostatic BP. Thus, there is increased fluid escaping from the capillaries and decreased resorption of fluid from tissues. Fluid tends to accumulate extravascularly, with generalized edema. *(Cotran, pp 87–92)*

549. **(B)** Radiation energy is a well-documented carcinogen. The sources of the radiation include sunlight and occupational and therapeutic exposure. Therapeutic radiation was previously used to treat many benign conditions as well as thyroid disease, and a 10- to 20-yr follow-up of patients who received this therapy shows an increased incidence of several types of cancer. People exposed to occupational irradiation also have a marked increase in carcinoma. Classic among these are employees who painted the faces of watches with radioactive paints and miners of radioactive ores. Survivors of atomic bombs show a markedly increased rate in the development of cancers and leukemias. The major biochemical theory of radiation-induced carcinogenesis is linked to damage of the cell's DNA. Radiation injures the DNA, inducing a mutation. The amount of cell damage is related to the dose, rate, quality, and length of total exposure to the radiation energy. Cells also have reparative capabilities for radiation damage, and they may repair or ignore the injured DNA. The exact mechanism of radiation-induced carcinogenesis is still unclear, but the existence of this phenomenon is well documented. *(Cotran, pp 258–264)*

550. **(E)** High doses of radiation delivered in utero to the embryo during its susceptible period may be a potent teratogen. Recognized abnormalities associated with high-dose radiation include microcephaly, mental retardation, and skeletal malformation. It is also believed to cause genetic mutations in fetal germ cells. Diagnostic doses of radiation, although not conclusively responsible for malformations, must be cautioned against, since the developing CNS is particularly sensitive to radiation injury. Masculinization of the female fetus is generally associated with maternal use of androgenic agents (e.g., progestogens) during pregnancy, not with radiation. *(Kissane, pp 268–269)*

551. **(D)** For any given area of skin, there is no significant difference in the number of melanocytes in blacks as compared with whites. Blacks do, however, have larger melanocytes that are reactive (as determined by dopa reactivity) and have more dendritic processes. In whites who are not exposed to UV light, melanocytic dopa activity is quite variable. After a single exposure to UV light, the melanocytes present demonstrate an increase in size and dopa activity. With repeated exposure to UV light, there is also an increase in the concentration of melanocytes. Studies of mice have shown sufficient mitotic activity in skin melanocytes repeatedly exposed to UV light to account for the increase in concentration. *(Rubin and Farber, pp 1196–1203)*

552. **(A)** Duchenne muscular dystrophy, also known as X-linked muscular dystrophy, is the most common of the muscular dystrophies. It usually occurs in early life, with symmetrical weakness and involvement of the pelvic girdle musculature. Later, the shoulder girdle muscles may be affected. As the disease progresses, pseudohypertrophy of the calves occurs and may be attributed to replacement of muscle by adipose tissue. This disease progresses rapidly and usually results in death by the age of 20 to 30 yr. A more benign form of the disease, known as Becker's muscular dystrophy, is considered a separate entity. It has its onset in the second decade of life and progresses slowly. Although many clinical features are shared by Duchenne and Becker's muscular dystrophy, the separation of the X-linked muscular dystrophies into these two subtypes is supported by certain factors: A given family demonstrates only one form of the disease, and linkage studies demonstrate differences. Serum CPK is elevated in the X-linked muscular dystrophies and may be used to help identify the carrier state. However, it is elevated in only 70 percent of carrier mothers. The latter have been defined as mothers with one son and one brother or two sons with the disease. *(Rubin and Farber, pp 1401–1403)*

553. **(C)** DES is a synthetic nonsteroidal estrogen that was administered in the 1940s to 1960s to pregnant women who were at high risk for miscarriage. Since 1970, there has been increasing

awareness of neoplastic and nonneoplastic changes in the daughters and sons of these women. The most significant pathologic change noted is the development of clear cell carcinoma of the vagina in women between the ages of 17 and 30 yr. The tumors invade the vagina and cervix, are small and polypoid, and are often asymptomatic. They are adenocarcinomas composed of large cells with clear cytoplasm or hobnail configuration. Other changes associated with DES include vaginal adenosis with glandular epithelium lining the upper third of the vagina, squamous metaplasia of the vagina or cervix, cervical ectropion, structural abnormalities of the uterus or fallopian tubes, or microglandular hyperplasia. The other pathologic changes listed in the question have no known association with DES exposure. *(Kissane, pp 1639–1640)*

554. (D) Gaucher's disease is an autosomal recessive disease caused by a deficiency of glucocerebrosidase, which is the enzyme that breaks down glucocerebroside in reticuloendothelial cells and neurons. A shortage of this enzyme interferes with the breakdown of glycolipids from dead WBCs and RBCs, so these metabolic products build up in phagocytic cells in the body. The reticuloendothelial cells of the spleen, liver, bone marrow, and lymph nodes are primarily affected. They fill up with glucocerebroside, obscuring the normal cell architecture. These distended cells are called Gaucher's cells, and they characteristically are large, with one or more small, dark eccentric nuclei in cytoplasm filled with eosinophilic fibrillar material resembling wrinkled tissue paper. Gaucher's cells grossly cause bone erosions, as well as enlargement of the spleen, liver, and lymph nodes. Gaucher's disease predominantly affects adult Jews of European descent, but juvenile and infantile forms also are described. Affected individuals show signs of splenomegaly and hepatomegaly, with bone pain and pancytopenia. *(Rubin and Farber, pp 1348–1350)*

555. (A) The disease designated as AIDS, associated with human immunodeficiency virus HIV type I, has now been well established as a serious disease entity, particularly in homosexual males in the USA and intravenous drug users in the USA and other western countries. The disease has been seen with an increased frequency recently in heterosexual males and in females and relatively infrequently in patients receiving blood transfusions with infected blood. AIDS also is prevalent in various parts of the world, including Central Africa, with the difference that it occurs in nonhomosexual males and females. The association with intravenous drug usage in Africa does not appear to be as strong as it is in the western world. Although there have been isolated cases of AIDS and positive serology in prostitutes in various parts of the world, this is still a relatively small proportion. *(Kissane, pp 1471–1474)*

556. (D) Carcinoma of the cervix has a diminishing frequency in the USA and other developed countries. If diagnosed in the early stages, either in the recognizable preinvasive stage or in stage I, it has a more than 90 percent cure rate. However, if it is left untreated to the advanced stage IV, with invasion of the pelvic organs and other sites, the prognosis is much worse. The disease is very common in developing countries of the world, particularly in black Africa, where it probably represents the major malignancy among females. *(Rubin and Farber, pp 957–959)*

557. (E) All of the statements are true of schistosomiasis in general, but *S. mansoni* primarily affects the gastrointestinal tract and liver, not the bladder. It is *Schistosoma haematobium* that affects the bladder and causes hematuria. *(Cotran, pp 424–427)*

558. (C) The anaphylactic reaction, or type I immunologic response, is a rapidly evolving immunologic reaction that occurs within minutes after reexposure to an antigen to which an individual has already been sensitized. The response is mediated by IgE antibody (not IgA), which interacts with or is bound to basophils and mast cells. The release of vasoactive amines (such as histamine, eosinophilic chemotactic factor, slow-reacting substance of anaphylaxis, and platelet-activating factor) from these cells occurs in reaction to cross-linking of the antibody and intracellular changes in cAMP. Tuberculin-type giant cells are a feature of type IV immunologic responses (delayed hypersensitivity) and play no active part in type I responses. *(Rubin and Farber, pp 105–116)*

559. (B) Neoplasms are tumors that may be either benign or malignant. They are composed of proliferating parenchymal cells (tumor cells) and stromal cells. Malignant tumors have the cell characteristics of anaplasia, with increased nucleus/cytoplasm ratios, hyperchromatic nuclei, and pleomorphic cells. There may also be multiple mitoses. High degrees of anaplasia are diagnostic of malignancy, but malignant tumors may mimic so closely the normal structures and be so well differentiated that they even elaborate the normal products of the cells and can be very difficult to diagnose on the basis of cytologic aspects alone. However, most tumors show some degree of anaplasia, and the architecture of the normal tissue is disorganized and destroyed. Malignant tumors have a rapid, erratic growth pattern, with abnormal mitoses. They tend to grow in an infiltrative pattern, invading local structures directly.

They never have structurally well-formed capsules. The most definitive criterion of malignancy is tumor invasion of blood and lymphatic vessels. Benign tumors do not metastasize, they are composed of cells resembling the tissue of origin, and they form structures typical of that organ. They grow slowly and expand, with few mitoses, and they have a well-formed capsule that completely surrounds the tumor. Cytologically benign tumors show no anaplastic changes, and the cells are innocuous and uniform, without malignant criteria. In rare cases, it is impossible to determine if the tumor is benign or malignant, since some tumors show histologic features of both malignant and benign neoplasms. These are borderline tumors, and their clinical course and treatment are usually intermediate between those of benign and malignant neoplasms. (Cotran, pp 243–249)

560. **(D)** Ectopic hormone production is sometimes seen in association with pulmonary neoplasms. Some tumor types may produce two or more different hormones. This is true, in particular, for oat cell carcinoma. Oat cell carcinoma may produce hyponatremia because of the ectopic production and inappropriate secretion of ADH. It, along with bronchial carcinoid tumors, also has been associated with Cushing's syndrome and the carcinoid syndrome. Squamous cell carcinoma is associated with hyperparathyroidism, and all types of lung tumors, including adenocarcinoma and large cell carcinoma, have been linked to gynecomastia secondary to the secretion of ectopic gonadotropin. In addition to endocrine abnormalities, oat cell carcinoma may also produce a confusional psychosis, encephalomyelitis, a sensory neuropathy, and muscular dysfunction. Clubbing of the fingers and hypertrophic pulmonary osteoarthropathy are manifestations of the proximity of the tumor to the pleural surface rather than to the specific type of tumor present and may, therefore, be seen in association with any of the various types of lung tumors. (Rubin and Farber, pp 559–560)

561. **(E)** Macrophages are derived from monocytes and are the major scavenger cells in the inflammatory process, especially in late stages of inflammation. They gather up and digest debris, dead cells, proteins, and foreign material, as well as release enzymes for degradation. They also release chemotactic and permeability factors, induce leukocytosis and fever, and secrete proteins important in defense, release factors to aid healing, and have a function in the immune-mediated response. Macrophages are large, long-lived cells with an eccentric nucleus and abundant cytoplasm, granules, and debris. They belong to the reticuloendothelial system (mononuclear phagocyte system) of cells, which are specialized for pinocytosis and phagocytosis. Neutrophils are the most important cells in the acute inflammatory response and are important in the initial engulfment and destruction of microorganisms and foreign material. Lymphocytes are inflammatory cells involved in chronic inflammation in immune reactions and delayed hypersensitivity responses. Plasma cells are modified lymphocytes involved in antibody production and secretion in immune-mediated inflammatory responses. Eosinophils are inflammatory cells whose true function is unknown. They are involved in hypersensitivity and allergic reactions as well as parasitic infections. (Cotran, pp 61–63)

562. **(A)** Liquefaction necrosis occurs characteristically in the brain from the action of powerful hydrolytic enzymes that favor autolysis and heterolysis of tissue rather than protein denaturation (coagulation necrosis). The heart, kidney, spleen, and small intestine are organs in which infarcts typically produce coagulation necrosis. (Cotran, p 18)

563. **(C)** Thrombogenesis, the formation of thrombi, is caused by injury to endothelial surfaces, alterations in normal blood flow, and hypercoagulable states. Injury to endothelium may expose vascular wall collagen and initiate clotting via the intrinsic pathway. Alterations in the normal laminar flow of blood in vessels leads to stasis and turbulence, with a concomitant increased risk of thrombosis. Hyperviscosity syndromes (such as polycythemia, cryoglobulinemia, or macroglobulinemia) increase resistance to flow, with resultant stasis. Hypercoagulable states include disseminated intravascular coagulation (DIC) and carcinomatosis. Treatment with warfarin, an anticoagulant, would inhibit clotting, making intravascular thrombogenesis unlikely. (Cotran, pp 99–105)

564. **(D)** The Tzanck test is a cytologic smear obtained by scraping the base of an early, freshly opened skin vesicle. The scrapings are smeared onto a glass slide and stained by either the Wright or Giemsa method. This technique allows a rapid, although preliminary, diagnosis of a vesicular skin rash that appears to be of the herpesvirus group. Definitive diagnosis should still rely on culture or direct immunofluorescence (IF) of a lesion and skin biopsy. The Tzanck test is nonspecific within the group of skin lesions that are caused by herpesviruses. Varicella (chickenpox), herpes zoster, and herpes simplex skin lesions all demonstrate the same cytologic changes in the Tzanck smear. The smear is examined for the presence of multinucleated acantholytic balloon cells from the floor of the vesicle. It should be noted that the biopsy specimens of all skin lesions of the herpesviruses show the same histology and cannot be differentiated from one another by biopsy alone. The history, physical examination, and culture would all aid in subtyping a particular herpesvirus skin lesion. The Tzanck test is of no value in the diagnosis of the skin lesions listed as alternative choices in the question. *(Rubin and Farber, pp 333–341)*

565–566. (565-B, 566-C) Light and electron microscopy (EM) and IF are complementary studies in the evaluation of renal biopsy specimens. The EM that accompanies the question demonstrates MGN. The changes to be noted include a thickened basement membrane (BM), subepithelial dense deposits (DD), and spike (SP) formation. The spike formation results from the remodeling of the basement membrane in response to the presence of the dense deposits. This remodeling may result in the eventual incorporation of the deposits into the substance of the basement membrane. The resultant projections of the basement membrane around the deposits give rise to the spiked appearance. Fusion of the epithelial foot processes is also noted. In general, all forms of glomerular disease listed in question 565, except AGN, may show fusion of the epithelial foot processes on EM. It is then necessary to evaluate the presence and distribution of electron-dense deposits to further classify the disease process. Of the entities listed in the question, MGN, MPGN, and AGN demonstrate dense deposits on EM. In MPGN, the deposits tend to be subendothelial in location. AGN renal biopsy specimens show subepithelial deposits described as "humps" but lack the fusion of the epithelial foot processes. It should be noted that MGN is subclassified into six stages depending on the extent of glomerular basement membrane reaction. In early (I) and late (VI) stages, the diagnosis may be difficult. MGN shows a male predominance of 2 : 1 or 3 : 1 and is most common between the ages of 50 and 70 years. At the time of diagnosis, 70 to 80 percent of patients have nephrotic syndrome. MGN accounts for 20 to 30 percent of cases of nephrotic syndrome in the adult population and is usually idiopathic.

IF is evaluated on the basis of the pattern (diffuse, granular, or linear) and type (IgG, IgA, IgM, complement, and antiglomerular basement membrane) of staining, if any. Idiopathic MGN is the most common cause of MGN and is the most appropriate diagnosis for an MGN that demonstrates IgG and complement IF staining. MGN characteristically shows diffuse and granular IF for IgG along the capillary walls corresponding to the subepithelial deposits. Diabetic nephropathy may also demonstrate IgG on IF but usually in a diffuse, linear pattern without the accompanying dense deposits on EM. Goodpasture's syndrome typically shows linear IF staining but with antiglomerular basement membrane antibody, a specific IgG. IgA nephropathy is a focal glomeru-

lonephritis with positive IF for IgA. AGN, despite its positive IF for IgG and complement, usually can be distinguished from MGN when the EM and clinical history are incorporated into the evaluation process. *(Kissane, pp 515–517)*

567. (E) The most common pituitary neoplasm is the pituitary adenoma, which arises from the endocrine-producing cells of the anterior pituitary. These tumors occur in the area of the sella turcica. They are solid or cystic and characteristically are composed of sheets or papillary clusters of uniform, round, benign-appearing cells. Based on H & E staining, the tumors have been classified as chromophobes (no staining), acidophils, or basophils. By immunohistochemical staining, electron microscopy (EM), and biochemical studies, they can be classified according to the types of hormones they secrete. Each tumor usually is composed of one type of hormone-secreting cell. Seven percent of pituitary adenomas secrete ACTH and cause Cushing's syndrome. These tumors arise in the anterior lobe and are usually chromophobes. By immunohistochemical staining, these tumors have ACTH granules, as demonstrated in the photomicrograph that accompanies the question. EM shows large, dense, secretory granules and microfilaments in the cells. Other pituitary adenomas may secrete thyroid-stimulating hormone (TSH), prolactin, or growth hormone. Pituitary granulomas are rare diseases usually secondary to tuberculosis, sarcoidosis, or histiocytosis X. Parapituitary gliomas are parapituitary astrocytomas with no endocrine activity. Craniopharyngiomas are pediatric tumors of the suprasellar region, are derived from Rathke's pouch remnants, and have no endocrine activity. Adrenocortical carcinomas are primary tumors of the adrenal gland that may be functioning, secreting cortisol, and causing Cushing's syndrome. These tumors are very rare, and it is extremely unusual for them to metastasize to the pituitary. *(Kissane, pp 1530–1535)*

568. (D) Auer rods are round, rod-shaped, or elongate cytoplasmic inclusions in the cytoplasm of immature, abnormal granulocytes or myeloblasts. They represent aberrant forms of the cytoplasmic azurophilic granules produced by abnormal cytoplasmic maturation in the leukemic blast cells. Although they may be seen in occasionally CML in blast crisis, they are most characteristic of AML. Erythroleukemia (DiGuglielmo's syndrome) is also considered one of the acute myeloid leukemias in the French-American-British classification (M-6) but is predominantly a disorder of erythroid precursors. At some stage of the disease, myeloid precursors may also be abnormal. In these instances, Auer rods may be seen when myeloblasts are present. ALL and CLL are leukemias of the lymphocyte cells and do not demonstrate Auer rod formation. *(Rubin and Farber, p 1075)*

569. **(E)** T cell lymphocytes can be enumerated by their ability to form rosettes with sheep erythrocytes. They are the crucial element of cellular immunity. Mycosis fungoides is a T cell lymphoproliferative disorder with prominent skin lesions include Pautrier's microabscesses and hyperchromic, atypical lymphocytes with marked convolutions called mycosis cells. Multiple myeloma and macroglobulinemia are lymphoproliferative disorders of B cells. AML and CML are neoplasms of nonlymphoid myeloid cells. *(Cotran, pp 716–717, 1293–1294)*

570. **(D)** CLL is common in the elderly population and uncommon in younger individuals. Affected patients may initially experience hepatosplenomegaly, lymphadenopathy, pancytopenia, malaise, and weight loss. Fever does not occur and is uncharacteristic of CLL unless there is a superimposed infectious process. About one fourth of patients are asymptomatic at the time of diagnosis, with the diagnosis having been made on the basis of an abnormal peripheral CBC. The diagnosis often can be made from the peripheral blood smear alone without the need for a bone marrow biopsy or aspirate. This tends to be true particularly when >15,000 mature lymphocytes are seen in the peripheral blood smear. The malignant lymphocytes are usually B cells that demonstrate small amounts of monoclonal surface immunoglobulin, usually IgM. Hypogammaglobulinemia affects at least 50 percent of patients and, in combination with neutropenia, may eventually render these patients susceptible to infection. Survival in CLL is long, with a median range of between 6 and 9 yr. Treatment is noncurative and is reserved for those patients who are symptomatic. Death is usually the result of infection, hemorrhage, or inanition. *(Kissane, pp 1396–1397)*

571. **(C)** The anemias are classified morphologically on the basis of RBC appearance, mean corpuscular volume (MCV), and mean corpuscular hemoglobin concentration (MCHC). Classically, iron deficiency anemia is characterized by a hypochromic microcytic anemia with MCV <80 g/100 ml and MCHC <31 g/100 ml. Vitamin B_{12} and folic acid deficiencies both produce macrocytic (MCV >94 g/100 ml and MCH >31 g/100 ml) megaloblastic anemia. Accelerated erythropoiesis also produces a macrocytic anemia, but of the nonmegaloblastic type. Megaloblastic changes refer to abnormalities in the maturation of the cell, usually nuclear. Recent blood loss, when sufficient to produce anemia, is generally of the normochromic-normocytic (MCV 82 to 92 mg/100 ml and MCHC >30 mg/100 ml) type. *(Cotran, pp 660–691)*

572. **(D)** LDH is the enzyme that catalyzes the conversion of pyruvate to lactate using nicotinamide adenine dinucleotide (NAD) as the cofactor. This enzyme is found in all tissues of the body and is a tetramer composed of two different peptic chains, identified as M and H. There are five different isoenzyme combinations of the M and H subunits. Various body tissues contain characteristic amounts of these isoenzymes, which can be separated and identified on the basis of different physical and chemical properties. Tissue damage and necrosis cause release of this intracellular enzyme into the circulating plasma. The amount and type of isoenzyme released reflect the organ or tissue injured. Normal circulating plasma contains primarily LDH_2, with small amounts of LDH_3, LDH_4, and LDH_5. The heart is primarily composed of LDH_1, the HHHH tetramer. With a myocardial infarct, there is a massive release of LDH_1, elevating its quantity in relation to LDH_2. An increase in total LDH with a relative increase in LDH_1 in relation to LDH_2 is consistent with a myocardial infarct—myocardial tissue injury. This pattern of elevated LDH_1 over LDH_2 is illustrated in the graph that accompanies the question. Liver and skeletal muscle are composed primarily of LDH_5, the MMMM tetramer, so their injury produces elevated serum LDH_5 levels. Pulmonary embolism is reflected in an increase in serum LDH_3 levels. Brain and cerebrospinal fluid contain relatively small amounts of LDH isoenzymes, so infection here is not correlated with increases in serum LDH levels. *(Cotran, p 613)*

573–575. **(573-B, 574-A, 575-E)** There are many compounds important chemically in mediating the acute inflammatory response. Histamine is an example of the vasoactive amines, which are principally important in the acute phase of increased vascular permeability. It causes vasodilatation and increased venular permeability. It is released from mast cells and platelets. The kinin system produces vasoactive peptides, of which bradykinin is the most potent. It causes vasodilatation, increased vascular permeability, smooth muscle contraction, and pain, but it is not chemotactic. It is derived from the clotting cascade from factor XII, the Hageman factor, through a kallikrein intermediate step. The complement system produces many compounds that help mediate the inflammatory response. These include C3 and C5a, which cause increased vascular permeability, and C5a and C567, which are chemotactic factors. Prostaglandins are arachidonic acid derivatives that are important in the inflammatory response. Prostaglandin E potentiates the permeability effect of the other chemical mediators and is also important in the production of pain, fever, and vasodilatation. The neutrophils themselves also release into the media lysosomal enzymes that are important chemical mediators. These compounds are released during phagocytosis, reverse endocytosis, or with neutrophil death. They consist of neutral proteases, which degrade such extracellular material as collagen, fibrin, and cartilage, acid proteases, which digest proteins, and cationic proteins. *(Cotran, pp 59–60)*

576–578. (576-C, 577-D, 578-E) Intermediate filaments can be used as immunomarkers to identify cell type. In tissue specimens, monoclonal antibodies—coupled with known visual tags (fluorescent or enzymatic)—are reacted with tumors to demonstrate the presence of certain intermediate filaments. The retained intermediate filaments can confirm the lineage of tumors. Epithelial cells, mesenchymal cells, smooth muscle cells, glial cells, and neurons possess the intermediate filaments of cytokeratin, vimentin, desmin, glial fibrillary acidic protein, and neurofilament, respectively. *(Rubin and Farber, pp 149–151)*

579–581. (579-E, 580-B, 581-D) Tularemia, pertussis, and plague are examples of bacterial diseases. Tularemia is caused by *Francisella tularensis,* a small gram-negative pleomorphic coccobacillus. Affected animals and arthropods serve as the vectors, of which wild rabbits and squirrels are the most common in the USA. Pertussis is caused by *Bordetella pertussis,* a gram-negative coccobacillus, and is transmitted via airborne droplets to the respiratory tract. Plague is transmitted through a number of animal vectors, the major reservoir being squirrels. The causative agent is *Y. pestis,* an encapsulated, gram-negative, pleomorphic bacillus. Rocky Mountain spotted fever is among the rickettsial diseases, caused by obligate intracellular microorganisms smaller than bacteria and larger than viruses. The vector is an infected tick. Lymphogranuloma venereum is a disease attributed to *Chlamydia* microorganisms, specifically *C. trachomatis.* Chlamydiae are also obligate intracellular microorganisms intermediate between bacteria and viruses but are transmitted through sexual contact (a venereal disease). *(Cotran, pp 326–328,350–351,362–363)*

582–584. (582-E, 583-D, 584-A) *Salmonella* species, *Shigella* species, and *V. cholerae* are all gram-negative rods that produce gastrointestinal disease. These organisms, however, may affect different sites and have various histologic manifestations. *Salmonella* species may produce typhoid fever, gastroenteritis, and septicemia. Typically, *Salmonella* species produce a marked reticuloendothelial hyperplasia in local, intestinal, and distant lymph nodes and in the spleen and liver. Erythrophagocytosis is highly suggestive of *Salmonella* infection, particularly of typhoid fever. *Salmonella* species may produce intestinal ulceration, generally in the small intestine. In contrast, *Shigella* species rarely produce bacteremia and elicit little, if any, reaction outside the intestinal tract. All *Shigella* species produce an endotoxin. Additionally, *Shigella dysenteriae* produces a potent exotoxin. The *Shigella* microorganisms tend to damage the colonic mucosa, producing mucosal ulcerations. Rarely, similar ulcerations may be seen in the ileum. *V. cholerae* produces both an endotoxin and an exotoxin. Voluminous amounts of watery diarrhea containing bits of mucus, and rice-water stool, are the result of the effects of the exotoxin. The organism is essentially noninvasive, does not produce bacteremia, and therefore elicits few anatomic changes and no mucosal ulceration in the bowel mucosa. The intestinal biopsy specimen in such a case would reveal an intact mucosa and only mild, nonspecific submucosal inflammatory changes. *(Cotran, pp 353–357)*

585–587. (585-B, 586-A, 587-E) Hashimoto's thyroiditis is an autoimmune disorder characterized by autoantibodies against thyroid stimulating hormone, thyroid microsomal fractions, and thyroglobulin. Chronic adrenocortical insufficiency, usually due to autoimmune destruction, is also termed Addison's disease. Cori's disease is a hereditary disorder of glycogen catabolism in which the debrancher enzyme activity is absent. Excess glucocorticoid production is termed Cushing's syndrome. De Quervain's thyroiditis is a subacute thyroid inflammation that may have a viral etiology. *(Rubin and Farber, pp 226–227,1138–1139, 1150)*

588–590. (588-E, 589-A, 590-B) In utero exposure to diethylstilbestrol is associated with an increased incidence of both vaginal adenosis and clear cell carcinoma of the vagina. The risk factors for developing cervical squamous cell carcinoma include multiple sexual partners, herpes simplex virus type 2 and human papilloma virus infections, cigarette smoking, and pre-existing dysplasia. The incidence of endometrial adenocarcinoma is increased in individuals with diabetes, obesity, nulliparity, preceding hyperplasia, breast cancer, hypertension, and late menopause. *(Rubin and Farber, pp 953–954,957–959,963–967)*

591–593. (591-D, 592-A, 593-E) The ductus arteriosus is a normal intrauterine vascular channel connecting the pulmonary artery to the aorta. It usually closes shortly after birth. Prolonged patency requires surgical correction or pharmacologic closure. The most common congenital heart anomaly is a ventricular septal defect. It accounts for about 30 percent of all congenital cardiac malformations. Truncus arteriosus arises from an incomplete separation of the aorta from the pulmonary artery. This anomaly is usually accompanied by other malformations including valvular defects, right aortic arch, and absence of the ductus arteriosus. *(Cotran, pp 620–624)*

594–596. **(594-C, 595-E, 596-B)** A large number of inhaled dust-like substances are able to produce pathologic changes in the respiratory system, which are generally referred to as pneumoconioses. Inhaled cotton fibers may produce an asthma-like disorder termed byssinosis. Inhalation of asbestos fibers is associated with an increased risk of developing malignant mesothelioma. Tin oxide miners may acquire a chronic fibrosing pulmonary disorder called stannosis. Silicosis is a pneumoconiosis caused by inhaled silica particles. Beryllium granulomatosis is seen with chronic beryllium inhalation. *(Cotran, pp 472–484)*

597–599. **(597-B, 598-C, 599-A)** Chagas's disease is caused by *Trypanosoma cruzi*, a protozoan organism. One of the hallmarks of the disease is destructive myocarditis. Dubin-Johnson syndrome is a familial disease characterized by intermittent jaundice and black pigment deposition in the liver. Goodpasture's syndrome is rapidly progressive glomerulonephritis and diffuse pulmonary hemorrhages, usually with autoantibodies to basement membrane material. Peutz-Jeghers syndrome is an autosomal dominant hereditary disorder consisting of intestinal polyps and mucocutaneous melanin pigmentation. Kawaski's disease (mucocutaneous lymph node syndrome) is an acute vasculitis of infancy and early childhood. *(Rubin and Farber, pp 402–405,484,582,681,402–405)*

600–602. **(600-C, 601-A, 602-B)** Hemophila A is an X-linked recessive hereditary disorder due to a deficiency of blood clotting factor VIII. Dwarfism (achondroplasia) is an autosomal dominant disease characterized by early ossification of the epiphyseal plate in the long bones. Normal head and truncal size, with significantly shortened extremities, are hallmarks of the disease. Ochronosis (alkaptonuria) is an autosomal recessive disorder due to a lack of the enzyme homogentisic oxidase. Homogentisic acid accumulates within collagen in connective tissue, tendons, and cartilage, imparting a blue-black discoloration. The articular cartilage is particularly damaged, with resultant severe arthritis. *(Cotran, pp 143–144,698,1319)*

603–605. **(603-E, 604-A, 606-E)** The lesion pictured is chronic infective endocarditis of the aortic valve. The presence of coronary ostia in a semilunar

valve allows the certain identification that the affected valve is aortic. Chronic infective endocarditis most commonly involves the aortic valve. The tricuspid valve is the least likely to be affected. Previously damaged valves, particularly post rheumatic valves, are likely candidates for chronic infective endocarditis. The most common organism cultured is *S. viridans*. The aortic valve is the usual site of origin of embolic endocarditic infarcts of the kidney. *(Cotran, pp 633–637)*

606–608. **(606-D, 607-B, 608-B)** The classic triad of ectopic gastrin production, excess gastric acid secretion, and persistent peptic ulcer disease comprise the Zollinger-Ellison syndrome. The majority of gastrinomas arise from either the pancreas or the duodenum. MEN IIa, also termed Sipple syndrome, is characterized by medullary carcinomas of the thyroid, parathyroid neoplasia, adrenocortical neoplasia or hyperplasia, and pheochromocytomas. The disorder is usually inherited in an autosomal dominant mode with incomplete penetrance. Stein-Leventhal syndrome includes polycystic ovaries, oligomenorrhea, hirsutism, and obesity. The major biochemical abnormality is low levels of follicle-stimulating hormone and androgens. Wedge resection of ovarian tissue is often curative. *(Cotran, pp 1007–1008,1157–1158)*

609–611. **(609-B, 610-A, 611-D)** Mycosis fungoides is a cutaneous T-helper cell lymphoma with epidermal infiltrates of atypical lymphocytes. Late in disease these cells may spill out into the peripheral blood (Sezary syndrome). Pemphigus is characterized by skin blister formation due to diminished cohesiveness of the keratinocytes. Autoantibodies to surface epidermal antigens is the primary etiology of pemphigus. Ichthyoses are hereditary disorders that show marked hypertrophy of the strateum corneum. Both autosomal dominant and X-linked recessive forms exist. *(Rubin and Farber, pp 1206–1207,1211–1214,1257–1258)*

612–614. **(612-E, 613-B, 614-A)** Pernicious anemia is due to a deficiency of vitamin B_{12} (cobalamin). Most instances of pernicious anemia are characterized by autoimmune destruction of gastric parietal cells leading to inadequate production of vitamin B_{12} absorption factor (intrinsic factor). Myelophthisic anemia is seen with bone marrow infiltrative disorders. The peripheral blood demonstrates a leukoerythroblastic pattern. Carcinoma with boney metastases is the most common cause of myelophthisic anemia. Thalassemia is a genetic disorder typified by defects in globin chain synthesis. The anemia is usually microcytic and hypochromic. *(Rubin and Farber, pp 1030–1042)*

615–617. (615-A, 616-C, 617-B) Acetaminophen is present in many over-the-counter analgesic preparations. Overdose causes massive hepatic necrosis via a toxic metabolite. Carbon monoxide poisons as a systemic asphyxiant by binding irreversibly to hemoglobin. Methyl alcohol exerts its prime poisoning effect on the retina and brain through its toxic metabolites, formaldehyde and formic acid. *(Cotran, pp 487–495)*

618–620. (618-D, 619-C, 620-E) Metaplasia is a reversible change in which one adult cell type is replaced by another adult cell type. It is an adaptive change, such as that seen in metaplastic bronchial squamous epithelium secondary to smoking. Atrophy is shrinkage of the cell size by loss of cell substance. Atrophy is most commonly seen with aging, ischemia, diminished workload, loss of innervation, or inadequate nutrition. Dysplasia is characterized by atypical cellular development that may be precancerous. Nuclear hyperchromatism, loss of cellular polarity, and impaired cellular maturation may all be features of dysplasia. *(Cotran, pp 30–34)*

621–626. (621-E, 622-I, 623-A, 624-J, 625-F, 626-B) Klinefelter's syndrome has a 47,XXY karyotype, testicular atrophy, eunuchoid tall habitus, gynecomastia, and a female distribution of hair. The normal female and male karyotypes are 46,XX and 46,XY, respectively. Down's syndrome is characterized by trisomy 21, congenital cardiac defects, epicanthic folds, mental retardation, dysplastic ears, and increased risk of developing leukemia. The multi-X female karyotype, particularly in the 47,XXX karyotype, is usually phenotypically normal. Turner's syndrome includes a 45,X karyotype, webbing of the neck, amenorrhea, streak gonads, cardiac defects, short stature, and a broad chest. Edwards' syndrome (trisomy 18) is seen in about 1 of 8000 live births and is characterized by mental retardation, prominent occiput, micrognathia, low-set ears, rocker bottom feet, and hypertonicity. *(Cotran, pp 127–135)*

627–630. (627-C, 628-H, 629-E, 630-G) Histoplasmosis is a granulomatous pulmonary disorder caused by the fungal organism, *Histoplasma capsulatum*. Old foci tend to become fibrotic and may be undistinguishable from pulmonary carcinoma by chest x-ray. Surgically removed nodules usually demonstrate small budding yeast forms with methenamine silver stains. Squamous cell carcinoma is associated with smoking and usually presents as a bronchogenic lesion. Metastases are first seen in the draining bronchial and hilar lymph nodes. Later, metastases may be found in the pleura, liver, adrenals, and brain. Secondary amyloidosis can be seen as a complication of myeloma or chronic infections. Histologically, the acellular material has apple green birefringence on polarized light examination after congo red staining. The characteristic electron microscopic feature of mesothelioma is abundant long microvilli. Most mesotheliomas are associated with asbestosis exposure. *(Cotran, pp 373–374,797–809)*

631–635. (631-J, 632-A, 633-E, 634-I, 635-D) Condyloma accuminatum is a sexually acquired warty growth with a predilection for the penile meatus, perianal skin, and cervix. Human papilloma viruses are the etiologic agent. Renal cell carcinoma is characteristically a variegated tumor of large size. Extension into the renal vein is a common finding. Endometriosis is more commonly found in the ovary or peritoneum, but may be present in the bladder. Endometriosis of the bladder is typified by benign endometrial glands and stroma in a hemorrhagic background. Hematuria is a common clinical complaint. Prostatic adenocarcinoma is a disease of elderly males. Bone metastases are common in the late stages of the disease. Prostate specific antigen is elevated in most patients with bony metastases. Glomerulonephritis following streptococcal infection is most often seen in a pediatric age group. Hematuria, edema, and hypertension are usual concomitant clinical findings. *(Rubin and Farber, pp 852–938)*

BIBLIOGRAPHY

Cotran RS, Kumar V, Robbins SL. *Robbins Pathologic Basis of Disease.* 4th ed. Philadelphia: WB Saunders Co; 1989

Kissane JM, ed. *Anderson's Pathology.* 9th ed. St. Louis: CV Mosby; 1990

Rubin E, Farber JL, eds. *Pathology.* Philadelphia: JB Lippincott Co; 1988

Subspecialty List: Pathology

Question Number and Subspecialty

509. Respiratory system
510. Cardiovascular system
511. Genetic syndromes and metabolic diseases
512. Inflammation
513. Liver
514. Immunopathology
515. Genetic syndromes and metabolic diseases
516. Processes of neoplasia
517. Nongenetic syndromes
518. Kidney and urinary system
519. Hemostasis and coagulation
520. Alimentary system
521. Inflammation
522. Immunopathology
523. Abnormal growth and development
524. Blood and lymphatic system
525. Immunopathology
526. Alimentary system
527. Kidney and urinary system
528. Alimentary system
529. Cutaneous, osseus, and muscle systems
530. Alimentary system
531. Blood and lymphatic system
532. Nervous system
533. Endocrine system
534. Processes of neoplasia
535. Miscellaneous
536. Inflammation
537. Inflammation
538. Inflammation
539. Processes of neoplasia
540. Processes of neoplasia
541. Alimentary system
542. Abnormal growth and development
543. Respiratory system
544. Respiratory system
545. Genetic syndromes and metabolic disorders
546. Circulatory system
547. Circulatory system
548. Circulatory system
549. Processes of neoplasia
550. Abnormal growth and development
551. Cell injury and response
552. Nervous system

553. Genital system
554. Genetic syndromes and metabolic diseases
555. Genital system
556. Genital system
557. Processes of infection
558. Immunopathology
559. Processes of neoplasia
560. Nongenetic syndromes
561. Inflammation
562. Healing and repair
563. Hemostasis and coagulation
564. Infectious diseases
565. Kidney and urinary system
566. Kidney and urinary system
567. Endocrine system
568. Blood and lymphatic system
569. Blood and lymphatic system
570. Blood and lymphatic system
571. Blood and lymphatic system
572. Miscellaneous
573. Inflammation
574. Inflammation
575. Inflammation
576. Processes of neoplasia
577. Processes of neoplasia
578. Processes of neoplasia
579. Infectious diseases
580. Infectious diseases
581. Infectious diseases
582. Infectious diseases
583. Infectious diseases
584. Infectious diseases
585. Endocrine system
586. Endocrine system
587. Genetic syndromes and metabolic disorders
588. Genital system
589. Genital system
590. Genital system
591. Cardiovascular system
592. Cardiovascular system
593. Cardiovascular system
594. Environmental pathology
595. Environmental pathology
596. Environmental pathology
597. Cardiovascular system
598. Genetic syndromes and metabolic disorders

599. Immunopathology
600. Blood and lymphatic system
601. Abnormal growth and development
602. Genetic syndromes and metabolic disorders
603. Cardiovascular system
604. Cardiovascular system
605. Cardiovascular system
606. Endocrine system
607. Endocrine system
608. Endocrine system
609. Blood and lymphatic system
610. Immunopathology
611. Immunopathology
612. Blood and lymphatic system
613. Blood and lymphatic system
614. Blood and lymphatic system
615. Environmental pathology
616. Environmental pathology
617. Environmental pathology
618. Abnormal growth and development
619. Abnormal growth and development
620. Abnormal growth and development
621. Genetic syndromes and metabolic disorders
622. Genetic syndromes and metabolic disorders
623. Genetic syndromes and metabolic disorders
624. Genetic syndromes and metabolic disorders
625. Genetic syndromes and metabolic disorders
626. Genetic syndromes and metabolic disorders
627. Respiratory system
628. Respiratory system
629. Respiratory system
630. Respiratory system
631. Kidney and urinary system
632. Kidney and urinary system
633. Kidney and urinary system
634. Kidney and urinary system
635. Kidney and urinary system

CHAPTER 6

Pharmacology
Questions

DIRECTIONS (Questions 636 through 685): Each of the numbered items or incomplete statements in this section is followed by answers or by completions of the statement. Select the ONE lettered answer or completion that is BEST in each case.

636. A hypothetical drug, when given as a single-bolus dose of 1 g to a 70-kg (154-lb) patient, results in peak plasma level of 20 µg/ml. The apparent volume of distribution is

(A) 0.05 L
(B) 5.00 L
(C) 14.20 L
(D) 50.00 L
(E) 500.00 L

637. A hypothetical drug follows first-order kinetics and has a half-life of 6 hr. A peak serum level obtained after a single IV dose of 100 mg is 8 µg/ml. After 12 hr, the serum level is expected to be

(A) 6 µg/ml
(B) 4 µg/ml
(C) 2 µg/ml
(D) 1 µg/ml
(E) none of the above

638. Warfarin exerts its anticoagulant effect by

(A) blocking calcium binding to clotting factors
(B) forming a complex with clotting factors
(C) breaking down thrombin
(D) inhibiting the formation of active clotting factors
(E) none of the above

639. All of the following sedatives have pharmacologically active metabolites EXCEPT

(A) prazepam
(B) chlordiazepoxide
(C) diazepam
(D) lorazepam
(E) chlorazepate

640. All of the following are important side effects of glucocorticoids when used as anti-inflammatory agents EXCEPT

(A) suppression of pituitary–adrenal function
(B) masculinization of female patients
(C) increased susceptibility to infections
(D) osteoporosis
(E) Cushing's habitus

641. Which of the following antineoplastic agents is associated with an increased incidence of severe pulmonary disease?

(A) methotrexate
(B) fluorouracil
(C) bleomycin
(D) vincristine
(E) cisplatin

642. Which of the following laxatives is a bulk-forming agent?

(A) docusate
(B) cascara sagrada
(C) magnesium citrate
(D) psyllium hydrophilic mucilloid
(E) bisacodyl

643. Use of magnesium-containing antacids is most likely to result in

(A) constipation
(B) diarrhea
(C) nausea
(D) headache
(E) neurologic impairment

644. Potassium supplementation often is necessary for patients taking

(A) spironolactone
(B) triamterene
(C) furosemide
(D) amiloride
(E) captopril

645. Hormonal side effects of estrogen excess related to oral contraceptive use may include all of the following EXCEPT

(A) weight gain
(B) headaches
(C) amenorrhea
(D) edema
(E) breast tenderness

646. A patient experiencing an initial attack of acute gout is most likely to respond to treatment with

(A) indomethacin
(B) tolmetin
(C) phenylbutazone
(D) colchicine
(E) ibuprofen

647. Severe bone marrow suppression can result with the concurrent administration of 6-mercaptopurine and

(A) phenobarbital
(B) chloramphenicol
(C) allopurinol
(D) phenytoin
(E) metronidazole

648. Lidocaine

(A) is a short-acting local anesthetic because it is metabolized by pseudocholinesterases
(B) has direct vasoconstrictor activities
(C) is inappropriate for use as a topical anesthetic
(D) is a local anesthetic and thus is devoid of CNS effects
(E) appears to block nerve conduction by preventing the large transient increase in sodium permeability produced by depolarization

649. The ideal hypnotic should be absorbed rapidly so that its pharmacologic effect can occur, it should be eliminated rapidly, and it should not be biotransformed to long-acting metabolites to avoid hangover effects. The hypnotic that most nearly achieves these criteria is

(A) triazolam
(B) temazepam
(C) flurazepam
(D) diazepam
(E) chlordiazepoxide

650. All of the following are fetal or neonatal side effects of β-sympathomimetic tocolytics EXCEPT

(A) tachycardia
(B) hyperglycemia
(C) ileus
(D) hypocalcemia
(E) hypotension

651. Cimetidine and ranitidine are pharmacologically classified as histamine receptor (H_2) antagonists. Which of the following disease entities is most likely to respond to the use of these agents?

(A) motion sickness
(B) seasonal rhinitis
(C) urticaria
(D) duodenal ulcer
(E) conjunctivitis

652. All of the following are factors that may increase the sensitivity of the myocardium to digoxin EXCEPT

(A) hypercalcemia
(B) hypoxia
(C) hypokalemia
(D) hyperthyroidism
(E) hypomagnesemia

653. Which of the following statements is correct regarding angiotensin-converting enzyme (ACE) inhibitors?

(A) chronic therapy with ACE inhibitors impairs hemodynamic response to exercise
(B) rebound hypertension after abrupt cessation of therapy is a frequent problem
(C) use of ACE inhibitors depresses renin activity
(D) therapy with ACE inhibitors appears useful in essential hypertension
(E) ACE inhibitors are of little value in therapy of congestive heart failure

654. All of the following drugs can decrease lower esophageal sphincter pressure EXCEPT

(A) dopamine
(B) morphine
(C) propranolol

(D) fentanyl

(E) theophylline

655. All of the following statements about rifampin are true EXCEPT

(A) it inhibits microbial RNA synthesis

(B) it is primarily excreted in the bile

(C) hepatotoxicity is a side effect

(D) it is used exclusively in the treatment of tuberculosis

(E) it reduces the effect of anticoagulants

656. Which of the following types of pulmonary dysfunction may follow heroin overdose?

(A) pulmonary fibrosis

(B) pulmonary edema

(C) bronchospasm

(D) pulmonary hypertension

(E) pneumonitis with eosinophilia

657. Which of the following statements regarding antidiuretic hormone (ADH) is correct?

(A) release of ADH is under the control of ADH-releasing factor, a hypothalamic hormone

(B) one of the main stimuli to ADH release is a decrease in plasma osmolality

(C) intranasal desmopressin (1-deamino-8-D-arginine vasopressin) is useful in treating diabetes insipidus

(D) ADH is one of at least 10 important hormones secreted by the anterior pituitary gland

(E) ADH can relax vascular smooth muscle

658. Of the following hypnotics, the safest is

(A) flurazepam

(B) chloral hydrate

(C) pentobarbital

(D) glutethimide

(E) paraldehyde

659. Since 1984, several new antiarrhythmic agents, including encainide, have become available for clinical use. Encainide is distinct from previous agents (procainamide or quinidine), since it is

(A) a member of the calcium channel blocker family

(B) useful in life-threatening sustained arrhythmia

(C) associated with prolonged repolarization (QT interval)

(D) capable of abolishing nonsustained ventricular arrhythmia with minimal cardiac toxicity [atrioventricular (AV) or sinoatrial (S-A) block]

(E) the only one available in a form for oral therapy

660. H_1 receptor antagonists are used to treat all of the following EXCEPT

(A) motion sickness

(B) allergic rhinitis

(C) sleep disorders

(D) bronchial asthma

(E) urticaria

661. All of the following are true about phenytoin EXCEPT that it

(A) is highly bound to plasma proteins

(B) is mainly excreted unchanged in the urine

(C) has dose-dependent elimination kinetics

(D) is effective in grand mal seizures

(E) induces the metabolism of certain drugs

662. Heparin anticoagulant therapy is associated with the following effects EXCEPT

(A) release of lipoprotein lipase

(B) breakdown of thrombin

(C) suppression of aldosterone secretion

(D) shortening of partial thromboplastin time (PTT)

(E) osteoporosis

663. Which of the following tricyclic antidepressants is most selective in blocking nerve reuptake of norepinephrine?

(A) doxepin

(B) desipramine

(C) amitriptyline

(D) imipramine

(E) nortriptyline

664. The onset and duration of sedative-hypnotic activity of the ultrashort-acting barbiturates may be influenced by all of the following EXCEPT

(A) serum elimination half-life

(B) lipid solubility

(C) cerebrovascular blood flow

(D) extent of tissue binding

(E) amount of body fat

665. All of the following pharmacologic effects may be associated with opiate use EXCEPT

(A) pupillary constriction
(B) emesis
(C) respiratory stimulation
(D) constriction of the lower end of the common bile duct
(E) urinary retention

666. All of the following are pharmacologic properties of the metabolically active form of vitamin D EXCEPT

(A) increased intestinal absorption of calcium
(B) decalcification of bone
(C) increased renal tubular reabsorption of calcium and phosphate
(D) suppression of peripheral conversion of androstenedione to testosterone
(E) suppression of production of parathyroid hormone

667. All of the following are factors that may influence transplacental transport of drugs EXCEPT

(A) molecular weight
(B) lipid solubility
(C) ionization
(D) maternal blood pressure (BP)
(E) protein binding

668. Significant movement into tubular urine (pH of 5) of a drug administered IV would be expected if the drug were

(A) a weak base
(B) a weak acid
(C) ionized throughout the pH range
(D) un-ionized throughout the pH range
(E) none of the above

669. All of the following antihypertensive agents act on the vascular smooth muscle EXCEPT

(A) hydralazine
(B) prazosin
(C) nitroprusside
(D) clonidine
(E) minoxidil

670. Hypokalemia is a likely result of therapy with all of the following drugs EXCEPT

(A) chlorothiazide
(B) furosemide
(C) spironolactone
(D) bumetanide
(E) theophylline

671. All of the following are appropriate for the treatment of hypercalcemia EXCEPT

(A) normal saline infusions
(B) furosemide
(C) prednisone
(D) mithramycin
(E) dihydrotachysterol

672. All of the following are pharmacologic effects of cocaine EXCEPT

(A) anesthesia
(B) CNS stimulation
(C) respiratory stimulation
(D) hypotension
(E) mydriasis

673. The most common problem associated with use of nonsteroidal anti-inflammatory agents, such as ibuprofen and naproxen, is

(A) toxic amblyopia
(B) fluid retention
(C) gastrointestinal complaints
(D) renal failure
(E) drowsiness

674. Levorphanol can be distinguished from morphine by

(A) lack of a depressant effect on respiration
(B) safe use in asthmatic patients
(C) fewer adverse gastrointestinal effects
(D) lower incidence of allergic reactions
(E) naloxone insensitivity

675. An early sign of phenytoin intoxication following oral dosing is

(A) nystagmus
(B) hyperexcitability
(C) loss of seizure control
(D) gastrointestinal complaints
(E) tremor

676. Cimetidine has been associated with all of the following side effects EXCEPT

(A) gynecomastia
(B) neural dysfunction
(C) reduction of sperm count
(D) relapse of ulcer symptoms on withdrawal
(E) increased hepatic drug-metabolizing capability

677. All of the following agents are useful in the treatment of bronchial asthma EXCEPT

(A) aminophylline

(B) isoproterenol

(C) ipratropium bromide

(D) cromolyn sodium

(E) propranolol

678. Epinephrine increases all of the following EXCEPT

(A) total peripheral resistance

(B) heart rate

(C) systolic arterial pressure

(D) oxygen consumption

(E) blood glucose

679. Which of the following statements regarding pharmacology of general anesthetics is correct?

(A) nitrous oxide alone may produce surgical levels of anesthesia

(B) enflurane may be considered more potent than halothane, since their respective minimum alveolar concentrations (MAC) are 1.68 and 0.75

(C) induction of anesthesia with methoxyflurane is much more rapid than with enflurane, since their partition coefficients are 12.0 and 1.8, respectively

(D) halothane is no longer used because it is associated with a high incidence of hepatitis

(E) halothane and all other fluorinated hydrocarbons used for anesthesia (isoflurane, enflurane, methoxyflurane) are associated with similar decreases in systemic blood pressure

680. Which of the following changes in the differential WBC count might occur in a patient receiving glucocorticoids?

(A) lymphocytosis

(B) neutrophilic leukocytosis

(C) eosinophilia

(D) monocytosis

(E) none of the above

681. Which dosage form of iron is preferred for the treatment of iron deficiency anemia?

(A) oral ferrous fumarate

(B) oral ferrous gluconate

(C) oral ferrous sulfate

(D) IM iron dextran

(E) IV iron dextran

682. Which of the following insulin preparations has the longest duration of action?

(A) semilente insulin

(B) globin zinc insulin

(C) NPH insulin

(D) regular insulin

(E) ultralente insulin

683. In combination chemotherapy for tuberculosis, the following are normally administered orally EXCEPT

(A) isoniazid

(B) rifampin

(C) streptomycin

(D) pyrazinamide

(E) ethambutol

684. Which of the following items correctly associates mechanism of action with the corresponding agent used in hyperlipidemia?

(A) nicotinic acid: altered excretion of bile acids

(B) clofibrate: decreased activity of lipoprotein lipase

(C) lovastatin (Mevinolin): inhibition of 3-hydroxy-3-methylglutaryl coenzyme A (HMG-CoA)

(D) cholestyramine: increased activity of lipoprotein lipase

(E) gemfibrozil: decreased plasma concentrations of high-density lipoprotein (HDL) by undetermined mechanism

685. Calcium disodium edetate is an antidote to poisoning with

(A) mercury

(B) atropine

(C) Paris green

(D) lead

(E) phosphorus

DIRECTIONS (Questions 686 through 735): Each set of matching questions in this section consists of a list of five lettered options followed by several numbered items. For each item, select the ONE lettered option that is most closely associated with it. *Each lettered heading may be selected once, more than once, or not at all.*

Questions 686 through 689

For each laxative agent, select the group in which it is classified.

(A) bulk-forming
(B) lubricant
(C) stimulant
(D) stool softener
(E) osmotic

686. Psyllium

687. Bisacodyl

688. Docusate

689. Lactulose

Questions 690 through 692

(A) inhibits formation of the bacterial wall
(B) inhibits protein synthesis by binding to ribosomes
(C) causes misreading of mRNA at the ribosome
(D) inhibits nucleic acid synthesis
(E) prevents the incorporation of para-aminobenzoic acid (PABA) into folic acid

690. Rifampin

691. Tetracycline

692. Vancomycin

Questions 693 through 696

For each agent listed below, select the site or mechanism of action with which it is most closely associated.

(A) releases norepinephrine from storage sites
(B) direct α-adrenergic agonist
(C) blocks β-adrenergic receptors
(D) agonist of β-adrenergic receptors
(E) blocks α-adrenergic receptors

693. Isoproterenol

694. Propranolol

695. Amphetamine

696. Methoxamine

Questions 697 through 701

For each chemotherapeutic agent listed below, choose the unique side effect with which it is associated.

(A) neuropathies
(B) pulmonary fibrosis
(C) hemorrhagic cystitis
(D) congestive heart failure
(E) ototoxicity

697. Cyclophosphamide

698. Vincristine

699. Doxorubicin

700. Bleomycin

701. Cisplatin

Questions 702 through 704

For each agent listed below, select the physiologic response with which it is most closely associated after clinically relevant doses of the agent are administered.

(A) tachycardia
(B) cholinesterase inhibition
(C) decreased intraocular pressure
(D) muscle paralysis
(E) sedation

702. Pilocarpine

703. Atropine

704. Succinylcholine

Questions 705 through 710

For each antineoplastic agent listed below, select the pharmacologic class in which it belongs.

(A) plant alkaloid
(B) antimetabolite
(C) alkylating agent
(D) antibiotic
(E) antiestrogen

705. Vincristine

706. Methotrexate

707. 5-Fluorouracil

708. Cyclophosphamide

709. Bleomycin

710. Tamoxifen

Questions 711 through 715

    (A) adenosine antagonist
    (B) nonselective adrenergic agonist
    (C) muscarinic antagonist
    (D) β_2-selective adrenergic agonist
    (E) β-selective adrenergic agonist

711. theophylline

712. isoproterenol

713. terbutaline

714. epinephrine

715. ipratropium bromide

Questions 716 through 720

    (A) cyclophosphamide
    (B) melphalan
    (C) methotrexate
    (D) prednisone
    (E) Tamoxifen

716. Must be activated by microsomal enzymes for its cytotoxic effect

717. Can produce hot flashes

718. Is cell cycle specific

719. Produces cystitis

720. Effective in management of hemolytic anemia associated with lymphomas

Questions 721 through 725

    (A) nitroglycerin (glyceryl trinitrate)
    (B) diltiazem
    (C) propranolol
    (D) digoxin
    (E) quinidine

721. Stimulates guanylyl cyclase

722. Blocks β-adrenoceptor mediated stimulation of adenylate cyclase

723. May induce reflex tachycardia

724. Mimics the effect of nitric oxide

725. Blocks calcium entry into smooth and cardiac myocytes

Questions 726 through 730

    (A) aspirin
    (B) acetaminophen
    (C) indomethacin
    (D) ibuprophen
    (E) phenylbutazone

726. Is effective in the treatment of patent ductus arteriosus

727. Does not have significant antiinflammatory activity

728. Tinnitus is a symptom of toxicity

729. Has replaced colchicine as the initial treatment for acute gout

730. Inhibits platelet aggregation

Questions 731 through 735

    (A) penicillin
    (B) tetracycline
    (C) clindamycin
    (D) sulfamethoxazole
    (E) dapsone

731. Binds to the 50 S subunit of bacterial ribosomes

732. Binds to the 30 S subunit of bacterial ribosomes

733. Has a β-lactam structure

734. Frequently combined with trimethoprim

735. Used in the treatment of leprosy

DIRECTIONS (Questions 736 through 762): Each of the numbered items or incomplete statements in this section is followed by answers or by completions of the statement. Select the ONE lettered answer or completion that is BEST in each case.

736. Which is the drug of choice for the prevention of ventricular fibrillation during acute myocardial infarction?

    (A) lidocaine
    (B) digoxin
    (C) quinidine
    (D) flecanide
    (E) propranolol

737. Agents that should be used initially in the management of *Ascaris* or *Enterobius vermicularis* include

    (A) thiabendazole
    (B) pyrantel pamoate
    (C) tetrachloroethylene
    (D) antimony potassium tartrate
    (E) diethylcarbamazine

738. Aminoglycoside antibiotics are associated with all of the following adverse side effects EXCEPT

    (A) ototoxicity
    (B) neuromuscular blockade
    (C) nephrotoxicity
    (D) hepatotoxicity
    (E) optic nerve dysfunction

739. All of the following statements concerning propranolol are true EXCEPT that it

    (A) competitively blocks β_1-adrenergic receptors
    (B) can be used as a prophylaxis for migraine
    (C) competitively blocks β_2-adrenergic receptors
    (D) can be safely used by asthma sufferers
    (E) can be used to treat atrial fibrillation

740. All of the following mechanisms are utilized to relieve angina EXCEPT

    (A) reduction of myocardial work
    (B) inhibition of platelet aggregation
    (C) increased extraction of oxygen from blood
    (D) decreased oxygen demand
    (E) selective coronary vessel dilation

741. One proposed mechanism for the antihypertensive effects of propranolol is

    (A) α-adrenergic receptor blockade
    (B) inhibition of renin release
    (C) depletion of amines in adrenergic nerves
    (D) blockade of norepinephrine reuptake into prejunctional neurons
    (E) down regulation of vascular β-adrenergic receptors

742. Which of the following drugs decreases the response of oral anticoagulants?

    (A) phenobarbital
    (B) aspirin
    (C) phenylbutazone
    (D) cimetidine
    (E) ibuprophen

743. Chronic lead poisoning is characterized by all of the following EXCEPT

    (A) gastrointestinal effects
    (B) muscle weakness
    (C) encephalopathy
    (D) impaired hemoglobin synthesis
    (E) skin rashes

744. Correct statements regarding multiple dosing therapeutics include all of the following EXCEPT that

    (A) the average plasma level after multiple dosing depends on clearance
    (B) the approach (rate) to steady-state (plateau) drug concentration depends only on the half-life of the drug
    (C) there is a greater mean plasma concentration for drugs administered via continuous infusion than by multiple dosing
    (D) an initial loading dose is often desirable when the time to reach steady-state is appreciable
    (E) halving both the dose and dosage interval reduces fluctuations but leaves mean steady-state plasma concentration unchanged

745. All of the following are advantages to combining carbidopa with levodopa EXCEPT

    (A) adverse effects of levodopa on the central nervous system are reduced
    (B) allows reduction of the dosage of levodopa
    (C) permits more rapid dosage titration
    (D) avoids pyridoxine antagonism of levodopa
    (E) causes fewer gastrointestinal side effects

746. Prostacyclin (PGI_2) has all of the following actions EXCEPT

    (A) potent vasodilation
    (B) inhibition of platelet aggregation
    (C) suppression of gastric ulceration

(D) reduces renal blood flow

(E) lowers the threshold of nociceptors at afferent nerve endings

747. Common ECG effects of <u>digitalis</u> glycosides include all of the following EXCEPT

(A) prolongation of the PR interval

(B) shortening of the QT interval

(C) widening of the QRS complex

(D) ST segment depression

(E) T wave inversion

748. The leukotrienes (LTC_4, LTD_4, and LTE_4)

(A) are important mediators in the pathophysiology of asthma

(B) have their biosynthesis greatly reduced by aspirin

(C) have few cardiovascular effects

(D) are stored in platelet granules for subsequent release

(E) are potent chemotactic agents for polymorphonuclear leukocytes

749. Which of the following agents used in the treatment of gout inhibits the enzyme xanthine oxidase?

(A) probenecid

(B) colchicine

(C) sulfinpyrazone

(D) allopurinol

(E) indomethacin

750. α-Adrenergic blocking effects are frequently observed after therapy with

(A) diazepam

(B) chlorpromazine

(C) meprobamate

(D) fluoxetine

(E) chlordiazepoxide

751. Potential mechanisms of resistance to antineoplastic drugs include all of the following EXCEPT

(A) quantitative increase in target enzyme

(B) decreased affinity of the target enzyme for the drug

(C) reduced cellular uptake of the drug

(D) enhanced active efflux of the drug

(E) decreased tumor cell heterogeneity

752. The mechanism of action of streptokinase is

(A) direct conversion of plasminogen to plasmin

(B) proteolytic breakdown of fibrin

(C) depletion of α_2-antiplasmin

(D) formation of a complex with plasminogen

(E) proteolytic breakdown of fibrinogen

753. Diazepam is effective in the treatment of convulsive disorders because it

(A) increases the binding of γ-aminobutyric acid (GABA) to its receptor

(B) blocks sodium channels

(C) stabilizes neuronal membranes

(D) depolarizes neurons

(E) competitively blocks binding of serotonin to its receptor

754. Inhibition of blood clotting by oral anticoagulants is due to interference with all of the following EXCEPT

(A) factor II

(B) factor III

(C) factor VII

(D) factor IX

(E) factor X

755. Bacterial resistance by enzymatic inactivation of amikacin occurs by

(A) phosphorylation

(B) sulfation

(C) adenylation

(D) hydroxylation

(E) acetylation

756. The mechanism of action of local anesthetics is related to

(A) ganglionic blockade

(B) inhibition of pain receptors

(C) inhibition of nerve conduction via blockade of Na^+ channels

(D) inhibition of nerve conduction via blockade of Ca^{2+} channels

(E) hyperpolarization of neurons via enhanced Cl^- influx

757. Acute poisoning with antihistamines is correctly described as

(A) treatable with histamine therapy

(B) characterized by fever and flushing in adults

(C) causing severe respiratory depression

(D) producing a state similar to atropine poisoning in children

(E) producing joint pain

758. An individual who has ingested a toxic dose of acetaminophen may experience all of the following EXCEPT

    (A) nausea and vomiting
    (B) hepatic enzyme elevation
    (C) impaired coagulation
    (D) tinnitus
    (E) abdominal pain

759. Chronic abusers of barbiturates will often display cross-tolerance to all of the following EXCEPT

    (A) diazepam
    (B) alcohol
    (C) morphine
    (D) methaqualone
    (E) chlordiazepoxide

760. The renal elimination of a drug that is a weak acid can be enhanced by

    (A) increasing the pH of the blood
    (B) decreasing the pH of the blood
    (C) increasing the pH of the urine
    (D) increasing the concentration of urinary organic acids
    (E) decreasing the pH of the urine

761. Renal failure occurring during gentamicin therapy is characterized by all of the following EXCEPT

    (A) the inability to concentrate urine
    (B) the presence of protein and casts in the urine
    (C) rising trough concentrations of the drug
    (D) reversibility
    (E) decreased plasma creatinine

762. Carbidopa is combined with levodopa in the treatment of Parkinson's disease because of the following EXCEPT that

    (A) lower doses of levodopa can be used
    (B) the peripheral side effects can be minimized
    (C) the CNS side effects can be minimized
    (D) dosage titration is more rapid
    (E) an increased fraction of the levodopa administered reaches the brain

Answers and Explanations

636. **(D)** In the example described in the question, the apparent volume of distribution is calculated as follows:

$$V_d = \frac{\text{total amount of drug in body}}{\text{concentration of drug in plasma}}$$

The total amount of drug in the body is the single-bolus dose of 1,000 mg and is calculated as follows:

$$V_d \neq \frac{1,000 \text{ mg}}{20 \text{ μg/ml}} = 50 \text{ L}$$

(Gilman et al, pp 23–25)

637. **(C)** The half-life for first-order kinetics is defined as the amount of time necessary for drug concentration to decrease by 50 percent. Six hours after a peak serum level of 8 μg/ml, the serum concentration of the drug described in the question should be 4 μg/ml. After 6 hr more (total of 12 hr), the serum level should be 2 μg/ml. *(Gilman et al, pp 25–28)*

638. **(D)** Warfarin blocks the vitamin K-dependent step in the synthesis of clotting factors. Carboxylation of the molecule descarboxyprothrombin to form prothrombin requires the reduced form of vitamin K (KH$_2$), which, in the process, is converted to vitamin K epoxide (KO). KH$_2$ is regenerated by an epoxide reductase requiring NADH. It is this step that is blocked by warfarin. *(Gilman et al, pp 1317–1319)*

639. **(D)** All benzodiazepines, with the exception of oxazepam and lorazepam, are converted via hepatic metabolic pathways. This usually occurs via *N*-alkylation or oxidation to metabolites that are pharmacologically active. This property may contribute to prolonged duration of action of the benzodiazepines. *(Gilman et al, pp 352–355)*

640. **(B)** Glucocorticoids are valuable adjuvants in anti-inflammatory therapy and inhibit all phases of inflammation (vascular, cellular, and connective tissue repair). Usual therapy involves a synthetic derivative (e.g., prednisolone, triamcinolone, desamethasone, betamethasone, beclomethasone) of the endogenous hormone, cortisol. Unfortunately, the biologic effects of glucocorticoids are myriad, and all effects aside from anti-inflammatory effects may become unwanted. Because of negative feedback from adrenal to pituitary gland, prolonged therapy with glucocorticoids can result in suppression of functions associated with this particular axis. Perhaps the most disastrous side effect is increased susceptibility to infection of all kinds secondary to effects of the drug on the immune system as well as inhibition of the inflammatory process. Decreased formation (decreased osteoblast activity) and increased resorption (secondary to elevated levels of parathyroid hormone due to decreased intestinal calcium absorption) of bone may lead to osteoporosis. Cushing's habitus, consisting of moonface, buffalo hump, enlargement of supraclavicular fat pads, central obesity, and other aspects of supraphysiologic affects of adrenal corticosteroids, also may occur. Masculinization of female patients is a common concern in androgen therapy. *(Gilman et al, pp 1448–1455)*

641. **(C)** Ten to twenty percent of patients receiving bleomycin develop a pulmonary interstitial fibrosis that severely compromises gas exchange and reduces diffusing capacity. This condition is most prevalent in older patients or those receiving a total bleomycin dose above 400 units. *(Craig and Stitzel, p 806)*

642. **(D)** Psyllium hydrophilic mucilloid, a bulk-forming laxative, exerts its therapeutic effect by increasing the mass and water content of stool and by speeding transit time in the colon. Bisacodyl and cascara sagrada are considered contact cathartics, which speed colonic transit time and alter water and electrolyte transport across the colonic mucosa. Magnesium citrate is a saline cathartic, which indirectly increases intestinal transit by its osmotic properties. Docusate, a stool-softening agent, is an anionic surfactant that presumably allows penetration of the fecal mass by water and fats. *(Gilman et al, pp 914–922)*

643. **(B)** The various magnesium salts act as saline cathartics and are sometimes used for this purpose. Hence, their use is commonly associated with the development of diarrhea. For this reason, various antacids contain an aluminum salt in addition to magnesium salts, which tends to counteract this effect. Neurologic sequelae develop when the small amount of absorbed magnesium cannot be excreted, as in moderate to severe renal insufficiency. *(Gilman et al, pp 914–922)*

644. **(C)** Spironolactone is a competitive antagonist of aldosterone and, therefore, may cause hyperkalemia if administered concomitantly with potassium supplements. Likewise, the potassium-sparing diuretics triamterene and amiloride cause potassium retention. Captopril inhibits production of angiotensin II and, therefore, inhibits aldosterone production. Furosemide promotes renal potassium excretion and often requires concomitant supplemental potassium administration. *(Gilman et al, pp 721–728)*

645. **(C)** Oral contraceptive agents with a high estrogen content can produce adverse effects reflective of excess estrogen. These effects include weight gain, headache, edema, and breast tenderness. ↑ bleeding Amenorrhea is associated with estrogen deficiency. *(Katzung, pp 571–573)*

646. **(D)** Colchicine is the drug of choice for an initial attack of acute gout because it provides symptomatic relief in more than 95 percent of cases. It also is a useful diagnostic tool because it is relatively specific for acute gout. The other choices listed in the question are nonsteroidal anti-inflammatory drugs that are used to treat acute gout if the side effects of colchicine are intolerable. *(Katzung, pp 507–508)*

647. **(C)** Allopurinol often is used in conjunction with oncolytic therapy to reduce the elevated serum and urinary uric acid levels associated with the degradation of nucleoprotein. Allopurinol works by inhibiting xanthine oxidase. The antineoplastic agent 6-mercaptopurine can lead to excess accumulation of allopurinol, resulting in severe bone marrow suppression. The remaining drugs listed in the question are all known to alter the hepatic mixed-function oxidase system, but they do not adversely interact with 6-mercaptopurine. *(Katzung, pp 509–510)*

648. **(E)** Lidocaine is a potent local anesthetic that also is useful in treatment of ventricular dysrhythmia. In contrast to ester-type local anesthetics (procaine), lidocaine and other amides are metabolized slowly in the liver and have moderate to long durations of action. Unlike cocaine, which is a vasoconstrictor, lidocaine can cause vasodilatation that results in absorption of the drug away from its intended local site. Local administration can be achieved by injection or topical application. Inadvertent introduction of lidocaine in large doses intravenously may result in significant CNS effects. If administered properly, these concerns as well as cardiac effects are minimal. Although the mechanism of action is not completely understood, lidocaine appears to enter the nerve cell and attach to a receptor at a site within the sodium channel, leading to inhibition of sodium conductance after depolarization of the nerve. *(Covino)*

649. **(A)** The benzodiazepine hypnotic triazolam most closely approximates the "ideal hypnotic" because of its rate of appearance in the blood after absorption, short elimination half-life, and lack of active metabolites. The other choices listed in the question are less than ideal. Temazepam has a slow onset, flurazepam has long-acting active metabolites, and diazepam and chlordiazepoxide have long half-lives and long-acting active metabolites. *(Craig and Stitzel, pp 441–445)*

650. **(B)** β-Sympathomimetic agents, such as terbutaline and ritodrine, are used in the management of premature labor. Fetal and neonatal abnormalities secondary to these agents may include tachycardia, hypotension, hypocalcemia, and ileus. Hypoglycemia (not hyperglycemia) usually occurs because of increases in umbilical cord insulin caused by maternal hyperglycemia. *(Gilman et al, pp 949–950)*

651. **(D)** Histamine receptor-blocking agents are classified as H_1 or H_2 blockers depending on what responses to histamine are prevented. H_2 receptors have been identified in numerous sites, including the stomach, uterus, ileum, and bronchial musculature. Gastric acid secretion involves activation of H_2 receptors, and disorders of acid secretion, such as duodenal ulcer, have responded to treatment with H_2 receptor antagonists. The remaining choices listed in the question do respond to conventional antihistamines (H_1-blocking drugs) but not to H_2 antagonists. *(Freston)*

652. **(D)** Several factors are known to sensitize the myocardium to digoxin, predisposing patients to digoxin toxicity. These factors include hypercalcemia, hypokalemia, hypomagnesemia, and hypoxia. Hypothyroidism (not hyperthyroidism) also makes patients more sensitive to the effects of digoxin. *(Gilman et al, p 834)*

653. **(D)** ACE inhibitors, such as captopril and enal-april, are effective agents in the treatment of systemic hypertension and congestive heart failure. Although initially perceived as being most useful for the therapy of renovascular disease and high renin hypertension, these drugs are now used routinely in many cases of essential hypertension. By inhibiting ACE, these drugs impair conversion of angiotensin I to angiotensin II while also prolonging the half-life of bradykinin, a vasodilator that normally is partially degraded by ACE. Accordingly, renin levels will rise as feedback inhibition via production of angiotensin II is removed. Unlike β-blockers, these drugs do not interfere with reflex sympathetic activity, and thus the response to exercise is unimpaired. Unlike centrally acting agents, such as clonidine, there is no indication of rebound hypertension. The drugs are being used more routinely as adjuvant therapy in congestive heart failure where a combination of decreased afterload and increased cardiac output is of great benefit to the patient. The mechanism underlying this effect is unclear. *(Lees)*

654. **(C)** Certain drugs have been shown to decrease lower esophageal sphincter pressure and predispose patients to gastroesophageal reflux. These drugs include the anticholinergics, dopamine, isoproterenol, morphine, fentanyl, and theophylline. Propranolol has not been shown to decrease lower esophageal sphincter pressure. *(Craig and Stitzel, pp 145,522,527)*

655. **(D)** Although rifampin is certainly a first-line drug in the treatment of tuberculosis, it is broadly antimicrobial and inhibits the growth of most gram-positive and gram-negative bacteria. More important, it is often part of the combined therapy used in the treatment of nontuberculous mycobacterial disease, where the causative organisms include *Mycobacterium leprae* or other species resistant to the other first-line antimycobacterial drugs, such as isoniazid. *(Gilman et al, pp 1149–1150)*

656. **(B)** Heroin overdose often is associated with pulmonary edema and carries a mortality rate of about 10 percent. Treatment is primarily supportive, with respiratory and oxygen therapy. The other choices listed in the question represent other drug-induced pulmonary syndromes. *(Katzung, p 845)*

657. **(C)** ADH and oxytocin are the major peptide hormones secreted by the posterior pituitary gland. Osmoreceptors in the hypothalamus, close to nuclei that synthesize and secrete ADH, are stimulated by an increase in plasma osmolality. ADH binds to receptors in the basolateral membrane of cells of the distal tubule and collecting ducts of the nephron, increasing permeability to water and thus aiding in the formation of hypertonic urine. These ADH receptors are distinct from those found on vascular smooth muscle that result in ADH-induced vasoconstriction. ADH is rapidly metabolized by peptidases, and thus desmopressin is used as an intranasal spray for the treatment of diabetes insipidus. This derivative is less susceptible to peptidase digestion, and the intranasal route avoids some aspects of degradation within the gastrointestinal system. Other uses of vasopressin include treatment of esophageal varices, since the vasoconstrictor effects of ADH appear to be marked in splanchnic circulation. *(Gilman et al, pp 732–740)*

658. **(A)** Benzodiazepines (such as flurazepam) are considered the hypnotics of choice. In comparison with chloral hydrate, barbiturates (pentobarbital), and glutethimide, they have better therapeutic indices, less likelihood of interacting with other drugs, less abuse liability, and less effect on respiration. Paraldehyde usually is unacceptable because of its unpleasant taste and odor. Some persons may develop hypersensitivity to benzodiazepines or may be unable to tolerate the hypnotic effects. The relative costs of these various medications also may be a factor. The manufacture of glutethimide recently has been halted. *(Gilman et al, pp 346–356)*

659. **(D)** Encainide is a structural analog of procainamide and is typical of the newly described class Ic antiarrhythmic drugs. Like quinidine or procainamide, it belongs to the family of drugs that block the fast inward sodium current in the heart. Unlike quinidine or procainamide, encainide does not alter the QT interval. Encainide is used for nonsustained arrythmia and is especially useful in conditions resistant to quinidine or procainamide, since encainide is without significant cardiac effects. Although some forms of life-threatening sustained arrhythmia may be treated with encainide, the drug has frequently been associated with exacerbation, rather than control, of these disorders. All three agents are available in oral form. Of note is that in many patients encainide is biotransformed to active metabolites under the control of a single hepatic cytochrome P_{450}. Encainide currently is under trial study to determine whether chronic antiarrhythmic treatment in postinfarction patients with arrhythmia reduces the risk of sudden death. *(Craig and Stitzel, pp 355–357)*

660. **(D)** Although histamine release is likely to be a part of the pathophysiology of asthma, antihistamines are ineffective in treating the disease. Nevertheless, their ability to block histamine binding is used in treating a variety of hypersensitivity reactions, of which urticaria is one. H_1 antagonists have anticholinergic properties that make them useful secondary agents in treating motion sickness. Their sedative effect is used to treat sleep disorders. *(Craig and Stitzel, pp 964–965)*

661. **(B)** Phenytoin is effective therapy for most types of epileptic seizures except absence (petit mal) seizures. It is approximately 90 percent bound to plasma proteins. Phenytoin is eliminated mainly through metabolism that is saturable at attainable serum concentrations. The dose-dependent (nonlinear) elimination of phenytoin often presents a clinical problem, since small changes in dosage may result in large increases in serum concentration and toxicity. Dosage adjustment in an individual patient is best accomplished through careful monitoring of serum concentrations and close observation for early signs of toxicity that include nystagmus, vertigo, ataxia, and drowsiness. *(Craig and Stitzel, pp 489–490)*

662. **(B)** Heparin inactivates thrombin; it does not cause its breakdown. Heparin achieves this effect in two ways: (1) by forming a complex with antithrombin III and the clotting factors, it promotes the action of antithrombin III in inhibiting the proteolytic conversion of prothrombin to thrombin, and (2) by directly and irreversibly inactivating thrombin. *(Gilman et al, p 1314)*

663. **(B)** Tricyclic antidepressants block reuptake of aminergic neurotransmitters into the presynaptic neurons. The result is a net increase in the amount of neurotransmitter in the synaptic cleft. These agents are relatively selective for certain neurotransmitters. Desipramine is the most selective agent for blocking uptake of norepinephrine, and amitriptyline is the most selective agent for blocking reuptake of serotonin. Imipramine, nortriptyline, and doxepin are intermediate in their selectivity. *(Hollister, 1978)*

664. **(A)** Barbiturates produce sedation through entry into the CNS. Ultrashort-acting agents are highly lipid soluble. The uptake of these agents by the CNS is rapid, with blood flow as the rate-limiting factor. The hypnotic activity of these agents is terminated by redistribution of drug from the CNS. Structural changes that affect various physiochemical properties of these agents influence the distribution of these agents into the CNS and, thus, their onset and duration of activity. Agents that are more lipid soluble (and are bound to tissues to a greater extent) have a rapid onset and short duration of action. Accumulation of these drugs in adipose tissue will affect the pharmacokinetics of these agents. Obese patients will require larger doses for sedative–hypnotic activity. Serum elimination half-life is not an important determi-

nant of onset or duration of activity with ultrashort-acting agents. *(Gilman et al, pp 358–361)*

665. **(C)** Opiates act as agonists at specific receptor sites with the CNS and other tissues. Opiates influence many organ systems and may be responsible for undesirable effects as well as desirable effects, such as analgesia. Miosis is often a prominent effect of opiates. Effects on the gastrointestinal tract include nausea and emesis resulting from direct stimulation of the chemoreceptor trigger zone. Biliary spasm due to constriction of the Oddi's sphincter often results in elevation of serum amylase and lipase levels in patients receiving certain opiates. Increased muscle tone at the vesical sphincter of the bladder may make urination difficult and result in urinary retention. Opiates act to depress respiration by directly affecting brain stem respiratory centers, reducing the responsiveness to carbon dioxide content in blood. *(Levine)*

666. **(D)** The metabolically active form of vitamin D (1,25-dihydroxycholecalciferol, or calcitriol) plays a major role in the control of calcium ion concentration in plasma. Calcitriol appears to enhance the intestinal absorption of calcium by stimulating formation of a calcium-binding protein that facilitates the absorption of calcium. Calcitriol also increases plasma calcium concentration through mobilization of calcium from bone. Parathyroid hormone appears to promote this action. Calcitriol's effect on the kidneys includes increased calcium and phosphate retention because of enhanced proximal tubular absorption. Negative feedback control of calcium homeostasis by calcitriol includes suppression of parathyroid hormone secretion and inhibition of renal activation of 25-hydroxycholecalciferol to calcitriol. Calcitriol has no effect on the formation or disposition of testosterone. *(DeLuca)*

667. **(D)** Placental transport of maternal substances is established by the fifth gestational week. Passage of substances occurs by simple passive diffusion. Substances that are of low molecular weight, high lipid solubility, and un-ionized are able to cross the placenta more rapidly. Protein binding determines the amount of drug available for diffusion. Drugs that are highly protein bound exhibit low concentrations in fetal tissues. Maternal BP does not influence transplacental transport of drugs. *(Craig and Stitzel, pp 37–38)*

668. **(A)** The un-ionized form of weak acids and bases undergoes passive reabsorption in the proximal and distal tubules. Because tubular cells are less permeable to the ionized form, reabsorption is pH dependent. When tubular urine is more acidic, weak bases are more ionized, passive reabsorption is reduced, and weak bases are excreted more rapidly. *(Craig and Stitzel, pp 21–24)*

669. **(D)** Clonidine stimulates α-adrenergic receptors centrally, causing a decrease in sympathetic outflow and a resultant decrease in blood pressure. The major action of hydralazine is direct relaxation of resistance vessels, with a greater effect on the arterioles than on the veins. Prazosin is an α-adrenergic blocking agent that acts on vascular smooth muscle and produces both venodilatation and arterial dilatation. Nitroprusside has a direct effect on vascular smooth muscle and dilates both resistance and capacitance vessels. Minoxidil relaxes vascular smooth muscle and produces vasodilatation. *(Craig and Stitzel, pp 276–298)*

670. **(C)** Spironolactone is a competitive antagonist of aldosterone. It binds to the receptor but evokes no response. Because aldosterone stimulates the reabsorption of Na^+ in exchange for K^+, the effect of the drug is to retain K^+. It is often used in combined therapy with other diuretics likely to cause hypokalemia. Theophylline is the only one of the drugs listed that is not used primarily as a diuretic, although this is one of its actions. *(Gilman et al, pp 725–726)*

671. **(E)** High serum calcium concentrations may produce metastic calcifications, renal damage, electrophysiologic disturbances, and various other nonspecific symptoms. Calcium excretion may be enhanced through increased sodium excretion. This may be accomplished through administration of normal saline or diuretics that promote calcium as well as sodium excretion (e.g., furosemide). Corticosteroids, such as prednisone, may correct hypercalcemia through decreasing vitamin D-mediated calcium absorption from the gastrointestinal tract. Mithramycin, an antitumor agent, inhibits bone resorption as well as exerts an anti-vitamin D effect. Dihydrotachysterol is a synthetic form of vitamin D. This agent would increase serum calcium concentrations. *(Lindeman and Papper)*

672. **(D)** Cocaine has two distinct pharmacologic actions. It is a potent local anesthetic as well as a CNS stimulant. Its local anesthetic activity makes this agent useful in surgical procedures involving the eyes and naso-oropharynx. Effects on the CNS progress from cortical excitement (resulting in euphoria, restlessness, and garrulousness) and respiratory stimulation with low doses to advanced stages of stimulation (e.g., tonic-clonic seizures) with high doses. Cardiovascular effects usually include a rise in blood pressure, particularly with higher doses. Mydriasis occurs presumably through potentiation of sympathetic stimulation. *(Gilman et al, p 319)*

673. **(C)** The most common and distressing side effect of nonsteroidal anti-inflammatory agents is gastrointestinal complaints. Of those persons taking ibuprofen, 5 to 15 percent have symptoms referable to the digestive system. A similar incidence has been observed for naproxen. Toxic amblyopia is an unusual complication of ibuprofen therapy. Edema formation and renal failure have uncommonly been associated with both drugs. Drowsiness is an extremely rare side effect. *(Craig and Stitzel, p 579)*

674. **(C)** In other respects, the action of levorphanol is similar to that of morphine. Thus, it depresses respiration, causes a histamine-mediated bronchoconstriction that makes it an inadvisable drug for asthmatics, produces a variety of allergic reactions, and like all opioid agonists, is blocked by naloxone. *(Gilman et al, p 504)*

675. **(A)** Therapeutic plasma phenytoin levels range from 10 to 20 μg/ml. Above 20 μg/ml, dose-related cerebellar–vestibular effects occur. At concentrations of 20 μg/ml, nystagmus is initially observed. Ataxia is observed at levels of 30 μg/ml, and at 40 μg/ml, lethargy is noted. Increased frequency of seizures also has occurred at very high plasma levels. *(Gilman et al, p 443)*

676. **(E)** The use of cimetidine has been associated with a decrease in the hepatic metabolism of various drugs, including warfarin, diazepam, and theophylline. Cimetidine has been noted to cause gynecomastia, presumably by elevating prolactin levels. Suppressed spermatogenesis also has been observed. A broad range of CNS problems, including dizziness, confusion, lethargy, and coma, has been observed, particularly in patients with pre-existing renal disease. Relapse of ulcer symptoms has prompted the use of low-dose maintenance cimetidine therapy in selected patients. *(Katzung, p 890)*

677. **(E)** Pharmacotherapy of the complex syndrome of bronchial asthma is aimed at reversing the bronchospasm, bronchial edema, and mucosal hypersecretion that are associated with the disease. Much of this pathophysiology is the result of altered autonomic control of the airways as well as contributions of chemical mediators from resident pulmonary and inflammatory cells. Airway smooth muscle appears to have a predominance of $β_2$-receptors, and such agents as isoproterenol are useful in dilating constricted airways and relieving some of the symptoms. Propranolol, a nonselective β-antagonist, is contraindicated in asthma. Recently developed β-agonists with improved selectivity for $β_2$-receptors include terbutaline and albuterol. Theophylline, or its more soluble derivative, aminophylline, also is useful in the treatment of asthma. Although xanthine derivatives are the drug of choice for many forms of asthma, their mechanisms remain obscure and probably involve (1) phosphodiesterase inhibition, (2) adenosine antagonism, (3) inhibition of other mediator release, and (4) increased sympathetic activity. Ipratropium bromide is a quaternary isopropyl derivative of atropine, which when administered by inhalation, relaxes bronchial smooth muscle by virtue of its antimuscarinic effects. Cromolyn sodium (disodium cromoglycate) is not a bronchodilator but is effective in asthma by preventing the release of chemical mediators from various cell types, including the mast cell. Cromolyn is effective only when used prophylactically and thus is of no value for reversal of acute episodes of asthma. *(Craig and Stitzel, pp 601–612)*

678. (A) In general, epinephrine decreases peripheral resistance because of the stimulation of β_2-receptors in skeletal muscle blood vessels, resulting in vasodilatation in these beds. Cardiac rate rises as a direct result of β_1 stimulation. Systolic blood pressure rises because of positive inotropic and chronotropic effects, as well as precapillary vasoconstriction. Myocardial stimulation increases oxygen consumption. Insulin secretion is inhibited as a result of β stimulation, and glucose levels rise. *(Gilman et al, pp 192–196)*

679. (E) Since the depth of anesthesia varies directly with tension of the agent in the CNS and since, for most agents, tension in the brain is always approaching tension in the arterial blood, several kinetic factors will influence the uptake and distribution of inhalational anesthetics. The more soluble an anesthetic is in blood, the slower is the approach of blood tension to that of inhaled gases. Therefore, methoxyflurane levels will rise slower than enflurane levels. At equilibrium, the partial pressure of drug in the lung is near that in the brain, and conventional dosage comparisons are made using MAC (minimal concentration of anesthetic at 1 atm that produces immobility in 50 percent of patients). Accordingly, a lower MAC value is indicative of a more potent drug. As a sole agent, nitrous oxide is used to provide some degree of analgesia (e.g., in dental procedures). However, at concentrations that are not associated with intolerable levels of tissue hypoxia, nitrous oxide by itself is not an effective anesthetic. Halothane hepatitis is a highly unusual toxic effect of the drug, which appears to be greater during repeated administrations of halothane over a short period of time. The incidence is extraordinarily low and has not precluded the use of this standard halogenated hydrocarbon for anesthetic purposes. Indeed, there is little real choice among halothane, enflurane, isoflurane, and methoxyflurane. All are associated with significant dose-de-

pendent decreases in systemic blood pressure. Enflurane was originally developed to avoid repeated administration of halothane and, for this and more subtle reasons, has become increasingly popular for anesthetic procedures. Isoflurane was introduced in 1981 and, aside from economic considerations, has become popular in anesthetic procedures, since depth of anesthesia can be adjusted rapidly, cardiac output is well maintained, and arrhythmias are uncommon. *(Gilman et al, pp 271–278)*

680. (B) Administration of glucocorticoids leads to an increase in the number of polymorphonuclear leukocytes in the blood, whereas the numbers of lymphocytes, eosinophils, monocytes, and basophils decreases. Neutrophilic leukocytosis is due to the release of mature neutrophils from the bone marrow. The lymphopenia associated with glucocorticoid use is due to a redistribution of the circulating lymphocytes to sites outside the intravascular compartment. Monocytopenia and eosinopenia are produced in the same fashion. *(Craig and Stitzel, pp 860–861)*

681. (C) The bioavailability of various oral ferrous salts is relatively similar, and the oral route is a reliable method of administration in most cases. Ferrous sulfate is less expensive than the other forms, however, and should be considered the treatment of choice. In those rare situations when the oral route cannot be used, parenteral iron dextran may be used. Its use is sometimes hampered by severe allergic and local reactions, precluding its routine use. *(Gilman et al, pp 1288–1292)*

682. (E) The duration of action of various insulin preparations is related to the rate of absorption from the SC injection site. Binding with various proteins, such as protamine or globin, results in slower absorption of insulin. Preparations with large insulin crystals and high zinc content are also slowly absorbed. Ultralente insulin has a particularly long duration of action (approximately 36 hr) for the latter reasons. Regular insulin and semilente insulin are fast-acting insulins, with duration of action ranging from 6 to 14 hr. Intermediate-acting preparations with duration of action of approximately 24 hr include NPH insulin, lente insulin, and globin zinc insulin. *(Gilman et al, pp 1475–1477)*

683. (C) Streptomycin is absorbed poorly by the gut mucosa and is usually administered by IV or IM injection. In the treatment of existing tuberculosis, a combination of drugs is used to offer continued protection should mycobacterial strains develop that are resistant to one drug. Although streptomycin has bacteriostatic, possibly even bactericidal, effects on the tubercle bacillus, its

mode of administration is a negative feature and, in long-term therapy, can lead to poor patient compliance. *(Gilman et al, pp 1153–1154)*

684. **(C)** Lovastatin (Mevinolin) is a recently approved drug that is a fungal inhibitor of cholesterol biosynthesis. It is a competitive, reversible, highly specific antagonist of HMG-CoA reductase, and in patients with heterozygous familial hypercholesterolemia, lovastatin lowers plasma low-density lipoprotein (LDL) by enhancing receptor-mediated degradation of lipoprotein. Nicotinic acid decreases the production of very low-density lipoprotein (VLDL), which in turn reduces production of its daughter particle, LDL. The mechanism by which this occurs is unclear and may be related to inhibition of lipolysis in adipose tissue, decreased esterification of triglycerides in the liver, and increased activity of lipoprotein lipase. Regardless, nicotinic acid does not affect synthesis of cholesterol or alter excretion of bile acids. Clofibrate reduces plasma triglyceride levels by lowering levels of VLDL. Although sites of action of clofibrate are only partially established, its primary effect is to increase the activity of lipoprotein lipase. Gemfibrozil is a congener of clofibrate that lowers VLDL in an undetermined manner but perhaps by hastening its secretion, since gemfibrozil does not affect lipoprotein lipase activity. Regardless of this lack of information, the net effect of gemfibrozil is to raise, not lower, HDL concentrations. Cholestyramine is a bile acid-binding resin that reduces the concentration of cholesterol in plasma by lowering the level of LDL. These resins are limited to an intestinal disposition where they hasten the excretion of neutral sterols as well as bile acids. Loss of these two substances results in compensatory changes in hepatic metabolism, including increase in number of cell-surface LDL receptors. This compensatory increase accounts for reduction in circulating concentrations of LDL. *(Gilman et al, pp 881–886)*

685. **(D)** The calcium in calcium disodium edetate is readily displaced by heavy metals, such as lead, forming stable complexes (chelates), which are excreted in the urine. Calcium disodium EDTA will bind in vivo any available divalent or trivalent metal that has a greater affinity for EDTA than has calcium. Mobilization and excretion of lead indicate that the metal is accessible to EDTA. Mercury poisoning does not respond to EDTA in vivo. *(Gilman et al, pp 1607–1608)*

686–689. **(686-A, 687-C, 688-D, 689-E)** Proprietary laxatives are traditionally classified into bulk laxatives, lubricants, stimulants, stool softeners, and osmotic laxatives. Bulk-forming preparations, which expand and soften the stool via their ability to retain water, include such preparations as bran and psyllium. Lubricants, such as mineral oil, have no pharmacologic effect on the gut and simply lubricate the passage of stool. Bisacodyl is a stimulant-type laxative. Its effect was believed to be due to the initiation of peristalsis in the colon but may be more closely related to the intraluminal accumulation of water. Additional stimulant-type laxatives include phenolphthalein, senna, cascara, danthron, and castor oil. Docusate is an anionic detergent that softens the stool by net water accumulation in the intestine. Osmotic laxatives are believed to hold water in the lumen by an osmotic action. Lactulose is a disaccharide compound that is broken down by colonic bacteria to form osmotically active molecules. Magnesium salts (magnesium sulfate and magnesium citrate) also act as osmotic laxatives. *(Thompson)*

690–692. **(690-D, 691-B, 692-A)** Rifampin inhibits DNA-dependent RNA polymerase and thus blocks RNA synthesis. The mechanism is only effective in prokaryotes, since nuclear RNA polymerase from eukaryotic cells does not bind rifampin. The tetracyclines bind to the 30S subunit of the ribosome and prevent access of tRNA to the mRNA–ribosome complex. Vancomycin inhibits formation of the bacterial cell wall by binding to the terminal carboxyl group on the D-alanyl-D-alanine terminus of the N-acetylglucosamine N-acetylmuramic acid peptide and prevents polymerization of the peptidoglycan. *(Gilman et al, pp 1118,1139,1150)*

693–696. **(693-D, 694-C, 695-A, 696-B)** Effector cells that are stimulated by the sympathetic nervous system contain α and β receptors. Agonists that affect these receptors themselves are termed direct agonists. Methoxamine is a direct agonist of α-adrenergic receptors. Isoproterenol is a direct β agonist. Some sympathomimetic agents act indirectly by displacing norepinephrine onto adrenergic receptors from storage sites in adrenergic nerve endings. Amphetamine acts in this way. α-Adrenergic and β-adrenergic blocking agents bind to adrenergic receptors and, therefore, interfere with the effects of sympathomimetic agents. Propranolol is the prototype β blocker, and phenoxybenzamine is an α blocker. *(Gilman et al, pp 187–240)*

697–701. **(697-C, 698-A, 699-D, 700-B, 701-E)** Cyclophosphamide causes hemorrhagic cystitis in 5 to 10 percent of users. This is probably caused by chemical irritation, and it is recommended that persons who take this drug have ample fluid intake and void frequently. The toxicity associated with vincristine characteristically involves neuropathies, including paresthesias, neuritic pain, loss of deep tendon reflexes, muscle weakness that may cause footdrop and inability to walk, headache, and double vision. Doxorubicin causes either acute or chronic cardiomyopathy. The acute form is characterized by abnormal ECG changes, including ST-T–wave alterations and arrhythmias. The chronic toxicity is a cumulative, dose-related toxicity manifested by congestive heart failure that is unresponsive to digitalis. The unique toxicity associated with bleomycin is pulmonary fibrosis, the incidence of which increases with doses larger than 400 units and in patients older than 70 yr who suffer underlying pulmonary disease. Cisplatin may cause unilateral or bilateral hearing loss or tinnitus. (Gilman et al, pp 1217–1253)

702–704.   (702-C, 703-A, 704-D) The agents listed affect cholinergic transmission in different manners, and their clinical use is in large part a manifestation of their cholinergic effect. Pilocarpine is a naturally occurring alkaloid that is cholinomimetic in effect and acts predominantly at muscarinic sites. In mimicking the effect of acetylcholine, it will cause pupillary constriction, spasm of accommodation, and a transient rise in intraocular pressure that is followed by a prolonged and greater decrease in intraocular pressure. Small doses of pilocarpine are associated with bradycardia and arousal. Atropine is the prototypic antimuscarinic agent, and by competitively blocking the effect of acetylcholine at muscarinic receptors, atropine usually is associated with tachycardia. Central effects of low doses of atropine usually include excitation. Atropine causes mydriasis and cycloplegia but does little to intraocular pressure, with the exception of increasing it in patients with narrow-angle glaucoma. Succinylcholine is the typical depolarizing neuromuscular blocker that produces fasciculation of muscle followed by total paralysis. Succinylcholine may raise intraocular pressure by contracting extraocular muscles and may cause bradycardia because of stimulation of vagal ganglion. Although tachycardia is possible (via stimulation of sympathetic ganglion) after succinylcholine, it is unlikely. None of the drugs listed have appreciable effects on the activity of acetylcholinesterase, the enzyme responsible for hydrolysis of acetylcholine as well as pilocarpine and succinylcholine. Typical inhibitors of cholinesterase are physostigmine, neostigmine, edrophonium, and diisopropyl fluorophosphate. (Gilman et al, pp 122–127)

705–710.   (705-A, 706-B, 707-B, 708-C, 709-D, 710-E) Antineoplastic agents are divided into several pharmacologic classes. The plant alkaloids are derived from the periwinkle plant, and they impair the synthesis of cellular microtubules. Vincristine and vinblastine are two clinically useful plant alkaloids. Antimetabolites interfere with the synthesis of new nucleic acids in actively dividing cells. Methotrexate, 5-fluorouracil, and 6-mercaptopurine are examples of antimetabolites. Alkylating agents form covalent bonds with nucleic acids, thus interfering with their action. Mechlorethamine, cyclophosphamide, chlorambucil, melphalan, and dacarbazine are examples of alkylating agents. Antibiotics, such as doxorubicin, mithramycin, and bleomycin, are useful anticancer agents because they can inhibit DNA and RNA synthesis. Tamoxifen is an antiestrogen used in treating breast cancer. (Gilman et al, pp 1209–1263)

711–715.   (711-A, 712-E, 713-D, 714-B, 715-C) Bronchodilator drugs are the mainstay of therapy for patients with bronchial asthma. Bronchodilators exert their antibronchoconstrictor effect via different mechanisms. β-Adrenergic receptor agonists such as epinephrine, isoproterenol, and terbutaline activate the enzyme adenylate cyclase, which increases the intracellular concentration of cyclic-AMP. The result is bronchodilation. Terbutaline has the advantage of being specific for β_2 adrenergic receptors and therefore produces less cardiac stimulation than epinephrine or isoproterenol. Theophylline is a methylxanthine derivative that inhibits the enzyme (phosphodiesterase) that metabolizes cyclic AMP. However, current studies suggest its mechanism of action may be inhibition of adenosine. Ipratropium bromide inhibits cholinergic receptors which play a role in initiating bronchoconstriction in response to irritant chemicals. (Craig and Stitzel, pp 604–609)

716–720.   (716-A, 717-E, 718-C, 719-A, 720-D) Cyclophosphamide must be activated by the P_{450} mixed function oxidase system in the liver to form 4-hydroxycyclophosphamide, which is in a steady state, and the acyclic tautomer, aldophosphamide. In cells, the latter is converted to acrolin, which is thought to result in damage to the bladder mucosa, leading to cystitis. Methotrexate, a folate analog, has as its mechanism of action the blockade of purine synthesis. Therefore, it is effective only during those phases of the cell growth cycle during which DNA synthesis occurs. One benefit of prednisone is that it is effective in treating hemolytic anemia and the hemorrhage associated with thrombocytopenia induced by malignant lymphomas and chronic lymphocytic leukemia. Hot flashes are associated with the antiestrogen effects of tamoxifen. (Gilman et al, pp 1209–1257)

721–725.   (721-A, 722-C, 723-A, 724-A, 725-B) Organic nitrates such as nitroglycerin, β-blockers such as propranolol, and calcium channel blockers including diltiazem are used in the management of angina pectoris. Nitrates mimic the actions of nitiric oxide in stimulating the enzyme gyanylyl cyclase, which, through a series of steps, facilitates the relaxation of vascular smooth muscle. Vasodilation decreases the preload and afterload of the heart, thus decreasing oxygen demand and consequently, angina. Decreased blood pressure in response to organic nitrates, however, may also result in reflex tachycardia. β-Blockers, such as propranolol, prevent the receptor mediated stimulation of adenylate cyclase, which ultimately results in a decrease in the force of contraction of the heart and hence decreased oxygen demand. Calcium is a key regulatory component for both smooth and cardiac muscle contraction. By blocking calcium entry, diltiazem can induce vasodilatation and also reduce myocardial contractility. *(Katzung, pp 162–173)*

726–730. (726-C, 727-B, 728-A, 729-C, 730-A) Nonsteroidal anti-inflammatory drugs (NSAID) have as their primary mechanism of action the inhibition of prostaglandin synthesis via inhibition of the enzyme cyclooxygenase. However, the particular agents differ in their potency, therapeutic effects, and toxicity. Indomethacin is one of the most potent NSAIDs. Its anti-inflammatory and analgesic properties has made it especially effective in the treatment of acute gout. Moreover, its application as an inhibitor of the prostaglandins responsible for maintaining the patency of ductus arteriosus in newborns has resulted in a significant reduction in the need for surgical repair of this lesion. Aspirin, the prototype for this class of drugs, through its ability to inhibit platelet TXA_2, prolongs bleeding time and is under investigation for the treatment of disorders associated with thrombi such as myocardial infarction and stroke. Aspirin toxicity is characterized by a syndrome, Salicylism, which includes ringing of the ears (tinnitus) as one of its symptoms. Acetaminophen has only weak activity as a prostaglandin synthesis inhibitor and, as a consequence, has no significant anti-inflammatory action. *(Smith and Reynard, pp 410–431)*

731–735. (731-C, 732-B, 733-A, 734-D, 735-E) Both clindamycin and tetracycline bind to bacterial ribosomes and inhibit protein synthesis of the bacteria. Clindamycin binds to the 50 S subunit where it inhibits a translocation step in peptide synthesis. Tetracycline binds to the 30 S subunit and prevents the addition of amino acids to peptide chains in the process of formation. Tetracycline requires an active transport mechanism to reach its site of action, and the inhibition of its transport is one mechanism of bacterial resistance to this drug. The β-lactam structure of penicillin plays a central role in the inhibition of the bacterial cell wall synthesis. Sulfamethoxazole is a competitive antagonist of para-aminobenzoic acid, a metabolic precursor of folic acid, which is required for purine synthesis. Sulfamethoxazole has

increased in use since it was found to be very effective when administered in combination with another antibiotic, trimethoprim. Dapsone is a drug with a mechanism of action similar to sulfamethoxazole, and is used in the treatment of leprosy. *(Gilman et al, pp 1065–1135,1159)*

736. (A) Lidocaine is beneficial in preventing ventricular arrhythmia during myocardial infarction (MI). Moreover, it is relatively safe for patients during the acute phase of this condition since it lacks significant depressant effects on the cardiovascular system and has a short duration of action. During acute MI, digoxin may promote arrhythmia; quinidine, fecanide, and propranolol are generally not used during the acute phase of MI. *(Craig and Stitzel, p 349)*

737. (B) Thiabendazole has a high degree of activity against a wide variety of nematodes, including those of the genera *Ascaris, Enterobius, Strongyloides,* and *Trichuris.* Although thiabendazole is useful in treating patients with multiple infections, it would not be the agent of choice in treating single infections with either *Ascaris* or *E. vermicularis* because of its potential for adverse reactions. Pyrantel pamoate is also a broad-spectrum anthelminthic that is effective against these nematodes. Side effects, which occur only occasionally, include gastrointestinal upset, headache, or dizziness. Tetrachloroethylene is useful in the treatment of hookworm but is seldom used, since more effective and less toxic agents are available. Trivalent antimonials such as antimony potassium tartrate are also not used because of unacceptable toxicity. Diethylcarbamazine is used primarily in the treatment of filariae of the genus *Wuchereria.* (Gilman et al, pp 971–974)

738. (D) Vestibular, auditory, and optic nerve toxicity have been reported as side effects of the administration of aminoglycosides. Although early toxicity may be reversible, once sensory cells are lost, regeneration does not occur. Moreover, high concentrations of aminoglycosides may accumulate in the renal cortex. Prolonged therapy with excessively high trough concentrations correlates with the development of both ototoxicity and nephrotoxicity. Nephrotoxicity usually is expressed as acute tubular necrosis, which first becomes detectable after 5 to 7 days of administration. Unlike ototoxicity and optic nerve damage, nephrotoxicity is usually reversible. Neuromuscular blockade has been reported following intrapleural and intraperitoneal instillation of aminoglycosides as well as from IV, IM, and oral administration. This symptom is seen most commonly in association with anesthesia or other neuroblocking agents. Streptomycin, in particular, may affect optic nerve function, and scotomas, which present as enlargement of the blind spot, have been reported. Hepatic failure has not been associated with the administration of this class of antibiotic. (Gilman et al, pp 1104–1108)

739. **(D)** Propranolol is a non-selective β-adrenergic antagonist blocking both β_1- and β_2-adrenergic receptor subtypes. As an antiarrhythmic drug, it is used primarily to treat arrhythmias of atrial origin such as supraventricular tachycardia, atrial fibrillation, or atrial flutter. The mechanism of this action is antagonism of adrenergic tone at the AV node, thereby increasing its refractoriness. Propranolol can also be effective in migraine prophylaxis, although the mechanism for this benefit is unknown. Seventy percent of patients with migraine experience fewer or less severe attacks following daily administration of propranolol. (Gilman et al, pp 865–866,946)

740. **(C)** A high proportion of oxygen (70 percent) is extracted from the coronary circulation under normal circumstances, and drugs have little effect on this component of oxygen utilization. The major benefit of antianginal drugs is their ability to reduce the oxygen demand of the heart by reducing cardiac work load. This is accomplished through vasodilation (organic nitrates, calcium channel blockers), or decreased heart rate and force of contraction (β-blockers, calcium channel blockers). Secondarily, angina can be alleviated by increasing the supply of oxygen to the heart by the selective dilation of large epicardial coronary blood vessels (nitrates). Finally, the ability of some nitrates to inhibit platelet aggregation may also result in a decrease in angina in some forms of ischemic heart disease. (Gilman et al, pp 764–781)

741. **(B)** The mechanism by which propranolol relieves hypertension is not fully understood, but is probably related to its blockade of β-receptors. The release of renin from the juxtaglomerular apparatus of the kidney is mediated by β-adrenergic receptors, and propranolol seems to be especially effective in patients with hypertension associated with elevated plasma renin levels. Propranolol in therapeutic doses does not significantly affect α-adrenergic receptors, depletion of amines, or the reuptake of norepinephrine. Propranolol would tend to induce up regulation of β-adrenergic receptors rather than down regulation. (Gilman et al, p 232)

742. **(A)** Barbiturates induce P_{450} microsomal enzymes of the liver and, thereby, increase the clearance of anticoagulants. Aspirin, phenylbutazone, and ibuprophen increase the response of oral anticoagulants by displacing them from plasma proteins. Cimetidine increases the potency of oral anticoag-

ulants by inhibiting the hepatic enzymes which metabolize them. (Craig and Stitzel, pp 376–377)

743. **(E)** The six major manifestations of plumbism (chronic lead poisoning) are gastrointestinal, neuromuscular, CNS, hematologic, renal, and miscellaneous symptoms. Intestinal symptoms consist of anorexia and constipation. Lead palsy, as the neuromuscular syndrome is sometimes called, is progressive, initially resulting in muscle weakness and fatigue and eventually producing paralysis. Encephalopathic symptoms, more common in children, include loss of motor skills, vertigo, ataxia, insomnia, restlessness, and, progressively, seizures. Punctate basophilic stippling is the hematologic hallmark of chronic lead ingestion. Progressive and irreversible renal insufficiency may result as well. Miscellaneous symptoms, such as pallor, gingival lead line, and emaciation, have been observed. Skin rashes are not noted. (Craig and Stitzel, pp 102–103)

744. **(C)** The rate at which a new plateau is reached is independent of dose administered and solely a function of the half-life of the drug. The actual plateau concentration depends only on clearance and the dosage administered per dosing interval and is independent of the half-life of the drug. Fluctuations in concentration during given intervals are proportional to the ratio of dosage interval to half-time; halving both the dose and dosage interval will produce a smoother rise to plateau concentration, with blunted fluctuations, but the actual plateau concentration will be unchanged. The mean plateau plasma concentration of a drug is a function of the dose administered and not whether it was administered in a constant infusion or multiple doses. (Gilman et al, pp 25–28)

745. **(A)** The major advantage of combining a decarboxylase inhibitor (carbidopa) with levodopa is that more levodopa is available for CNS penetration. In addition, far fewer gastrointestinal effects are observed, and interference by pyridoxine is avoided. The time for titration is reduced, since the limiting gastrointestinal side effects are diminished. Adverse cardiovascular effects of levodopa are also decreased. However, CNS side effects remain and may even develop earlier in the course of treatment and be more pronounced. (Gilman et al, p 471)

746. **(D)** Prostacyclin is a short-lived product of arachidonic acid metabolism. Prostacyclin is a very potent vasodilator in most systemic vascular beds and therefore increases renal blood flow. It is also an inhibitor of platelet aggregation. Since vascular endothelium is capable of synthesizing PGI_2, it has been suggested that it plays a role in maintaining vascular patency via these 2 mechanisms.

In addition, PGI_2 is cytoprotective and is capable of inhibiting gastric ulceration by inhibiting the volume of secretion, acidity, and pepsin content. This effect is useful in counteracting the gastrointestinal ulcerative effects of nonsteroidal anti-inflammatory drugs. *(Gilman et al, pp 605–607)*

747. **(C)** ECG effects of digitalis glycosides include prolongation of the PR interval, T wave inversion, ST segment depression, and shortening of the QT interval. The QRS complex duration does not increase, even during toxicity. If this should occur, other causes, such as conduction defects, should be sought. *(Gilman et al, p 824)*

748. **(A)** Leukotrienes are thiolether-linked lipoxygenase metabolites of arachidonic acid. They appear to play a critical role in bronchospasm, edema, and mucous hypersecretion common to many forms of asthma. Among their profound cardiovascular effects is their ability to constrict coronary arteries, supporting a potential role for leukotrienes in shock and myocardial ischemia. Most commonly used nonsteroidal anti-inflammatory drugs, such as aspirin, do not affect lipoxygenase activity, and there are suggestions that by inhibiting cyclooxygenase activity, aspirin's net effect is to direct arachidonic acid through the lipoxygenase pathway. Platelets do not contain 5'-lipoxygenase (although they do contain 12'-lipoxygenase), and leukotrienes are not stored in platelet granules. The cyclooxygenase product of arachidonic acid, TXA_2, is critical in platelet physiology, and acetylation of this enzyme by aspirin accounts for the effect of this drug in inhibiting platelet function. LTB_4 is a potent chemotactic agent for polymorphonuclear leukocytes, but not for the other leukotrienes. *(Gilman et al, pp 605–610)*

749. **(D)** Agents used in the treatment of gout may be classified by their ability to decrease the production of uric acid or increase its excretion. Allopurinol and its metabolite, oxypurinol, inhibit the enzyme xanthine oxidase. This enzyme is responsible for the conversion of hypoxanthine and xanthine to uric acid. Probenecid and sulfinpyrazone are uricosuric agents that promote renal excretion of uric acid. Cholchicine inhibits the migration of granulocytes into acutely inflamed gouty tissue. Indomethacin does not affect uric acid levels, but its anti-inflammatory and analgesic properties are useful in relieving the symptoms of this condition. *(Craig and Stitzel, pp 594–600)*

750. **(B)** α-Adrenergic blocking effects are frequently observed after therapy with the phenothiazine or butyrophenone antipsychotic agents. Chlorpromazine may cause orthostatic hypotension or reflex tachycardia because of the combination of α-adrenergic blockade and central actions of the drug. Meprobamate, benzodiazepines, or fluoxetine have little or no α-adrenergic blocking activity. *(Gilman et al, pp 393)*

751. **(E)** Tumors have a wide range of mechanisms by which they can resist the effects of antineoplastic agent. Among these are increases in target enzymes or alterations in the structure of target enzymes, which decreases the affinity of the drug for the enzyme. This mechanism is seen most frequently with antimetabolite drugs such as methotrexate. Some tumor cells have genes that decrease the uptake or enhance the elimination of anticancer drugs. This form of resistance is termed pleiotropic, or multidrug resistance, and is effective against such drugs as the anthracyclines, vinca alkaloids, and dactinomycin. Tumors that are heterogeneous tend to be more resistant to drug therapy because a wide variety of cell types tends to increase the probability of cells with resistant mechanisms. *(Craig and Stitzel, pp 779–780)*

752. **(D)** Streptokinase forms a complex with plasminogen, activating the protease to form plasmin. Plasmin is a protease that digests fibrin clots. Increased plasmin can also cause the depletion of α_2-antiplasmin, an inhibitor of plasmin. *(Gilman et al, p 1323)*

753. **(A)** GABA is the major inhibitory neurotransmitter in the CNS. Diazepam enhances the action of GABA in a number of ways. It increases the binding of GABA to its receptor. This receptor, and the binding site of diazepam, are both associated with the GABA-gated chloride channel and modulate it, causing an influx of chloride ions that results in hyperpolarization of the cell. By these mechanisms, and possibly others, diazepam reduces repetitive neuronal firing. It has no action on serotonin binding. *(Katzung, pp 311–312)*

754. **(B)** Oral anticoagulants interfere with hepatic synthesis of the vitamin-K dependent clotting factors. These factors (II, VII, IX, and X) appear in the form of their biologically inactive precursors after the administration of oral anticoagulants. In this precursor form, they are unable to bind calcium or phospholipid, which is the usual site of activation. *(Gilman et al, 1317–1319)*

755. **(E)** Most bacterial resistance to aminoglycosides occurs by enzymatic inactivation by multiple enzymes located in the bacterial membrane. These enzymes inactivate aminoglycosides by phosphorylation, acetylation, or adenylation. Amikacin, however, is resistant to inactivation, with acetylation being the only mechanism of bacterial enzymatic resistance. *(Gilman et al, p 1101)*

756. (C) Local anesthetics inhibit sensory nerve conduction via blockade of voltage sensitive sodium channels. As a result of this blockade, the threshold of excitability of the nerve is increased and the ability of the nerve to propagate an action potential is decreased. Ultimately, the transmission of sensory stimuli to the CNS is suppressed. *(Gilman et al, 312–313)*

757. (D) In an individual severely poisoned by antihistamines, the central effects, both the depressant and stimulant actions, cause the greatest danger. There is no specific therapy for poisoning, and treatment is usually supportive. In a child, the dominant effect is excitation, and hallucinations, ataxia, incoordination, athetosis, and convulsions may occur. Symptoms such as fixed and dilated pupils, a flushed face, and fever are common and markedly resemble those of atropine poisoning. Deepening coma and cardiorespiratory collapse characterize terminal poisoning. Fever and flushing generally are not manifestations of antihistamine poisoning in adults. *(Gilman et al, pp 586–587)*

758. (D) The course of acute acetaminophen overdose follows a fairly consistent pattern. During the initial 24 hr, nausea, vomiting, anorexia, and abdominal pain occur. Indications of hepatic damage become evident, biochemically, within 2 to 6 days of ingestion of toxic doses. Prominent increases in alkaline phosphatase are common. The hepatotoxicity may precipitate jaundice and coagulation disorders and progress to encephalopathy, coma, and death. Tinnitus, or ringing in the ears, is a feature of chronic salicylate intoxication and is not encountered in acetaminophen overdose. *(Gilman et al, pp 658–659)*

759. (C) Chronic abuse of sedative-hypnotics (e.g., barbiturates) results in drug tolerance to other agents within this class by (1) enhanced metabolism of similar agents and (2) cross-pharmacodynamic tolerance. Cross-tolerance by a pharmacodynamic mechanism has implications in the clinical management of withdrawal symptoms or detoxification. Patients who chronically abuse short-acting barbiturates, benzodiazepines (e.g., secobarbital, diazepam), or alcohol may undergo detoxification using a longer-acting agent, such as phenobarbital. Cross-tolerance does not extend to opiates. Sedative-hypnotics may be useful in symptomatic management of symptoms associated with withdrawal from opiates. *(Khantzian and McKenna)*

760. (C) The elimination of drugs that are weak acids or bases can be enhanced by altering the pH of the urine to cause the drug to shift to its ionized form. Thus, for drugs that are weak acids, raising the pH of the urine via the administration of bicarbonate would enhance elimination. The blood, however, is well buffered and it would be difficult (and medically unwise) to alter its pH. Increasing the concentration of organic acids in the urine would lower its pH and would therefore retard the elimination of a weak acid. *(Smith and Reynard, p 29)*

761. (E) Nephrotoxicity associated with gentamicin therapy resembles acute tubular necrosis. Manifestations include the inability to concentrate urine, proteinuria, casts in the urine, and increased plasma creatine. Rising trough concentrations appear to be an early indicator of renal damage. If gentamicin is discontinued, damage is reversible. *(Gilman et al, p 1106)*

762. (C) Parkinson's disease appears to be caused by a relative deficiency of dopamine in the basal ganglia of the brain. Levodopa, a precursor of dopamine, is transported into the CNS, where it is decarboxylated to form dopamine. Peripheral decarboxylation wastes a significant amount of absorbed levodopa and also causes peripheral side effects (e.g., cardiac arrhythmias, nausea, and vomiting). Although levodopa is effective when used alone, peripheral conversion to dopamine may be inhibited by administration of carbidopa, a dopa-decarboxylase inhibitor. Carbidopa does not cross the blood-brain barrier and thus has no effect on conversion of levodopa to dopamine in the brain. Inhibition of peripheral destruction of levodopa allows a larger and more predictable proportion to enter the brain. *(Boshes)*

BIBLIOGRAPHY

Boshes BB. Sinemet and the treatment of Parkinson's. *Ann Intern Med.* March 1981; 364–370

Covino BJ. Pharmacology of local anesthetics. *Rational Drug Ther.* 1987; 21:1–8

Craig CR, Stitzel RE, eds. *Modern Pharmacology.* 3rd ed. Boston: Little, Brown and Co; 1990

DeLuca HF. Vitamin D metabolism and function. *Arch Intern Med.* 1978; 138:836

Freston JW. Cimetidine. I. Developments, pharmacology, and efficacy. *Ann Intern Med.* October 1982; 573–580

Gilman AG, Goodman RW, Nies AS, Taylor P, eds. *The Pharmacological Basis of Therapeutics.* 8th ed. New York: Pergamon; 1990

Hollister LE. Treatment of depression with drugs. *Ann Intern Med.* July 1978; 78–84

Hollister LE. Perspectives and summary of aspirin/acetaminophen symposium. *Arch Intern Med.* February 23, 1981; 404–406

Katzung BG, ed. *Basic & Clinical Pharmacology.* 5th ed. Norwalk, CT: Appleton & Lange; 1992

Khantzian EJ, McKenna GJ. Acute toxic and withdrawal reactions associated with drug use and abuse. *Ann Intern Med.* 1979; 90:361

Lees KR. Angiotensin-converting enzyme inhibitors. *Rational Drug Ther.* 1988; 22:1–6

Levine J. Pain and analgesia: The outlook for more rational treatment. *Ann Intern Med.* February 1984; 269–276

Lewis JH, Zimmerman HJ, Ishak KG, Mullick FG. Enflurance hepatotoxicity: A clinicopathologic study of 24 cases. *Ann Intern Med.* June 1983; 984–992

Lindeman RD, Papper S. Therapy of fluid and electrolyte disorders. *Ann Intern Med.* January 1975; 64–70

Smith CM, Reynard AM, eds. *Textbook of Pharmacology.* Philadelphia: Saunders; 1992

Thompson WG. Laxatives: Clinical pharmacology and rational use. *Drugs.* January 1980; 49–58

Subspecialty List: Pharmacology

705. Chemotherapeutic agents (topical and systemic)
Antineoplastic and immunosuppressive drugs
706. Chemotherapeutic agents (topical and systemic)
Antineoplastic and immunosuppressive drugs
707. Chemotherapeutic agents (topical and systemic)
Antineoplastic and immunosuppressive drugs
708. Chemotherapeutic agents (topical and systemic)
Antineoplastic and immunosuppressive drugs
709. Chemotherapeutic agents (topical and systemic)
Antineoplastic and immunosuppressive drugs
710. Chemotherapeutic agents (topical and systemic)
Antineoplastic and immunosuppressive drugs
711. Respiratory system
712. Respiratory system
713. Respiratory system
714. Respiratory system
715. Respiratory system
716. Chemotherapeutic agents
Antineoplastic drugs
717. Chemotherapeutic agents
Antineoplastic drugs
718. Chemotherapeutic agents
Antineoplastic drugs
719. Chemotherapeutic agents
Antineoplastic drugs
720. Chemotherapeutic agents
Antineoplastic drugs
721. Cardiovascular and respiratory systems
722. Cardiovascular and respiratory systems
723. Cardiovascular and respiratory systems
724. Cardiovascular and respiratory systems
725. Cardiovascular and respiratory systems
726. Nonnarcotic analgesia
727. Nonnarcotic analgesia
728. Nonnarcotic analgesia
729. Nonnarcotic analgesia
730. Nonnarcotic analgesia
731. Antibiotics
732. Antibiotics
733. Antibiotics
734. Antibiotics
735. Antibiotics
736. Cardiovascular and respiratory systems
Antiarrhythmic agents
737. Chemotherapeutic agents
738. Chemotherapeutic agents
739. Cardiovascular and respiratory systems
740. Cardiovascular and respiratory systems
741. Cardiovascular system
742. Blood and blood-forming organs
743. Poisoning and therapy of intoxication
744. General principles
745. Central and peripheral nervous systems
746. Autacoids and prostaglandins
747. Cardiovascular and respiratory systems
748. Autacoids and prostaglandins
749. Kidneys, bladder, fluids, and electrolytes
Uricosurics
750. Central and peripheral nervous systems
751. Chemotherapeutic agents
752. Blood and blood-forming organs
753. CNS agents
754. Blood and blood-forming organs
755. Chemotherapeutic agents
756. Central and peripheral nervous systems
757. Poisoning and therapy of intoxication
758. Poisoning
759. CNS agents
760. General principles
761. Chemotherapeutic agents
Antibacterial drugs
762. CNS agents

Behavioral Sciences
Questions

DIRECTIONS (Questions 763 through 792): Each of the numbered items or incomplete statements in this section is followed by answers or by completions of the statement. Select the ONE lettered answer or completion that is BEST in each case.

763. A patient who is afraid of insects is first shown a picture of a butterfly. Next session, he is put in the same room as a bottle containing ants. This procedure may be an example of

   (A) biofeedback
   (B) shaping
   (C) desensitization
   (D) operant conditioning
   (E) stimulus generalization

764. The functions of the ego include all of the following EXCEPT

   (A) psychologic defense mechanisms
   (B) reality testing
   (C) thinking
   (D) perception
   (E) instinctual drives

765. In a prospective randomized study comparing drug A to placebo, by the luck of the draw, 80 of the 120 patients assigned to placebo were young and had relatively minor disease severity, whereas 80 of the 120 patients in the group assigned to drug A were older and more severely diseased. The authors report that 95 placebo-treated patients and 98 patients treated with drug A are alive at the end of 5 years. They calculate chi-square and report that drug A is no better than placebo. Which of the following statements is true?

   (A) Drug A is no more effective than placebo.
   (B) Matched pair analysis might demonstrate that drug A is better than placebo.
   (C) Since the patients were assigned by random allocation, it is not possible that the two

groups would vary so much in baseline characteristics.

   (D) Stratified analysis of the data might demonstrate that drug A is more effective than the placebo.
   (E) This is an example of β error.

766. In general, medical students experience all of the following EXCEPT

   (A) increasing identification with the medical profession
   (B) exposure to students from diverse backgrounds
   (C) increasing idealism throughout medical school
   (D) anxiety concerning evaluations and examinations
   (E) tendency for specialization

767. Which of the following statements concerning psychotherapy is correct?

   (A) Psychotherapy can be performed only by professionals with special training in an accredited psychoanalytic institute.
   (B) Reliving childhood experience is the fundamental objective of psychotherapy.
   (C) Physical examination may be psychotherapeutic.
   (D) Giving advice is countertherapeutic.
   (E) Insight is always the goal in psychotherapy.

768. A delusion may be distinguished from a hallucination on the basis of

   (A) consensual validation
   (B) perceptual experience
   (C) grandiosity
   (D) laboratory tests
   (E) intelligence tests

769. All of the following statements concerning the drug treatment of elderly patients is true EXCEPT that

(A) drug clearance may be delayed because of increased fat/muscle ratio

(B) there may be increased toxicity due to decreased plasma albumin levels

(C) excretion half-life of drugs may be increased because of decreased liver function

(D) there may be decreased extrapyramidal side effects with neuroleptics because of decreased nigrostriatal dopamine

(E) there may be increased sensitivity to anticholinergic drugs due to decreased CNS cholinergic functioning

770. Goslings that are exposed to humans early in life may follow them as if humans were their mothers. This conduct is an example of

(A) instrumental conditioning

(B) imprinting

(C) cognitive map

(D) instinctual behavior

(E) counterphobic behavior

771. The double line of authority in the hospital is most likely to cause a conflict between professional and administrative roles for

(A) physicians

(B) hospital administrators

(C) nurses

(D) patients

(E) hospital security officers

772. Assuming that 98 percent of all people with a particular illness, such as depression, will have positive results on a hypothetical new screening test and that 90 percent of all people without the illness will have a negative result, which of the following statements will be true when the test is used to screen a general population?

(A) Someone having a positive result has a 98 percent chance of having the illness.

(B) Someone having a negative result has a 2 percent chance of having the illness.

(C) Someone having a positive result has a 90 percent chance of having the illness.

(D) Ten percent of the people with negative results will have the illness.

(E) none of the above

773. During human development, the capacity to discriminate between different sounds can first be demonstrated

(A) in the newborn

(B) at 3 mo

(C) at 6 mo

(D) at 9 mo

(E) at 12 mo

774. Approximately what percentage of deaths among persons between 15 and 24 years of age is attributable to accidents, murder, and suicide?

(A) 10

(B) 20

(C) 40

(D) 60

(E) 75

775. The suicide rate is highest among

(A) boys between the ages of 11 and 14 yr

(B) girls between the ages of 15 and 19 yr

(C) boys between the ages of 15 and 19 yr

(D) girls between the ages of 11 and 14 yr

(E) women between the ages of 20 and 25 yr

776. Thirty seventh-grade students who scored in the lowest tenth percentile of their class on a reading examination are assigned to a special education class in reading for a year. At the end of the year, the reading scores of these students are significantly improved in comparison with the rest of the class. Which of the following threats to internal validity is most likely to account for the improvement?

(A) history

(B) testing

(C) statistical regression

(D) instrumentation

(E) maturation

777. Among children who are severely retarded, the percentage that shows some type of psychiatric disorder is

(A) 10

(B) 20

(C) 30

(D) 50

(E) 75

778. In a case-control study of the relationship between exposure to a suspected toxic substance and the development of a rare type of cancer, 16 of 20 cases were exposed to the substance, whereas only 20 of 80 controls were exposed. The relative risk of developing the cancer among exposed subjects is best estimated to be

(A) 0.32

(B) 3.20

(C) 12.00

(D) 12.80

(E) none of the above

779. The most effective antidepressant therapy is

(A) tricyclic antidepressants

(B) monoamine oxidase inhibitors

(C) lithium carbonate

(D) psychotherapy

(E) electroconvulsive therapy (ECT)

780. All of the following are examples of biofeedback EXCEPT

(A) electric shock given to a person when antisocial behavior is manifested

(B) electronic display of skin temperature

(C) a physician's telling a patient that, as a result of a diet, the patient's blood pressure (BP) is reduced

(D) electroconvulsive therapy (ECT) given to a depressed patient

(E) tension headache treated with electromyogram

781. Tardive dyskinesia may be caused by all of the following EXCEPT

(A) perphenazine

(B) amoxapine

(C) trifluoperazine

(D) clorazepate

(E) haloperidol

782. A 38-year-old woman tells her physician that for several months she has been experiencing palpitations, shortness of breath, and a feeling of impending doom. She also has episodes of dizziness and a feeling that she is going to drop dead. The physician's first course of action should be to

(A) provide psychotherapy

(B) treat the patient with benzodiazepines

(C) perform a physical examination

(D) refer the patient to a psychiatrist

(E) teach the patient self-hypnosis

783. A patient is convinced that an IV injection he received has made him immortal. This is an example of

(A) illusion

(B) delusion

(C) hallucination

(D) delirium

(E) euphoria

784. Drugs used in the treatment of schizophrenia have in common their ability to

(A) block α-adrenergic receptors in the locus ceruleus

(B) block dopamine receptors in the brain

(C) sensitize the dopamine receptors in the locus ceruleus

(D) increase functional levels of norepinephrine in the synapses

(E) increase serotonin synthesis in the CNS

785. All of the following have been implicated as possible neurotransmitters EXCEPT

(A) norepinephrine

(B) endorphins

(C) γ-aminobutyric acid (GABA)

(D) serum pepsinogen

(E) glycine

Questions 786 through 789

A 35-year-old man is admitted to the hospital for an elective operation. After a week's stay in the hospital, during which various examinations are performed, he receives general anesthesia for an abdominal operation. Two days after the operation, he becomes agitated, visibly tremulous, and seems to be hallucinating. He also accuses the nurses of being unsympathetic and uncaring, just like his own mother.

786. In relation to this patient's agitation and hallucination, a history of which of the following would have most immediate relevance in management plans?

(A) schizophrenic family members

(B) alcoholism

(C) LSD use

(D) depression

(E) traumatic early childhood

787. This patient's accusatory behavior toward the nurses may be attributed to all of the following EXCEPT

(A) transference

(B) displacement

(C) sublimation

(D) regression

(E) organic brain syndrome

788. If this patient's hallucinations are predominantly visual, the likelihood of which of the following diagnoses is increased?

(A) organic brain syndrome

(B) schizophrenia

(C) depressive syndrome

(D) anxiety neurosis

(E) transference neurosis

789. Which of the following is LEAST likely to be essential in formulating effective management plans for this patient?

(A) laboratory studies, e.g., electrolytes, blood urea nitrogen (BUN)

(B) chart review to determine intraoperative complications

(C) interview with the patient's mother to determine the quality of interaction in childhood

(D) interview with the patient to get a good description of the hallucinations

(E) interview with the patient's girl friend to determine drug and alcohol history

790. In the Isle of Wight study, the percentage of children who scored more than 2 standard deviations below the norm on the Wechsler Intelligence Scale for Children (WISC) was

(A) 1.25

(B) 2.51

(C) 5.12

(D) 8.40

(E) 12.05

791. An example of rapid-eye-movement (REM) sleep disorder may be

(A) narcolepsy

(B) epilepsy

(C) catalepsy

(D) polydipsia

(E) cachexia

792. All of the following are examples of biologic rhythms EXCEPT

(A) rapid-eye-movement (REM) sleep

(B) menstrual cycle

(C) vernal equinox

(D) basic rest–activity cycle

(E) depressive mood swings

DIRECTIONS (Questions 793 through 854): Each set of matching questions in this section consists of a list of up to six lettered options followed by several numbered items. For each item, select the ONE lettered option that is most closely associated with it. Each lettered heading may be selected once, more than once, or not at all.

Questions 793 through 801

For each item listed below, choose the brain wave or phenomenon with which it is usually associated.

(A) α wave

(B) β wave

(C) Δ wave

(D) rapid-eye-movement (REM) sleep

(E) cataplexy

793. Concentrating on mental arithmetic

794. Sudden loss of muscle tone

795. Non-REM (NREM) sleep

796. Sleepwalking

797. Irregular pulse rate and respiration

798. Visual dreams

799. Narcolepsy

800. Comatose state

801. Relaxed, awake state

Questions 802 through 804

For each study design described below, choose the major flaw or bias in its construction.

(A) selection bias or confounding

(B) Berkson's bias

(C) overmatching

(D) recall bias

(E) no bias, no flaws

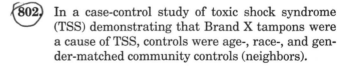

802. In a case-control study of toxic shock syndrome (TSS) demonstrating that Brand X tampons were a cause of TSS, controls were age-, race-, and gender-matched community controls (neighbors).

803. In a case-control study of the relationship between diethylstilbestrol (DES) use during pregnancy and the subsequent development of vaginal cancer in the offspring, controls were chosen from the birth records (controls were the next recorded female birth from the same hospital at which the patient was born). Use of DES during pregnancy was ascertained by inspection of the medical records of prenatal and obstetric care. During the period under study, DES was used for high-risk pregnancies or threatened abortions.

804. In a case-control study investigating the reputed importance of exposure to benzene as a cause of leukemia, controls were chosen from the workmates of cases.

Questions 805 through 808

For each experiment or research design described below, select the statistical test that would be most appropriate for the analysis of the data.

    (A) correlation coefficient
    (B) chi-square
    (C) Student's *t*-test
    (D) paired Student's *t*-test
    (E) Wilcoxon matched-pairs signed rank test

805. Sixty patients with a certain disease are randomly assigned to receive treatment A or placebo. Condition after 1 year for each patient is rated as improved, no change, or deteriorated.

806. Two surgically similar wounds were inflicted on each of 10 rats. One wound was sutured; the other was taped. At the end of 10 days, tensile strength was measured using a spring scale that was judged to be accurate to about 10 lb/in².

807. To determine whether there is any relationship between blood pressure (BP) and serum cholesterol levels, BP and serum cholesterol levels are measured in a cross-sectional study of hypertensive patients.

808. Forty patients with hypertension are treated with active drug for 1 month and placebo for 1 month using a sophisticated cross-over design and washout period (to mitigate against the effects of secular trend or drug carryover). Blood pressure (BP) for each patient is determined during treatment with active drug and placebo according to a prearranged plan.

Questions 809 through 815

For each description below, choose the defense mechanism with which it is most closely associated.

    (A) repression
    (B) projection
    (C) isolation
    (D) regression
    (E) identification

809. A patient described, without showing any emotion, the details of an automobile accident in which his closest friend died.

810. A 6-year-old child was brought to the doctor for bedwetting. He had been successfully toilet trained previously. The mother is expecting a baby soon.

811. Free association may be effective against this.

812. Paranoid patients often manifest this.

813. Persons who had been abused as children often become child abusers.

814. This may explain why so many people think the old days were so good.

815. A psychotic patient is found in bed in the fetal position.

Questions 816 through 823

For each description below, choose the neurotransmitter with which it is usually associated.

    (A) serotonin
    (B) norepinephrine
    (C) dopamine
    (D) acetylcholine
    (E) γ-aminobutyric acid (GABA)

816. Much of this substance in the brain is produced by the locus ceruleus.

817. This substance opens the chloride channel.

818. Blockers of this substance are effective in schizophrenia.

819. An indoleamine

820. Decreased in Alzheimer's disease

821. Ingestion of L-tryptophan increases the levels of this substance in the brain.

822. Dryness of mouth, constipation, and blurred vision are side effects of many antidepressants caused by the blocking of the effects of this substance.

823. A depletion of this substance in the brain often results in muscular rigidity and tremors.

Questions 824 through 827

For each developmental phase described below, select the age at which it is most likely to occur.

    (A) 0 to 2 mo
    (B) 2 to 8 mo
    (C) 9 to 10 mo
    (D) 10 to 17 mo
    (E) 18 to 36 mo

824. Normal autistic phase

825. Separation-individuation phase

826. Normal symbiotic phase

827. Object constancy

Questions 828 through 831

For each of the following studies or problems, choose the most appropriate multivariable method of analysis.

    (A) discriminant function analysis
    (B) log linear modeling
    (C) factor analysis
    (D) analysis of variance
    (E) analysis of covariance

828. One hundred mildly to severely hypertensive patients are randomly assigned to one of two treatment regimens. Blood pressure (BP) is determined for each patient before treatment and after 1 mo of treatment. Treatments are to be compared.

829. It is necessary to determine two indices, one measuring demoralization and the other measuring somatization, based on the information obtained from four separate questionnaires that were administered to 200 people and that initially were designed to assess depression, anxiety, anger, and psychophysiologic symptoms.

830. It is to be determined which items measured on a 21-item life stress checklist predict the onset of illness during the 6 months following health screening.

831. It is necessary to evaluate the effects of gender, socioeconomic status, and marital status on a happiness scale.

Questions 832 through 835

For an investigation of each situation described below, choose the study design that is most appropriate.

    (A) retrospective case control
    (B) randomized controlled clinical trial

    (C) observational cohort
    (D) cross-sectional survey
    (E) prospective single-case study

832. The causes of or risk factors for a rare disease

833. An association between two diseases

834. The efficacy of a new intervention

835. The hazards of occupational or environmental exposure

Questions 836 and 837

For each of the following hypothetical situations, choose the most appropriate control population.

    (A) community control
    (B) hospital control
    (C) matched control
    (D) historical control
    (E) no control necessary

836. A new case-control study designed to rebut criticisms that a previous study was flawed by Berkson's bias.

837. Investigation of a new treatment for a uniformly fatal disease.

Questions 838 through 846

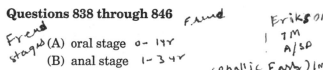

    (A) oral stage
    (B) anal stage
    (C) phallic stage
    (D) genital stage
    (E) sensorimotor stage
    (F) latency

838. Problems in this stage may lead to excessive dependency.

839. Problems in this stage may lead to parsimony and/or obsessive traits.

840. This is NOT a developmental stage described by Sigmund Freud.

841. Pleasure in this stage revolves around sucking.

842. Oedipal complex occurs during this stage.

843. Corresponds to Erikson's developmental stage of Industry vs Guilt

844. Usually engages in play with peers of the same gender

845. Autonomy is of paramount importance.

846. Love and sexual intimacy can be achieved during this stage.

Questions 847 through 854

(A) β-endorphin
(B) serotonin
(C) norepinephrine
(D) cholecystokinine
(E) morphine
(F) dopamine

847. A substance made by the human body whose effect can be blocked by naloxone

848. Antipsychotic medications block its receptors

849. An alkaloid

850. A drug used to control pain

851. This substance is secreted together with corticotropin, cleaved from a larger molecule that also contains the moiety for melatonin.

852. Locus ceruleus is a major source of this substance in the brain.

853. This substance contains the indole ring.

854. Fluoxetine (Prozac) is a potent re-uptake blocker of this substance.

DIRECTIONS (Questions 855 through 859): Each of the numbered items or incomplete statements in this section is followed by answers or by completions of the statement. Select the ONE lettered answer or completion that is BEST in each case.

855. Depressive symptoms are LEAST LIKELY associated with

(A) levodopa
(B) cancer of the pancreas
(C) hypothyroidism
(D) viral infection
(E) cocaine abuse

856. A 30-year-old woman complains of episodic faintness, tingling sensation in her hands, shortness of breath, and severe anxiety. Thorough medical workup reveals no pathologic condition. During an episode of these symptoms, chemical analysis of the serum will probably reveal

(A) decreased chloride
(B) increased blood urea nitrogen (BUN)

(C) decreased protein
(D) increased serum amylase
(E) increased pH

Questions 857 through 859

A 42-year-old widow complains of persistent burning pain in her right forearm. The patient has a history of recurrent depression. Her husband died of a myocardial infarction within the past year.

857. Possible diagnoses include

(A) causalgia
(B) depressive equivalent
(C) psychogenic pain
(D) myocardial infarction
(E) all of the above

858. If the patient described has difficulty falling asleep and frequently awakens from sleep because of pain, all of the following statements are true EXCEPT that

(A) depression is possible
(B) causalgia is possible
(C) the pain is not likely to have an organic basis
(D) the symptoms may indicate the presence of anxiety
(E) bereavement may contribute to the symptoms

859. Values of serum normitase (a fictitious substance) have been determined on 10,000 hospitalized patients by the hospital laboratory. Fortunately, the values follow a normal distribution, with a mean normitase level of 6.3 units and a standard deviation of 2.2 units. A valid conclusion that can be reached from these data is that

(A) a serum normitase level of 12.8 units is incompatible with life
(B) 95 percent of the serum normitase values fall between 1.9 and 10.5 units
(C) the range of normal serum normitase level is 4.1 to 8.5
(D) approximately half of the patients tested have a serum normitase level of 6.3 units
(E) all of the above are correct statements

DIRECTIONS (Questions 860 through 880): Each set of matching questions in this section consists of a list of up to eight lettered options followed by several numbered items. For each item, select the ONE lettered option that is most closely associated with it. <u>Each lettered heading may be selected once, more than once, or not at all.</u>

Questions 860 through 862

(A) rooting reflex
(B) Moro reflex
(C) 0–1-month-old infant
(D) symbiotic stage of development
(E) passive, undifferentiated organism
(F) active, stimulus-seeking organism
(G) 2–3-month-old infant
(H) 4–5-month-old infant

860. Seen in newborn babies when the cheek is touched; aids feeding

861. The newborn baby

862. The infant begins to smile selectively and recognizes its mother.

Questions 863 through 867

(A) transitional object
(B) a function of the ego
(C) Harry Harlow's together-together animals
(D) executive monkeys
(E) The study of behavior change in animals depending on contingents
(F) The study of instinctual and acquired animal behavior
(G) Castration anxiety

863. Ethology

864. A rhesus monkey is isolated from its mother and raised with a peer.

865. Object relationships

866. Serves as a substitute for mother

867. The "Phallic Phase" of development

Questions 868 through 875

(A) Alzheimer's disease
(B) multi-infarct dementia
(C) delirium
(D) Wernicke's syndrome
(E) pseudodementia
(F) dementia praecox
(G) normal pressure hydrocephalus
(H) subcortical dementia

868. Verbal and perceptuomotor abilities are largely preserved. It may be seen in Parkinson's disease.

869. Clouding of consciousness is a prominent feature

870. Usually associated with hypertension and atherosclerosis

871. Secondary to depression

872. Chromosomal abnormalities (e.g., autosome 21), cholinergic abnormalities, and infectious etiologies have been postulated for this syndrome.

873. Most common form of dementia in the elderly

874. A severe amnestic disorder often follows this neurologic entity.

875. An older term for schizophrenia

Questions 876 through 880

(A) free association
(B) squeeze technique
(C) sensate focus exercise
(D) reciprocal inhibition
(E) positive reinforcement

876. Nondemanding, mutually pleasurable explorations of one another's bodies without sexual intercourse

877. A person has difficulty achieving sexual arousal under conditions of duress.

878. Used to treat premature ejaculation

879. The primary technique of psychoanalysis

880. A spouse becomes sexually enthusiastic after a complement from the other spouse.

Answers and Explanations

763. (C) Desensitization is a procedure in which a phobic object (insect, in this case) is presented to the patient repeatedly in a nonthreatening way in gradual increments so that extinction of the conditioned response (fear) might occur. *(Leigh and Reiser, pp 41–78; Kaplan and Sadock, pp 262–271)*

764. (E) The ego functions include emotions, defense mechanisms, cognitive and perceptual functions, movement, and so forth. The ego is the agent of the personality system that mediates between the demands of the id, which is the reservoir of instinctual drives, and the demands of the superego, which represents parental and societal values. The ego also mediates between the personality system and external reality. *(Kaplan and Sadock, pp 372–373)*

765. (D) Despite randomization, the two groups described in the question differed in baseline susceptibility, and drug A may be more effective than placebo. Matching must be performed before randomization and is probably logistically impossible. Stratified analysis would allow comparison of groups stratified according to equivalent baseline susceptibility—outcome for young and relatively healthy patients in one group would be compared with outcome for young and relatively healthy patients in the other group. Similarly, outcome for older and more severely diseased patients would be compared for each treatment. β Error (or type II error), which refers to the failure to reject the null hypothesis when the experimental hypothesis is true, results from not having a large enough sample size to demonstrate a particular level or magnitude of difference. *(MacMahon and Pugh, pp 278–281)*

766. (C) Medical students experience an increasing identification with the medical profession. The student is exposed to persons from different backgrounds. There is generally much anxiety concerning evaluations and examinations. Unfortunately, the idealism that students originally the group would be expected to regress toward the mean score, even in the absence of any intervention. Although historical factors, changes in the test (instrumentation), testing (learning from the test), and maturation might all affect performance on the second test, these factors would be likely to affect both the students who received special education and those who did not. *(Campbell and Stanley)*

767. (C) Physical examination is a potent psychotherapeutic tool in that it can reduce the patient's anxiety and provide effective reassurance. Psychotherapy may be performed by any clinician, knowingly or not. Whereas insight is the goal of depth psychotherapy, increase in coping ability is often the goal in supportive and other types of phychotherapy. *(Leigh and Reiser, pp 421–436)*

768. (B) Both hallucination and delusion lack consensual validation. Delusion is a fixed idea or belief that is not based on reality. Hallucinations are perceptual experiences that are not based on stimulus from reality and that cannot be substantiated by normal observers. *(Leigh and Reiser, pp 145–178)*

769. (D) With increasing age, there is decreased nigrostriatal dopamine, resulting in an increase rather than decrease in extrapyramidal side effects with neuroleptics. Other age-related changes include delayed absorption because of the antacids, milk of magnesia, or anticholinergic drugs that many elderly patients take, decreased first-pass effect with age and congestive heart failure, decreased hepatic function in general, decrease in renal function causing decreased lithium clearance and delay in reaching steady-state of lithium, and increased CNS sensitivity to benzodiazepines. *(Leigh and Reiser, pp 179–209)*

770. (B) Imprinting refers to early learning that occurs during a critical period. It is characterized by rapidity and specificity. Instinctual behavior refers to preprogrammed, unlearned behavior. *(Kaplan and Saddock, pp 424–443)*

771. **(C)** The nurses in a hospital are directly responsible to the hospital administration and also to the physicians concerning clinical matters. The physicians are responsible only to other physicians in a hierarchy usually apart from the administrative hierarchy of the hospital. Other staff personnel, including clerks and security guards, are responsible only to the hospital administration. *(Leigh and Reiser, pp 401–420)*

772. **(E)** The percentage of people having positive (or negative) test results who have (or do not have) an illness (e.g., depression) will depend on the prevalence of that illness in the population studied. For example, if the prevalence of depression is 1 in 10,000 and 1,000,000 people are studied, 100 people will have the illness, 10 percent of the 999,900 people without it will have positive results (99,990 false positives), and 98 percent of the 100 people affected will have positive results (98 true positives). In this situation, only 98 of 100,088 people with positive results will have depression (less than 1 percent). Alternatively, if the population consisted only of people with the illness, 100 percent of the people with positive results would have depression. *(Feinstein, pp 215–226)*

773. **(A)** Infants appear to be programmed to move in rhythm to the human voice. Observations have shown that they will orient with eyes, head, and body to animated sound stimuli. Within a few weeks after birth, infants are able to differentiate between sounds and make more appropriate responses. Obviously, this ability increases with maturity during the first year. *(Friedlander)*

774. **(E)** Deaths due to violent causes are more common in the age group between 15 and 24 years than among younger persons. Accidents and homicides constitute the major portion of these deaths, followed by suicides. Children younger than 12 years rarely commit suicide, but thereafter the incidence increases through age 24. *(Department of Health and Human Services)*

775. **(C)** The ratio of attempted suicide increases by a factor of 10 between the ages of 15 and 19 years, compared with the rate between the ages of 10 and 14 years. At the same time, the ratio of boys to girls who commit suicide is 3:1. In 1979, suicide was the fourth cause of death among adolescents and rose to the second cause of death in 1982, surpassed only by accidents. *(Committee on Adolescence, American Academy of Pediatrics)*

776. **(C)** A variety of random factors, including measurement error, transient illness, or random sloppiness, might account for low reading scores of many of the students assigned to a special education class. Since these random factors might ac-

count for the low scores, on retesting 1 year later, the group would be expected to regress toward the mean score, even in the absence of any intervention. Although historical factors, changes in the test (instrumentation), testing (learning from the test), and maturation might all affect performance on the second test, these factors would be likely to affect both the students who received special education and those who did not. *(Campbell and Stanley)*

777. **(D)** The rate of psychiatric disorders among mentally retarded children is 50 percent. The rate found among the general population is 37 percent. There is nothing particularly characteristic about the kind of psychiatric disorder found among retarded children. *(Rutter et al)*

778. **(C)** In a case-control study, the odds ratio serves as a good estimate of the relative risk. The odds ratio is defined as the ratio of cases to controls in the exposed group divided by the ratio of cases to controls in the unexposed group (in this example, [16/20]/[4/60] = 12). Since incidence rates of the disease for the exposed and nonexposed population are not calculated, the true relative risk can only be estimated. *(MacMahon and Pugh, pp 269–273)*

779. **(E)** Although antidepressant drugs usually are used before ECT is considered, ECT remains the most effective (meaning that the response rate to ECT is higher than to other modalities) treatment for depression. ECT is indicated for patients who fail to respond to drug treatment. *(Leigh, p 134)*

780. **(D)** Although biofeedback usually involves modern electronic instrumentation, the essence of the technique is the feedback of biologic information. ECT does involve the use of an electrical instrument, but there is no feedback element in this treatment. Although no sophisticated instrumentation is involved, a physician's telling the patient that the BP has been reduced entails all aspects of biofeedback, including a reward for desirable behavior (diet). *(Kaplan and Sadock, pp 1024–1025)*

781. **(D)** Tardive dyskinesia is caused by neuroleptics that are dopamine receptor blockers (phenothiazines and butyrophenones). Amoxapine is an antidepressant that has dopamine-blocking function and has similar side effects as neuroleptics. Clorazepate is a benzodiazepine and is a muscle relaxant antianxiety agent. *(Leigh and Reiser, pp 441–455)*

782. **(C)** The symptoms of the patient described in the question may result from anxiety alone, but a number of other causes must be ruled out first. These include hyperthyroidism, drug-induced states, and CNS-depressant withdrawal states. Physical examination and routine laboratory tests must be performed on all patients with anxiety symptoms before a specific course of treatment can be considered. *(Leigh and Reiser, pp 41–78)*

783. **(B)** Delusion is a fixed idea or belief that does not correspond to reality. Hallucination is perception without stimulus. Illusion is distorted perception in the presence of stimulus. Delirium involves an alteration of the sensorium, with confusion and disorientation. Euphoria refers to expansive, exalted mood. *(Leigh and Reiser, p 147)*

784. **(B)** All antipsychotic agents except rauwolfia alkaloids block dopamine receptors in the brain. Locus ceruleus is the site of most noradrenergic neurons in the brain. The dopaminergic neurons in the brain are primarily found in three areas—the basal ganglia (nigrostriatal tract), the midbrain (mesolimbic tract), and the hypothalamus. *(Leigh and Reiser, pp 437–455)*

785. **(D)** Putative neurotransmitters include biogenic amines, such as norepinephrine, dopamine, and serotonin. Peptides such as endorphins are also neurotransmitters. GABA is a general inhibitory neurotransmitter. Glycine and substance P are also neurotransmitters. Serum pepsinogen is an enzyme. *(Leigh and Reiser, pp 49–62)*

786. **(B)** The tremor and hallucinations experienced by the patient described in the question indicate the presence of delirium tremens. Physicians should be aware that alcoholic patients often do drink in the hospital. Following an operation, however, the patient is often allowed nothing by mouth, which may precipitate an alcoholic withdrawal state. *(Leigh and Reiser, pp 305–324)*

787. **(C)** Transference may play a role in accusatory behavior, especially since the patient described in the question accused the nurses of being like his own mother. Regression results in the patient's feeling and thinking as though he were a child, which may in turn contribute to impulsiveness and increased transference feelings. His feelings concerning the nurses may be displacements from his mother. Organic brain syndrome, through reduction of higher cortical inhibitory functions, may increase distortion and impulsive behavior. Sublimation is the channeling of unacceptable impulses into acceptable and creative channels. *(Leigh and Reiser, pp 79–100)*

788. **(A)** Visual hallucinations are more common in patients with organic brain syndrome as opposed to schizophrenia. Visual hallucinations are particularly common in delirium tremens. Schizophre-

nia usually is characterized by auditory hallucinations. *(Leigh and Reiser, pp 145–178)*

789. **(C)** Intraoperative factors may be important in causing postoperative organic brain syndrome. Laboratory tests may document a metabolic derangement that may account for the organic brain syndrome. Drug and alcohol history are important in considering withdrawal states. The patient's own description of the hallucinations is important in determining the possible cause of the syndrome; patient interview also is important to document the mental status. Early developmental history is of secondary importance in the management of acute organic brain syndrome. *(Leigh and Reiser, pp 179–209,325–340)*

790. **(B)** In the Isle of Wight study, 2.51 percent of children aged 9, 10, and 11 years were found to be intellectually retarded. Among these children, 30 to 100 percent also were found to be behaviorally disturbed. This rate of disturbance is three to four times greater than the rate found in a control group. *(Rutter et al)*

791. **(A)** Narcolepsy may be an REM sleep disorder. Hypnagogic hallucinations and cataplexy (sudden loss of muscle tone), often seen in patients with narcolepsy, may be caused by the dissociation of REM phenomena from sleep. Catalepsy refers to the waxy flexibility seen in patients with catatonic syndrome. *(Leigh and Reiser, pp 271–302)*

792. **(C)** Biologic rhythms include ultradian, diurnal, and circadian rhythms. REM–non-REM (NREM)cycles, hormonal cycles (e.g., cortisol), and even pathologic cycles such as manic-depressive cycles are examples of biologic rhythms. Biologic rhythms are a subset of periodic phenomena, such as the vernal equinox, which is related to the earth's rotation around the sun. *(Leigh and Reiser, pp 271–302)*

793–801. **(793-B, 794-E, 795-C, 796-C, 797-D, 798-D, 799-E, 800-C, 801-A)** α Waves are associated with a relaxed, awake state in which the subject's eyes are closed. Concentration, as during mental arithmetic, is associated with faster, β waves. Δ Waves (3 or less cycles per sec) are associated with NREM sleep (stages 3 and 4). Sleepwalking and night terrors occur during Δ wave sleep. Δ Waves are also prominent in comatose patients (the EEG tracing may be flat in very deeply comatose patients). REM sleep is characterized by visual dreams, relaxation of skeletal muscles, irregular respiration and pulse, and physiologic arousal, such as erection. Cataplexy is the sudden loss of muscle tone that occurs in narcolepsy. *(Leigh and Reiser, pp 271–302)*

802–804.   (802-D, 803-A, 804-C) The major flaw in the study design of question 802 is the possibility that women with TSS will be more likely to remember using a particular brand of tampon (especially one that the news media have already implicated) than will women who did not have TSS. Reports about the brand of tampon used need to be validated, although this may be quite difficult to accomplish. Berkson's bias, which refers to the differential rate of detection of disease in patients with and without the reputed risk factor, and confounding would not be problematic in this study.

In the study design of question 803, recall bias was avoided by the use of hospital records. The major flaw is the possibility that high-risk pregnancy or threatened abortion may be the cause or marker for the subsequent development of vaginal cancer as well as the cause of DES use. Rather than overmatched, the controls were undermatched, since they were less likely to have been high-risk pregnancies or threatened abortions.

In an attempt to avoid selection bias or possible confounding, the investigators in question 804 have ensured that the controls will have the same occupational exposure as the cases. Because both groups were exposed to benzene, benzene exposure could not be demonstrated as a risk factor for the occurrence of leukemia in this design, even if it were a significant risk factor (which it is). Controls should have an equivalent susceptibility to the development of the disease as the cases and an equivalent susceptibility to exposure as the cases, but they should not be overmatched to ensure that they have the same exposure history. *(MacMahon and Pugh, pp 207–282)*

805–808.   (805-B, 806-E, 807-A, 808-D) Chi-square is a nonparametric statistic that is particularly useful for analysis of categorical data (data measured nominally). In the situation described in question 805, outcome was measured in one of three categories. Chi-square is calculated by determining the difference between the observed frequency for each category (e.g., placebo-improved) and the expected frequency under the assumption that the treatment does not affect outcome.

Since the scale described in question 806 is not a true interval scale but is an ordinal scale and since we do not know anything about the underlying distribution of scores on the test, a nonparametric test should be used to analyze the data. The Wilcoxon matched-pairs signed rank test can be used on matched pairs in which measurements are made on an ordinal scale. The test is based on a ranking of the difference between scores obtained for each matched pair.

The correlation coefficient is particularly useful to describe the degree of association between two mutually dependent variables, as in question

807. The correlation coefficient (the product moment correlation or Pearson's coefficient of correlation) is unitless and varies between –1 and +1. A perfect correlation (+1 or –1) implies that the two variables are completely interdependent, whereas a zero correlation indicates that none of the variance of one variable can be explained by the other variable.

As described in question 808, each patient serves as his or her own control so that a paired Student's *t*-test is appropriate and has the greatest statistical power to demonstrate an association. Both the paired Student's *t*-test and the Student's *t*-test for independent samples compare the mean scores of the two groups and determine the probability of obtaining as large a difference (or larger) between the means if the two groups actually come from the same population. The probability will depend on the magnitude of the difference and the variance of the scores. *(Colton, pp 101–230)*

809–815.   (809-C, 810-D, 811-A, 812-B, 813-E, 814-A, 815-D) Isolation is the process by which painful emotions are selectively detached from factual memory, which may allow for factual report of a very traumatic event, such as an accident, without an emotional outburst. Regression is a pervasive change in personality to assume the attributes of an earlier age and, in severe form, is characteristic of severely ill schizophrenic patients. In less severe form, a child may unconsciously use this mechanism for increased attention. Repression relegates memories of conflictual or painful experiences into the unconscious, thus making the past appear to be better than it was. Free association may reveal the unconscious material by decreasing the alertness of the critical or sensoring function (superego) of the mind. Projection is a distortion of perception in which a characteristic of the self is attributed to someone else. Exaggerated projection leads to feelings of persecution (projected hostility) and paranoid symptoms. Identification is a process by which a person becomes like the person who is either admired or hated ("identification with the aggressor" as in case of a child abuser.) *(Leigh and Reiser, pp 79–100)*

816–823.   (816-B, 817-E, 818-C, 819-A, 820-D, 821-A, 822-D, 823-C) The amino acid L-tryptophan is the precursor for serotonin, which is a neurotransmitter needed for non-rapid-eye-movement (NREM) sleep as well as for mood and pain modulation. Up to 70 to 90 percent of brain norepinephrine is produced in the pontine nucleus, locus ceruleus. Dopamine is implicated in schizophrenia and also is an important neurotransmitter for the extrapyramidal system. Depletion of this substance, as in parkinsonism, causes muscular rigidity and tremors. Acetylcholine is the neurotransmitter associated with higher cortical functioning and is depleted in Alzheimer's disease. Acetylcholine also is an important neurotransmitter for the autonomic nervous system (parasympathetic system and the sympathetic nerves to the sweat glands). Many antidepressants have an anticholinergic action, thus dryness of mouth, constipation, and blurred vision. GABA is an important inhibitory transmitter that opens the chloride channels directly associated with the GABA receptors, hyperpolarizing the cell. *(Simons, pp 553–564; Leigh and Reiser, pp 59–61,114–120,157–165, 184–188)*

824–827. (824-A, 825-C, 826-B, 827-E) The stages listed in the question form part of the developmental line that psychoanalytic theorists describe as occurring from dependency to adult object relationships. This sequence leads from the newborn's dependence on maternal care to the adult's emotional and material independence and self-reliance. The following eight steps, or stages, are described: period of biologic unity, part-object stage, stage of object constancy, preoedipal ambivalent stage, object-centered phallic-oedipal stage, latency period, preadolescent period, and adolescent stage. *(Freud)*

828–831. (828-E, 829-C, 830-A, 831-D) Analysis of covariance is used to describe the relationship between a dependent variable and one or more nominal independent variables, controlling for other continuous variables. Analysis of covariance might be used to demonstrate that post-treatment BP, when adjusted for pretreatment BP, is significantly less for one treatment than for another.

Factor analysis is a multivariable method that is used to reduce or explain the relationships among many intercorrelated variables to a few meaningful and relatively independent factors. In the example, four separate scales were reputed to measure four separate factors, but when the scales were administered to the same 200 individuals, they were found to be highly intercorrelated. By the use of factor analysis, two relatively independent factors could be identified that summarized the four original scales.

Discriminant analysis is used to determine how one or several independent variables can differentiate (or distinguish) among the different categories of a dependent variable. Discriminant analysis will provide a "discriminant function" that allows the prediction of illness onset based on knowledge of the values of the independent variables.

In question 831, analysis of variance is used to assess how several nominal independent variables (gender, socioeconomic status, marital status) affect a continuous dependent variable. In effect, analysis of variance compares the mean value of the dependent variable (happiness) for each of the cross-classified independent variables (i.e., compares the mean happiness for single males of one socioeconomic status to the mean happiness for married males of the same socioeconomic status, and so forth). *(Kleinbaum and Kupper)*

832–835. (832-A, 833-D, 834-B, 835-C) Retrospective case-control studies are particularly well suited for the investigation of the causes of rare diseases. If a disease is sufficiently rare, the odds ratio determined from a retrospective case-control study provides a good approximation of the relative risk. Prospective studies would require extremely large initial populations in order to ensure an adequate number of cases, especially if the disease occurs rarely. Cross-sectional surveys will not provide information regarding causes, since associations are measured only at one point in time. Under certain circumstances, observational cohorts could be used to investigate the significance of a risk factor for the subsequent development of a disease, but the initial cohort would have to be very large, and the logistics of the investigation would be difficult.

Cross-sectional surveys measure two or more variables at a single moment in time. The strength of association between two variables can be determined, but temporality of the relationship (does the occurrence of variable 1 precede the occurrence of variable 2) cannot be determined from a cross-sectional survey. Relative risk may be determined on the basis of a cross-sectional survey, but causality cannot be inferred.

Randomized controlled clinical trials are state of the art for demonstrating the efficacy of a new intervention. Randomization helps ensure that the groups are equivalent, so that outcome is less likely to be biased by initial susceptibility. Randomized controlled trials may be costly and time-consuming and are not always feasible to use.

Observational cohorts, studied either retrospectively or prospectively, allow an estimation of the incidence or rate of occurrence of a specified outcome in a group with special exposure. Although retrospective case-control studies can be used also to investigate the relationship between prior exposure and disease onset, case-control studies start by identifying cases of specific disease (rather than exposed persons) and are less useful than observational cohorts for determining the effects of a given exposure. Classic examples of observational cohort studies are the numerous studies of occupational exposures (e.g., bladder cancer in workers exposed to dyes or scrotal cancer in chimney sweeps). *(MacMahon and Pugh, pp 207–300)*

836–837. (836-A, 837-D) Berkson's bias, a form of selection bias, may result when the exposure factor or other characteristic of interest differentially affects the probability of admission to a hospital for those persons with the disease and those without the disease. Berkson's bias occurs when cases are hospitalized patients with the disease of interest and controls are hospitalized patients with another illness (with a different rate of admission than that for the disease of interest) and when the exposure factor affects these rates of admission. In order to avoid Berkson's bias, controls could be drawn from the community.

The situation described in question 837 is one in which the use of historical controls may provide compelling evidence for the efficacy of a new treatment. Usually, historical controls are considered inadequate to demonstrate efficacy, since numerous factors (including the severity of the illness in the patients studied or other changes that have occurred over time in the management or treatment of patients) are not adequately controlled. If a disease has been fatal in nearly 100 percent of all previous cases, successful treatment of a small series of patients with the disease is extremely unlikely unless the new treatment is efficacious. The value of insulin in treating diabetic coma was demonstrated in comparison with historical controls. *(Lilienfeld and Lilienfeld, pp 199–202, 260–268)*

838. **(A)** The oral stage of development, during the first year of life, is characterized by gratification related to the activities of the mouth and nurturance, including dependency needs. A fixation at this stage results in dependent character traits. *(Leigh and Reiser, pp 358–361)*

839. **(B)** The anal stage of development occurs during the second year of life with toilet training. Control of bowel movement is an important task. Fixation in this stage may lead to parsimony, rigidity, sadistic tendencies, and obsessive-compulsiveness. *(Leigh and Reiser, pp 358–361)*

840. **(E)** The sensorimotor stage or period is a developmental stage described by Jean Piaget. This period denotes the first 18 months to two years of life during which the infant learns through repetition—initially, from blind imitative repetition to repetition in anticipation of results and invention of new methods. Response-feedback loops called "circular reactions" form an important part of the experience. *(Leigh and Reiser, p 363)*

841. **(A)** During the oral stage of development, pleasure is concentrated on oral activities such as sucking and, later, biting. *(Leigh and Reiser, pp 358–361)*

842. **(C)** The phallic stage takes place between the ages of 3 and 6. During this stage, erotic sensation concentrates in the genital organs, and the child experiences strong love toward the parent of the opposite sex. The boy, during this stage, feels an intense desire to possess the mother and replace the father as her primary lover—the Oedipus complex. The boy gradually relinquishes this wish, due to the fear of the father's anger (castration anxiety), and, instead, identifies with the father. *(Leigh and Reiser, pp 358–361)*

843. **(F)** The latency period, ages 7 till adolescence, is characterized by a relative absence of intense sexual interest. Children tend to identify with the parent of the same sex. *(Leigh and Reiser, pp 358–361)*

844. **(F)** During the latency period, children tend to play with playmates of the same sex, perhaps due to their intense identification with the parent of the same sex and general turning away from sexuality. *(Leigh and Reiser, pp 358–361)*

845. **(B)** During the anal stage of development, bowel control is the major task. This stage corresponds to Erikson's stage of Autonomy vs Shame and Doubt, and a sense of mastery if the stage is successfully completed. *(Leigh and Reiser, pp 361, 358–361)*

846. **(D)** According to the Freudian stages of development, the genital stage of adult sexuality is achieved when a person successfully completes adolescence and finds a partner for mature sexuality. *(Leigh and Reiser, pp 358–361)*

847. **(A)** Endorphins including β-endorphin are endogenous peptides that have morphine-like biological effects including analgesia, respiratory depression, and potential for addiction. Their effects are blocked by opiate antagonists such as naloxone. *(Leigh and Reiser, pp 222–223)*

848. **(F)** Most drugs that have an antipsychotic effect have the property of blocking one or more types of dopamine receptors in the brain. The dopamine-blocking effect of antipsychotics is also responsible for their extrapyramidal side effects, including rigidity and tremor. *(Leigh and Reiser, pp 160–161)*

849. **(E)** Morphine is an alkaloid obtained from the poppy plant. Although the biologic effects are similar, endorphins and morphine have entirely different chemical structures. *(Leigh and Reiser, pp 222–223)*

850. **(E)** Morphine is a drug used to control pain, while endorphins are endogenous substances released by the body. Endorphins are thus not drugs. *(Leigh and Reiser, pp 222–223)*

851. **(A)** β-endorphin is a part of pro-opiomelanocortin molecule (POMC). POMC is cleaved in the anterior pituitary gland into β-endorphin, corticotropin (ACTH), and melanocyte stimulating hormone (MSH). *(Kaplan and Sadock, pp 52–57)*

852. **(C)** The locus ceruleus is located in the pons and provides the principal noradrenergic input into the brain. The stimulation of locus ceruleus in animals results in typical anxiety-fear behaviors, and most antianxiety drugs inhibit locus ceruleus. *(Leigh and Reiser, pp 59–61)*

853. **(B)** Serotonin (5-hydroxytryptamine, 5-HT) is synthesized from the essential amino acid, tryptophan, with tryptophan hydroxylase serving as the initial and rate-limiting enzyme. Serotonin is degraded by monoamine oxidase (MAO) to 5-hydroxy-indole-acetic acid (5HIAA). *(Kaplan and Sadock, p 49)*

854. **(B)** After being released from the presynaptic membrane, serotonin is normally reabsorbed into the presynaptic neuron. Fluoxetine potently blocks this reuptake, resulting in a functional increase of available serotonin at the synaptic junction. *(Leigh and Reiser, pp 444–448)*

855. **(A)** Many cancers, especially cancer of the tail of the pancreas, all endocrine disorders, and viral infections are known to be associated with depressive symptoms. Cocaine abuse may result in severe withdrawal depression. Levodopa, on the other hand, is often associated with manic symptoms and seldom with depression. *(Leigh and Reiser, p 127)*

856. **(E)** Anxiety, coupled with shortness of breath, tingling sensations in the hands, and faintness in the absence of an underlying physical condition, suggests hyperventilation syndrome. Hyperventilation causes respiratory alkalosis (reduced PCO_2 and thus increased pH). The increased blood pH leads to decreased ionization of calcium, causing tingling sensations. *(Leigh and Reiser, p 64)*

857. **(E)** The amount of information is not sufficient to rule out any of the possible etiologies for pain listed. The history of depression and recent bereavement rule in the possibility of depressive equivalent, psychogenic pain, as well as myocardial infarction, as bereavement often contributes to morbidity from any cause. *(Leigh and Reiser, pp 110–112,211–243)*

858. **(C)** Sleep disturbance often indicates the presence of anxiety and/or depression. Being awakened by pain is often indicative of an organic basis for pain. *(Leigh and Reiser, pp 211–243)*

859. **(B)** In a normal distribution curve, 95 percent of the values fall within two standard deviations (in this example, 6.3 ± 4.4). The physiologic effect of

normitase level cannot be determined from the data. Normal range for normitase cannot be determined because the sample was exclusively hospitalized patients, not the normal population. *(Kaplan and Sadock, pp 340–355)*

860. **(A)** The rooting reflex denotes the turning of the face (and mouth) toward the object that touches the infant's cheek. This reflex, as well as the Moro or startle reflex, palmar grasp reflex, and positive Babinski reflex, is seen typically in infancy, and gradually disappears. *(Simons and Pardes, p 167)*

861. **(F)** Contrary to the old notion that a newborn baby is a relatively passive, undifferentiated organism who behaves primarily to reduce tension and stimulation, modern observations have shown that the newborn is, in fact, active, stimulus-seeking, and creative in the ways it begins to construct its world. *(Simons and Pardes, p 168)*

862. **(G)** By the time an infant reaches 2–3 months of age, it will begin to smile selectively, recognizing the mother. This is sometimes called a "social smile," which is particularly pleasurable to parents. This indicates that the child is emerging from an "autistic stage" of life into one that recognizes an external world. *(Simons and Pardes, pp 170–171)*

863. **(F)** Ethology refers to the study of instinctual and acquired behavior patterns in animals, usually in their natural habitat. Such concepts as imprinting and aggression have been studied extensively by ethologists. *(Simons and Pardes, pp 198–199)*

864. **(C)** Harlow described the "together-together" animals, isolated from their mother and raised together with each other. These animals typically cling to each other and do not show the normal developmental pattern of increasing social and physical interaction with the outside environment. *(Simons and Pardes, p 204)*

865. **(B)** The formation and modulation of relationships and interchanges with other persons is an important aspect of the ego function. Other ego functions include a sense of self, control of drives, as well as perception, memory, thinking, emotions, motor activity, and speech. *(Simons and Pardes, pp 179–180)*

866. **(A)** Many infants, toward the end of the first year, become attached to a specific object, such as a blanket, and carry it wherever they go. These objects are considered to represent the mother, allowing the infant to move away from the mother with the help of the substitute. *(Simons and Pardes, pp 176–177)*

867. **(G)** According to the Freudian scheme of psychosexual development, the ages 3–6 years are characterized by a fear of bodily injury that may be derived from the "castration anxiety." Castration anxiety refers to the fear of boys of possible retaliation by the father for his forbidden incestuous wishes toward his mother. In girls, there may be a fantasy that they were somehow damaged, and thus do not have a penis. *(Simons and Pardes, pp 215–218)*

868. **(H)** Subcortical dementia denotes dementia associated with lesions of the subcortical structures, such as the basal ganglia, with relative sparing of the cortical neurons. There is impairment of memory, abstractions, personality change, and marked slowing of thought processes with relative sparing of verbal and perceptuomotor abilities. *(Leigh and Reiser, p 183)*

869. **(C)** In delirium, clouding of consciousness or reduction in awareness of the environment are prominent features. The patient is disoriented and shows major deficits in attention and concentration as well as in memory. *(Leigh and Reiser, pp 181–182)*

870. **(B)** Multi-infact dementia is secondary to cerebrovascular changes, often due to hypertension and atherosclerosis. The brain shows multiple and extensive areas of softening. Multi-infact dementia is more common among men than women, and most common between the ages of 40 and 60. *(Leigh and Reiser, p 188)*

871. **(E)** Cognitive difficulties, including inability to concentrate, indecisiveness, and slowed thinking processes, are common in patients with major depression. These cognitive difficulties occurring in depression are called "pseudodementia" and are associated with other symptoms of depression when carefully questioned. *(Leigh and Reiser, p 194)*

872. **(A)** A familial form of Alzheimer's disease has been associated with chromosome 21 abnormalities, and there is a loss of cholinergic neurons in this syndrome. Viral infection has also been suspected in some cases of Alzheimer's disease as many viral encephalitides cause late-onset dementia, and certain slow-virus infections such as Crcutzfeld-Jakob disease have histological and clinical features similar to Alzheimer's disease. *(Leigh and Reiser, pp 186–188)*

873. **(A)** Primary degenerative dementias, such as Alzheimer's and Pick's disease, account for more than 50 percent of dementia in persons over 65 years of age. The most common dementing conditions of the elderly, Alzheimer's disease and multi-infact dementia, account for some 75 percent of the dementias in the elderly. *(Leigh and Reiser, p 190)*

874. **(D)** Wernicke's syndrome, caused by thiamine deficiency associated with alcoholism, is characterized by confusion, ataxia, gaze palsies, nystagmus, and other neurologic signs. These signs gradually subside, but a major impairment of memory, Alcohol Amnestic Syndrome (Korsakoff's psychosis), remains. *(DSM III-R, p 133)*

875. **(F)** The German psychiatrist, Emil Kraepelin, in 1896 systematically described in his book, Psychiatry, 5th Edition, under the rubric of "Dementia Praecox," the signs and symptoms of psychotic illnesses that seemed to have a progressively downhill course, later known as schizophrenia. Dementia Praecox means "premature losing of mind" as opposed to senile dementia. *(Leigh and Reiser, p 150)*

876. **(C)** Sensate focus exercises are a key factor in most brief sex therapies. Initially, genital touching is excluded, and attention is focused on giving and receiving pleasure without performance demands. *(Simons and Pardes, p 364)*

877. **(D)** Reciprocal inhibition denotes that the elicitation of certain emotional states will inhibit the experience of another mutually incompatible emotional state. The emotions of fear, arising under conditions of duress, may be incompatible with the emotional state of sexual arousal. This principle is often used in the treatment of anxiety, especially phobias, by inducing states of relaxation through training or hypnosis in the presence of the phobic object, thus inhibiting the development of the incompatible emotion of anxiety. *(Kaplan and Sadock, p 112)*

878. **(B)** In this Masters and Johnson technique to treat premature ejaculation, the woman squeezes the coronal area of the penis just before the man reaches orgasm. The erection is lost, and stimulation is begun again. This technique, together with the Stop-Start technique, is an effective means of controlling ejaculation. *(Simons and Pardes, pp 371–373)*

879. **(A)** Free association, the cornerstone of psychoanalytic technique, refers to the patient's saying aloud anything that passes through his or her mind. Its functions, besides providing content for the analysis, include induction of the necessary regression and passive dependence that facilitate the development of the transference neurosis. *(Kaplan and Sadock, p 396)*

880. **(E)** Positive reinforcement refers to the process by which certain consequences of a behavior increase the probability that the behavior will occur

again. In this case, the increased sexual enthusiasm is likely to increase the probability that the spouse will pay more compliments. *(Kaplan and Sadock, p 264)*

BIBLIOGRAPHY

American Psychiatric Association. *Diagnostic and Statistical Manual of Mental Disorders.* 3rd ed. rev. (DSM-III-R). Washington, DC: American Psychiatric Association; 1987

Balis GU, ed. *The Behavioral and Social Sciences and the Practice of Medicine.* Vol. II. *The Psychiatric Foundations of Medicine.* Stoneham, Mass.: Butterworth Publishers, Inc.; 1978

Erikson EH. *Identity and the Life Cycle.* Vol. I. *Psychological Issues.* New York: International Universities Press; 1959

Hine FR, Carson RC, Maddox GL, Thompson RJ, Williams RB. *Introduction to Behavioral Science in Medicine.* New York: Springer-Verlag New York, Inc.; 1983

Kaplan HI, Sadock BJ, eds. *Comprehensive Textbook of Psychiatry.* 5th ed. Baltimore: Williams & Wilkins Co.; 1989

Leigh H, Reiser MF. *The Patient. Biological, Psychological, and Social Dimensions of Medical Practice.* 3rd ed. New York: Plenum Publishing Corp.; 1992

Lennenberg EH. *Biological Foundations of Language.* New York: John Wiley & Sons, Inc.; 1967

Lindemann E. Symptomatology and management of acute grief. *Am J Psychiatry.* May 1944; 141–148

MacMahon B, Pugh T. *Epidemiology, Principles and Methods.* Boston: Little, Brown & Co.; 1970

Mechanic D. Social psychologic factors affecting the presentation of bodily complaints. *N Engl J Med.* May 5, 1972; 1132–1139

Rutter M, Tizard J, Whitmore K. *Education, Health, and Behavior.* London: Longman Group, Ltd; 1970

Scheiber SC, Doyle BB. *The Impaired Physician.* New York: Plenum Publishing Co.; 1983

Simons RC, ed. *Understanding Human Behavior in Health and Illness.* 3rd ed. Baltimore: Williams & Wilkins Co.; 1985

Agoraphobia → fear of being alone like on a bridge or alone in public places like shopping mall.

claust claustrophobia → fear of closed spaces.

Subspecialty List: Behavioral Sciences

Question Number and Subspecialty

763. Emotions/anxiety disorder
764. Personality/psychodynamics
765. Epidemiology
766. Ethics, norms, values
767. Doctor-patient relationship psychotherapy
768. Psychological assessment/psychodynamics
769. Life cycle/organic mental syndromes
770. Correlates of animal and human behavior
771. Hospital community
772. Epidemiology
773. Life cycle/psychodynamics
774. Life cycle/psychodynamics
775. Life cycle/psychodynamics
776. Epidemiology
777. Life cycle/psychodynamics
778. Epidemiology
779. Pharmacological correlates of behavior
780. Physiological correlates of behavior/learning theory
781. Pharmacological correlates of behavior
782. Emotions/anxiety disorder
783. Psychological assessment/psychodynamics
784. Psychological assessment/psychodynamics
785. Nervous system and behavior
786. Biochemical correlates of behavior/substance abuse disorder
787. Biochemical correlates of behavior/substance abuse disorder
788. Biochemical correlates of behavior/substance abuse disorder
789. Biochemical correlates of behavior/substance abuse disorder
790. Life cycle/psychodynamics
791. Sleep
792. Physiological correlates of behavior
793. Sleep/nervous system and behavior
794. Sleep/nervous system and behavior
795. Sleep/nervous system and behavior
796. Sleep/nervous system and behavior
797. Sleep/nervous system and behavior
798. Sleep/nervous system and behavior
799. Sleep/nervous system and behavior
800. Sleep/nervous system and behavior
801. Sleep/nervous system and behavior
802. Epidemiology
803. Epidemiology
804. Epidemiology
805. Biostatistics
806. Biostatistics
807. Biostatistics
808. Biostatistics
809. Personality/psychodynamics
810. Personality/psychodynamics
811. Personality/psychodynamics
812. Personality/psychodynamics
813. Personality/psychodynamics
814. Personality/psychodynamics
815. Personality/psychodynamics
816. Nervous system and behavior
817. Nervous system and behavior
818. Nervous system and behavior psychosis
819. Nervous system and behavior
820. Nervous system and behavior life cycle/organic mental syndromes
821. Nervous system and behavior pharmacological correlates of behavior
822. Pharmacological correlates of behavior
823. Nervous system and behavior
824. Life cycle
825. Life cycle
826. Life cycle
827. Life cycle
828. Biostatistics
829. Biostatistics
830. Biostatistics
831. Biostatistics
832. Epidemiology
833. Epidemiology
834. Epidemiology
835. Epidemiology
836. Epidemiology
837. Epidemiology
838. Personality and psychodynamics
839. Personality and psychodynamics
840. Life cycle
841. Sexual development and behavior
842. Personality and psychodynamics/sexual development and behavior
843. Life cycle/personality and psychodynamics

844. Life cycle/personality and psychodynamics
845. Life cycle/personality and psychodynamics
846. Life cycle/sexual development and behavior
847. Biochemical correlates of behavior/pharmacological correlates of behavior
848. Biochemical correlates of behavior/pharmacological correlates of behavior
849. Pharmacological correlates of behavior
850. Pharmacological correlates of behavior
851. Biochemical correlates of behavior/physiological correlates of behavior
852. Biochemical correlates of behavior/pharmacological correlates of behavior
853. Biochemical correlates of behavior/physiological correlates of behavior
854. Pharmacological correlates of behavior
855. Physiological correlates of behavior/pharmacological correlates of behavior
856. Emotions, motivations, perception, cognition, and memory
857. Stress and adaptation/psychological assessment
858. Stress and adaptation/psychological assessment
859. Biostatistics/social epidemiology
860. Life cycle/child development
861. Life cycle/child development/child psychology
862. Life cycle/child development/child rearing practice
863. Correlates of animal and human behavior
864. Correlates of animal and human behavior
865. Personality and psychodynamics
866. Life cycle/child development/child psychology
867. Life cycle/child development/psychodynamics/child psychology
868. Cognitive and behavioral disorders/organic mental disorders/anatomic correlates of behavior
869. Organic mental disorders/psychological assessment
870. Organic mental disorders/anatomic correlates of behavior
871. Cognitive and behavioral disorders/emotions/cognition/mood disorder
872. Genetic correlates of behavior/degenerative disorders of the nervous system/Alzheimer's disease
873. Degenerative disorders of the nervous system/Alzheimer's disease/medical epidemiology
874. Cognitive and behavioral disorders/alcohol abuse/psychological assessment/vitamin deficiency
875. Schizophrenia
876. Sexual development and behavior
877. Learning theory/emotions, anxiety
878. Sexual development and behavior
879. Personality and psychodynamics
880. Learning theory, including behavior modification

CHAPTER 8
Practice Test

Carefully read the following instructions before taking the Practice Test.

1. This examination consists of 311 questions that are from each of the subject areas you will encounter on the actual examination. They are integrated in an effort to simulate the examination style.
2. Remember that the examination allows approximately 50 seconds for each item.
3. The test items are explained in the Introduction to this book. We suggest you read the entire Introduction prior to taking this practice test.
4. Be sure you have an adequate number of pencils and erasers, a clock, a comfortable setting, and enough distraction-free time to complete the test.
5. Use the answer sheet on pages 265 and 266 when recording your answers. This simulates the actual practice you will experience when taking the USMLE Step 1.
6. Once you complete the practice test, be sure to check your answers and assess your areas of weakness against the subspecialty lists on pages 260–263.

Practice Test
Questions

DIRECTIONS (Questions 1 through 143): Each of the numbered items or incomplete statements in this section is followed by answers or by completions of the statement. Select the ONE lettered answer or completion that is BEST in each case.

1. What is the approximate weight of the average adult human brain?

   (A) 1,000 grams
   (B) 1,400 grams
   (C) 2,000 grams
   (D) 2,200 grams
   (E) 3,600 grams

2. Which of the following fatty acids can be the precursor of prostaglandins in humans?

   (A) oleic
   (B) palmitic
   (C) stearic
   (D) arachidonic
   (E) palmitoleic

3. All of the following are associated with primary hyperparathyroidism EXCEPT

   (A) parathyroid adenoma
   (B) nephrolithiasis
   (C) bone disease
   (D) hyperphosphatemia
   (E) chief cell hyperplasia

4. The cell bodies of the first-order sensory neurons are located in which of the following structures?

   (A) cerebellum
   (B) cortex
   (C) dorsal root ganglia
   (D) superior cervical sympathetic ganglion
   (E) thalamus

5. Vitamin B_{12} is needed for the reduction of the C-2′ atom of ribonucleoside triphosphate to produce the corresponding 2′-deoxyribonucleoside. The mineral necessary for the ring system of vitamin B_{12} is

   (A) iron
   (B) cobalt
   (C) calcium
   (D) manganese
   (E) magnesium

6. Squamous cell carcinoma of the lung shows all of the following features EXCEPT

   (A) increasing incidence in women
   (B) most common type of bronchogenic carcinoma
   (C) peripheral location in the lung
   (D) high association with a history of smoking
   (E) greater predilection for men than women

7. Bipolar cells are located in which of the following structures?

   (A) spinal cord
   (B) retina
   (C) dorsal root ganglia
   (D) olfactory bulb
   (E) semilunar ganglion

8. A solution of acetic acid (pK_a 4.75) is titrated with sodium hydroxide until 80 percent of the acetic acid has been converted to sodium acetate. What is the pH of the solution?

   (A) 4.15
   (B) 5.35
   (C) 4.75
   (D) 8.75
   (E) 2.35

9. The occurrence of malignant mesothelioma has been correlated with industrial exposure to

   (A) beryllium
   (B) silica
   (C) coal dust
   (D) asbestos
   (E) nitrogen dioxide

10. All of the following are important compensatory mechanisms in hemorrhagic shock EXCEPT

   (A) tachycardia
   (B) venoconstriction
   (C) decreased peripheral vascular resistance
   (D) absorption of fluid from interstitial space
   (E) formation of angiotensin II

11. The sinuatrial node is located at the superior end of which of the following structures?

   (A) interventricular septum
   (B) septomarginal bundle
   (C) conus arterosus
   (D) crista terminalis
   (E) orifice of the coronary sinus

12. Temporary occlusion of both common carotid arteries is promptly accompanied by

   (A) vasodilatation throughout the peripheral circulation
   (B) an increase in the number of impulses from the carotid sinus nerve
   (C) an increase in venous capacity
   (D) an increase in arterial pressure
   (E) a decrease in heart rate

13. Under normal metabolic conditions, the energy produced from 1 g of glycogen is approximately

   (A) 0.8 kcal
   (B) 1.0 kcal
   (C) 4.2 kcal
   (D) 8.2 kcal
   (E) 9.5 kcal

14. A skin biopsy showing the following features: hyperkeratosis, parakeratosis, thickening of the epidermis and club-shaped papillae, and collections of neutrophil leukocytes in clusters in the upper layers of the epidermis is most characteristic of which of the following conditions?

   (A) basal cell carcinoma
   (B) malignant melanoma
   (C) squamous cell carcinoma
   (D) pemphigus vulgaris
   (E) psoriasis

15. Which of the following statements concerning the atrioventricular node is correct?

   (A) It is the natural pacemaker of the heart.
   (B) It is composed of specialized cardiac muscle cells.
   (C) It is located in the interventricular septum.
   (D) It initiates the impulses for contraction.
   (E) It may be located by following the nodal artery from the right coronary artery.

16. Long-term regulation of arterial blood pressure (BP) is primarily a function of

   (A) the CNS
   (B) the sympathetic nervous system
   (C) peripheral baroreceptors
   (D) urine output and fluid intake
   (E) total peripheral vascular resistance

17. The major amino acid precursor for gluconeogenesis is

   (A) alanine
   (B) aspartate
   (C) cysteine
   (D) glutamate
   (E) serine

18. Constrictive pericarditis with dense fibrosis and calcification of the pericardium is most likely to be associated with which of the following conditions?

   (A) acute rheumatic fever
   (B) acute staphylococcal infection
   (C) uremia
   (D) tuberculosis
   (E) lupus erythematosus

19. If in a medical school department it is observed that most of the junior faculty and residents dress and speak like the department's chairperson, this phenomenon may be an example of

   (A) sublimation
   (B) projection
   (C) denial
   (D) reaction formation
   (E) identification

20. The transversalis fascia forms all of the following EXCEPT the

   (A) femoral sheath
   (B) deep inguinal ring

(C) internal spermatic fascia

(D) psoas fascia

(E) extraperitoneal fat

21. Atrial fibrillation is a common arrhythmia that accompanies several forms of heart disease. During atrial fibrillation, the atria do not contract sequentially and thus do not contribute to ventricular filling. Which of the following statements best describes this pathophysiologic condition?

(A) On ECG, the P waves usually are normal in atrial fibrillation.

(B) A drug such as quinidine, which acts in part by prolonging the effective refractory period of conducting tissue, is useful therapy.

(C) The interval between QRS complexes remains constant.

(D) Atrial fibrillation is life threatening and usually requires application of strong electric current to place the entire myocardium in refractory period.

(E) Since the atria contribute little to ventricular function, the pulse is usually extremely regular in spite of the abnormality.

22. Which one of the following statements about the peptide of Val-Ala-Pro-Glu-Gly is true?

(A) Its isoelectric point will be found at a high pH.

(B) It has an overall positive charge at pH 11.

(C) It has an overall positive charge at pH 7.

(D) It has an overall negative charge at pH 7.

(E) It has an overall negative charge at pH 1.

23. Glomerular wire-loop lesions are most often found in renal biopsy specimens of patients with

(A) diabetes mellitus

(B) systemic lupus erythematosus

(C) hypertension

(D) hepatorenal syndrome

(E) acute tubular necrosis

24. All of the following are common examples of society's sick-role expectations EXCEPT that

(A) individuals are exempt from normal responsibilities

(B) individuals are responsible for maintenance of health

(C) being sick is an undesirable state

(D) a sick person cannot be expected to get well by "pulling himself together"

(E) a sick person should seek help from a competent professional

25. An indirect inguinal hernia leaves the abdominal cavity lateral to which of the following structures?

(A) anterior superior iliac spine

(B) deep inguinal ring

(C) inferior epigastric artery

(D) superficial circumflex iliac vessels

(E) crest of the ilium

26. Numerous ion channels are involved in the generation of the cardiac action potential. The ion channel most closely associated with the plateau phase of the cardiac action potential is

(A) voltage-gated sodium channel

(B) voltage-gated potassium channel

(C) calcium-gated potassium channels

(D) voltage-gated calcium channels

(E) phosphoptidyl inositol-gated calcium channels

27. Which of the following amino acids is purely ketogenic?

(A) cysteine

(B) serine

(C) glycine

(D) leucine

(E) alanine

28. Activator of the alternate complement pathway is

(A) interleukin 1 (IL-1)

(B) β-interferon

(C) lipoproteins

(D) endotoxin

(E) complement component C1

29. A red infarct would be most likely to occur in the

(A) heart

(B) spleen

(C) kidneys

(D) lungs

(E) pancreas

30. Which of the following is LEAST effective as an anti-inflammatory agent?

(A) indomethacin

(B) aspirin

(C) acetaminophen

(D) phenylbutazone

(E) tolmetin

31. If a bell rings each time a dog is given food, the dog will soon salivate at the sound of the bell. This phenomenon is called

    (A) operant conditioning
    (B) classical conditioning
    (C) cognitive learning
    (D) shaping
    (E) instinctual behavior

32. All of the following structures are formed from the aponeurosis of the external abdominal oblique EXCEPT the

    (A) linea alba
    (B) inguinal ligament
    (C) lacunar ligament
    (D) arcuate line
    (E) superficial inguinal ligament

33. Certain tumors produce a substance closely resembling PTH in its biologic activity. The physiologic effects of this substance would include all of the following EXCEPT

    (A) stimulation of bone resorption
    (B) decreased renal phosphate excretion
    (C) increased serum calcium
    (D) increased metabolism of vitamin D to the 1,25-OH form
    (E) increased serum calcitonin levels

34. The steroid compound of greatest potency in the control of plasma sodium ion concentration is

    (A) pregnenolone
    (B) progesterone
    (C) aldosterone
    (D) cortisol
    (E) cortisone

35. The microbicidal oxygen-dependent mechanisms of phagocytes depend on all of the following EXCEPT

    (A) superoxide radical
    (B) singlet oxygen
    (C) ferrous ions
    (D) hydrogen peroxide
    (E) hydroxyl radicals

36. The biology of chemical induction of carcinoma includes all of the following principles EXCEPT

    (A) irreversible dose dependency
    (B) dependency on hormonal promoters

    (C) fixed latency period
    (D) transmission to daughter cells
    (E) enhancement by cell proliferation

37. Propylthiouracil is useful in the treatment of

    (A) derangement toxicosis
    (B) hyperthyroidism
    (C) thyroiditis
    (D) hypoparathyroidism
    (E) hypothyroidism

38. The functions of the limbic system include all of the following EXCEPT

    (A) cognition
    (B) emotion
    (C) reproduction
    (D) nutrition
    (E) aggression

39. Which of the following structures are retroperitoneal?

    (A) kidney
    (B) transverse colon
    (C) stomach
    (D) spleen
    (E) sigmoid colon

40. The stimulation in salivary gland acini results in a loss of intracellular and a rise in extracellular potassium ions. The efflux of potassium ions is believed to be primarily due to the action of

    (A) a Na^+-K^+ exchange mechanism
    (B) voltage-dependent nonspecific cation channels
    (C) calcium-activated potassium channels
    (D) Na^+-K^+-Cl^- cotransport
    (E) an ouabain-sensitive pump

41. All of the following bonding reactions are important in the stabilization of the tertiary structure of proteins EXCEPT

    (A) peptide bonds
    (B) hydrogen bonds between peptide groups
    (C) ionic bonds
    (D) hydrophobic interactions
    (E) hydrogen bonds between side chains of amino acids

42. The figure below represents the antibiotic

(A) streptomycin
(B) cephalothin
(C) erythromycin
(D) penicillin
(E) gentamicin

43. Adrenocortical carcinoma is a rare malignant tumor that is

(A) most common among children
(B) a small occult lesion
(C) associated with Cushing's syndrome
(D) of neural crest origin
(E) usually bilateral

44. Within 48 to 72 hr after the last dose of heroin, an addicted individual may experience

(A) anorexia, hypotension, and paralysis of the respiratory muscles
(B) severe irritability, insomnia, anorexia, nausea, and vomiting
(C) yawning, hypothermia, and excruciating pain
(D) mild discomfort with more severe symptoms peaking earlier, 12 to 24 hr after the last dose
(E) mild discomfort with more severe symptoms peaking 4 to 5 days after the last dose

45. All of the following are associated with the use of benzodiazepines EXCEPT

(A) antianxiety effects
(B) addictive effects
(C) anticonvulsant effects
(D) impaired conditioned avoidance learning
(E) additive action with alcohol

46. Which of the following ligaments is part of the lesser omentum?

(A) gastrocolic
(B) gastrosplenic
(C) gastrophrenic
(D) hepatoduodenal
(E) falciform

47. In the pathways for the synthesis of steroids, a deficiency of the enzymes 21β-hydroxylase or 11β-hydroxylase may result in abnormally high levels of circulating androgens. A major factor that contributes to this increase is

(A) loss of inhibition of androgen synthesis by corticosteroids
(B) increased synthesis of testosterone within the gonads
(C) decreased conversion of androgens to estrogen
(D) increased release of ACTH
(E) increased release of luteinizing hormone (LH)

48. Which of the following events takes place during the complete biosynthesis of collagen?

(A) Biosynthesis is completed within fibroblasts.
(B) Procollagen is secreted by fibroblasts.
(C) Triple-helix formation occurs from procollagen.
(D) Tropocollagen is secreted by fibroblasts.
(E) Conversion of proline to hydroxyproline occurs after secretion of collagen precursors.

49. The virulence of *Streptococcus pneumoniae* is primarily associated with the presence of

(A) cell wall teichoic acid
(B) pneumolysin
(C) polysaccharide capsule
(D) M protein
(E) peptidoglycan

50. Which of the following descriptions of the histology of non-Hodgkin's lymphoma best describes the least aggressive or lowest grade of tumor?

(A) nodular: small cell with cleaved nuclei
(B) diffuse: large cell with noncleaved nuclei
(C) nodular: large cell with cleaved nuclei
(D) diffuse: small cell with noncleaved nuclei
(E) diffuse: immunoblastic

51. The following effects are associated with phenothiazine administration EXCEPT

(A) antiemetic
(B) release of prolactin
(C) prevention of parkinsonism
(D) gynecomastia
(E) antihistaminic

52. All of the following statements are true concerning aggression EXCEPT

    (A) XYY syndrome may contribute to aggression.
    (B) Males are more likely to commit homicide, battery, or rape than females.
    (C) Aggression is more common toward unfamiliar, strange persons than to familiar persons.
    (D) The sex ratio for domestic violence is about equal between males and females.
    (E) Psychiatric inpatients have a higher rate of aggression than the general population.

53. Spinal nerves contain fibers that carry all of the following functional components EXCEPT

    (A) special visceral efferent
    (B) general somatic afferent
    (C) general visceral afferent
    (D) general somatic efferent
    (E) general visceral efferent

54. One effect of androgens is to promote linear bone growth. This effect is transient because

    (A) androgens cause epiphyseal closure
    (B) androgens slow the synthesis of collagen
    (C) receptors for androgens are down regulated
    (D) androgens increase the excretion rate of calcium and phosphate ions
    (E) androgens stimulate bone resorption

55. All of the following are true concerning the formation of a δ-aminolevulinic acid EXCEPT that it

    (A) requires glycine
    (B) is prerequisite to the formation of porphobilinogen
    (C) requires succinyl-coenzyme A (CoA)
    (D) is catalyzed by δ-aminolevulinate dehydrogenase
    (E) is the rate-limiting step in the formation of heme

56. Retroviruses are unique among all viruses in that

    (A) the mature virus contains a strand of RNA and a strand of DNA
    (B) they can carry out replication of their genomes extracellularly within intact vesicles
    (C) they contain reverse transcriptase in the virion
    (D) they are nonantigenic
    (E) the mature virus contains no nucleic acid

57. The changes seen in the kidney shown in the photograph below may be produced by

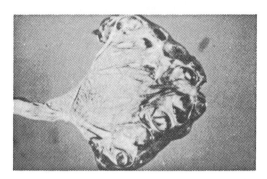

    (A) postrenal obstruction
    (B) renal infarct
    (C) hypertension
    (D) renal cell carcinoma
    (E) abuse of analgesics

58. Bacterial resistance to penicillin usually occurs by

    (A) thickening of the bacterial wall
    (B) changes in the activity of the transpeptidase required for wall formation
    (C) reduced requirement for folic acid
    (D) enzymatic hydrolysis of the β-lactam ring
    (E) decreased affinity of the ribosomal subunit for the drug

59. An attenuated form of anxiety that plays an important role in psychologic defense mechanisms is

    (A) signal anxiety
    (B) actual anxiety
    (C) neurotic anxiety
    (D) panic anxiety
    (E) psychotic anxiety

60. First-order sensory neurons for pain and temperature are located in which of the following structures?

    (A) anterior gray column
    (B) dorsal gray column
    (C) thalamus
    (D) dorsal root ganglion
    (E) lateral funiculus

61. In normal adult men, the major source of circulating estradiol is provided by

    (A) secretion from the Leydig's cells in the testes
    (B) secretion from the Sertoli's cells in the testes
    (C) the action of aromatase on circulating androgens
    (D) the action of aromatase on circulating estrone
    (E) release from the inner layers of the adrenal cortex

62. Which of the following is present only in the intrinsic pathway of clotting?

    (A) fibrinogen (factor I)
    (B) accelerin (factor V)
    (C) prothrombin (factor II)
    (D) antihemophilic factor (factor VIII)
    (E) Stuart factor (factor X)

63. All of the following are DNA viruses EXCEPT

    (A) variola
    (B) herpes simplex
    (C) molluscum contagiosum
    (D) papova
    (E) measles

64. Down's syndrome is characterized by the karyotype

    (A) trisomy 13
    (B) trisomy 18
    (C) trisomy 21
    (D) XO
    (E) XXY

65. The most common serious side effect of a single dose of one aspirin tablet is

    (A) infertility
    (B) hepatotoxicity
    (C) nephrotoxicity
    (D) allergic asthma
    (E) hemolytic anemia

66. A physician neglected to discuss with a patient potential complications of proposed surgery. When a colleague pointed this out, the physician claimed that the patient did not want to know it anyway. This may be an example of

    (A) reaction formation
    (B) denial
    (C) organic brain syndrome
    (D) rationalization
    (E) sublimation

67. Which of the following pathways is concerned with the conduction of pain and temperature modalities?

    (A) corticospinal
    (B) fasciculus gracilis
    (C) dorsal spinocerebellar
    (D) fasciculus cuneatus
    (E) lateral spinothalamic

68. Tumors of acidophilic cells in the anterior pituitary of adults are most likely to lead to

    (A) dwarfism
    (B) acromegaly
    (C) Cushing's syndrome
    (D) gigantism
    (E) adrenogenital syndrome

69. The blood protein thrombin is known to

    (A) have an enzymatic specificity similar to trypsin
    (B) form clots by complexing with fibrin
    (C) be an oligomeric protein
    (D) require vitamin K in its activated form
    (E) contain γ-carboxyglutamate residues

70. A 3-year-old child has a temperature of 38.3°C (101°F). On examination, discrete vesiculoulcerative lesions (Koplik's spots) are noted on the mucous membranes of the mouth. The most probable diagnosis is

    (A) rubella
    (B) herpangina
    (C) measles
    (D) herpetic gingivostomatitis
    (E) scarlet fever

71. Which of the following is NOT characteristic of the process of atherosclerosis?

    (A) primarily and initially an intimal disease
    (B) associated with elevated serum cholesterol levels
    (C) monoclonal proliferation of smooth muscle cells in the intima
    (D) associated with increase in serum lipids of the low-density lipoprotein (LDL) class
    (E) associated with increase in serum high-density lipoproteins (HDL)

72. In most individuals, endogenous cortisol plasma concentrations may be described as

    (A) highest in the early morning
    (B) lowest in the late morning and early afternoon
    (C) lowest in the late afternoon
    (D) highest in the late afternoon
    (E) nonvariable throughout the day

73. Which of the following statements correctly characterizes unsuccessful attempts at suicide?

    (A) Advanced age is usually a factor.
    (B) Females are more likely than males to attempt suicide.
    (C) Subsequent successful suicide attempts are unlikely.
    (D) Interpersonal difficulties usually are not a factor.
    (E) Such attempts are infrequent among Catholics.

74. Second-order sensory neurons for pain and temperature of the face are located in which of the following structures?

    (A) trigeminal ganglion
    (B) nucleus of the spinal tract of the trigeminal
    (C) main sensory nucleus of the trigeminal nerve
    (D) mesencephalic root of the trigeminal nerve
    (E) spinal tract of the trigeminal nerve

75. A circadian rhythm in the synthesis and release of melatonin occurs primarily in the

    (A) suprachiasmatic nuclei
    (B) adrenal medulla
    (C) raphe nuclei
    (D) pineal gland
    (E) skin

76. The number of moles of ATP produced by complete mitochondrial oxidation of 1 mol of pyruvate to CO_2 and water is

    (A) 1
    (B) 6
    (C) 12
    (D) 15
    (E) 24

77. The DiGeorge syndrome is characterized by

    (A) a depletion of lymph node lymphocytes in both T- and B-dependent areas
    (B) defective development of the third and fourth pharyngeal pouches
    (C) an absence of isohemagglutinins
    (D) a defect in neutrophil chemotaxis
    (E) a depletion of B-dependent areas in lymph nodes

78. All of the following are signs of local inflammation EXCEPT

    (A) redness
    (B) heat
    (C) numbness
    (D) pain
    (E) swelling

79. In anticoagulant therapy, an increased response would be expected with

    (A) barbiturates
    (B) rifampin
    (C) phenylbutazone
    (D) cholestyramine
    (E) glutethimide

80. Which of the following are considered to be pain receptors?

    (A) Meissner's corpuscles
    (B) Vater-Pacini corpuscles
    (C) basal cells
    (D) rods
    (E) free nerve endings

81. The fibers terminating in the nucleus gracilis originate in which of the following areas?

    (A) face
    (B) lower extremities
    (C) upper extremities
    (D) neck
    (E) head

82. In the absence of hormone replacement therapy, adrenalectomy may result in death within a few days. This is most likely to be caused by the loss of the adrenal hormone

    (A) cortisol
    (B) corticosterone
    (C) aldosterone
    (D) dehydroepiandrosterone
    (E) epinephrine

83. All of the atoms composing urea are contained within

    (A) aspartate and ornithine
    (B) carbamoyl phosphate and citrulline
    (C) ornithine and citrulline
    (D) aspartate
    (E) argininosuccinate

84. Sterilization of surgical instruments that are sensitive to heat can best be accomplished by

    (A) the autoclave
    (B) ionizing radiation
    (C) ethylene oxide
    (D) phenol
    (E) ethyl alcohol

85. The characteristic pathologic lesion of sarcoid is

    (A) fibroblastic proliferation
    (B) noncaseating granuloma
    (C) pyogenic abscess
    (D) mucoid cyst
    (E) hyaline membrane formation

86. Propranolol is beneficial in the treatment of angina because it

    (A) dilates capacitance vessels
    (B) increases coronary blood flow
    (C) increases oxygen delivery
    (D) decreases contractile force
    (E) reduces oxygen requirements

87. Lithium salts are most effective in

    (A) generalized anxiety disorder
    (B) unipolar depression
    (C) panic disorder
    (D) acute mania
    (E) schizophrenia

88. With a lesion of the lemniscal pathway, all of the following occur EXCEPT a

    (A) loss of position sense
    (B) loss of two-point discrimination
    (C) loss of the ability to recognize objects by feel and palpation
    (D) loss of vibratory sense
    (E) loss of pain

89. The secretion of glucagon from α cells of pancreatic islets is

    (A) inhibited by elevated amino acid concentrations in plasma
    (B) inhibited by elevated cyclic AMP levels
    (C) stimulated by elevated plasma glucose
    (D) stimulated by insulin
    (E) enhanced by sympathetic stimulation

90. In mammals, all of the following can serve as a substrate for the net synthesis of glucose EXCEPT

    (A) glycerol
    (B) β-hydroxybutyric acid
    (C) oxaloacetic acid
    (D) glutamic acid
    (E) propionic acid

91. In a positive viral hemagglutination inhibition test, hemagglutination is inhibited by which of the following substances in the serum?

    (A) antiviral antibody
    (B) latex agglutinins
    (C) Rh antibody
    (D) hemolysin
    (E) virus

92. Malignant melanomas may do all of the following EXCEPT

    (A) metastasize via the lymphatic vessels
    (B) metastasize hematogenously
    (C) arise in sun-exposed areas of skin
    (D) arise in the papillary dermis
    (E) arise de novo

93. In persons suffering from severe anaphylactic shock, the drug of choice for restoring circulation and relaxing bronchial smooth muscle is

    (A) epinephrine
    (B) norepinephrine
    (C) isoproterenol
    (D) phenylephrine
    (E) dopamine

94. All of the following statements concerning suicide are true EXCEPT that

    (A) most people who commit suicide give definite warnings about their intent
    (B) suicide may occur when the patient's mood seems to be lifting
    (C) people who habitually talk of suicide seldom commit suicide
    (D) most people who commit suicide see a physician before the suicidal act
    (E) suicide is more common among professional persons than individuals in lower economic groups

95. Cell bodies of lower motor neurons in the spinal cord are located in which of the following structures?

(A) posterior funiculus
(B) corticospinal tract
(C) anterior gray column
(D) dorsal root ganglion
(E) ventral root

96. The most active form of thyroid hormone in the stimulation of oxygen use is

(A) thyroxine
(B) thyroglobulin
(C) triiodothyronine
(D) reverse triiodothyronine
(E) monoiodotyrosine

97. Symptoms of von Gierke's disease include massive enlargement of the liver, severe hypoglycemia, ketosis, hyperlipemia, and hyperuricemia. Biopsy of the tissues of an affected person would show that the liver had a specific deficiency of the enzyme

(A) glucokinase
(B) hexokinase
(C) glucose 6-phosphatase
(D) phosphofructokinase
(E) α-1,4-glucosidase

98. In an influenza virus complement-fixation procedure, the indicator system consists of sheep RBCs plus

(A) ^{51}Cr-labeled sheep RBCs
(B) antibody to influenza virus
(C) fluorescent-tagged virus
(D) antibody to sheep RBCs
(E) complement

99. The photomicrograph below is from a breast biopsy in a 35-year-old female. Which of the following most characteristically describes the lesion?

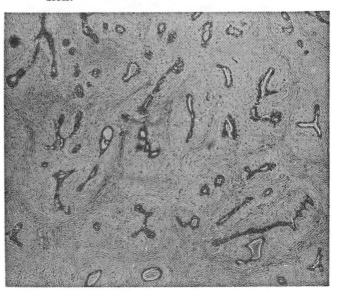

(A) medullary carcinoma
(B) fibroadenoma
(C) Paget's disease
(D) intraductal carcinoma
(E) scirrhous carcinoma

100. Atropine, at normal dosages, blocks the effects of acetylcholine by

(A) inhibiting the synthesis of acetylcholine
(B) competing at the muscarinic receptor sites
(C) blocking the release of acetylcholine from storage sites
(D) enhancing the effects of acetylcholinesterase
(E) competing at the nicotinic receptor sites

101. All of the following occur during the rapid-eye-movement (REM) sleep EXCEPT

(A) rapid eye movements
(B) sleepwalking
(C) visual dreams
(D) penile and clitoral erection
(E) irregular heart rate

102. The linea semilunaris indicates the lateral border of which of the following structures?

(A) sternum
(B) rectus abdominis muscle
(C) inguinal ligament

(D) infrasternal angle

(E) external abdominal aponeurosis

103. Damage to Wernicke's area in the cerebral cortex is associated with

(A) impaired vocalization

(B) impaired comprehension of speech

(C) impaired recognition of visual forms

(D) dyslexia

(E) loss of short-term memory

104. The figure shown below demonstrates enzyme kinetics of

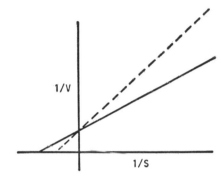

Double-reciprocal plot of enzyme kinetics.

(A) a competitively inhibited enzyme

(B) a noncompetitively inhibited enzyme

(C) an allosteric enzyme with and without effector

(D) two enzymes, each with a different Vmax

(E) an irreversibly inhibited enzyme

105. A graft-versus-host reaction may occur

(A) because the graft is contaminated with gram-negative microorganisms

(B) only when tumor tissues are grafted

(C) when immunocompetent lymphoid cells are present in the graft and the recipient is immunosuppressed

(D) because the graft has histocompatibility antigens not found in the recipient

(E) when a histocompatible graft is irradiated before engraftment

106. A primary adenocarcinoma of the colon that has invaded the muscle wall but not the serosa, has no local spread, and has invaded local lymph nodes is regarded as stage

(A) T1,N1,M0

(B) T2,N0,M1

(C) T2,N1,M0

(D) T3,N1,M1

(E) T4,N1,M1

107. The uptake and elimination of inhalational anesthetics may be affected by all of the following EXCEPT

(A) pulmonary ventilation

(B) blood flow

(C) the extent of liver metabolism

(D) the solubility of gas in blood

(E) the solubility of gas in tissue

108. Insight-oriented psychotherapy is an example of which of the following models of doctor–patient relationships?

(A) activity–passivity

(B) exploitive

(C) guidance–cooperation

(D) mutual participation

(E) authoritarian

109. Which of the following arteries is a branch of the external iliac artery?

(A) inferior epigastric

(B) external pudendal

(C) superficial epigastric

(D) superficial circumflex iliac

(E) superior epigastric

110. All of the following statements about the skeletal muscle circulation of experimental animals are true EXCEPT that

(A) it contributes significantly to the maintenance of systemic arterial blood pressure (BP)

(B) blood flow within a given group of muscles is relatively homogeneous

(C) an increase in carotid sinus pressure produces vasodilatation of the vascular bed of most muscles

(D) contracting muscle can be shown to autoregulate

(E) stimulation of a pathway from the cortex and hypothalamus may produce vasodilatation

111. All of the following statements concerning mutations are correct EXCEPT that

    (A) substitutions of base pairs may cause mutations
    (B) transition or transversion may cause mutations
    (C) insertion of base pairs may cause mutations
    (D) deletions of base pairs may cause mutations
    (E) most mutations are caused by thymine dimers

112. Tissue grafts in which the same individual acts as both donor and recipient are termed

    (A) allografts
    (B) autografts
    (C) xenografts
    (D) isografts
    (E) homografts

113. The tetrology of Fallot most characteristically includes all of the following EXCEPT

    (A) pulmonary stenosis
    (B) ventricular septal defect
    (C) coarctation of the aorta
    (D) right ventricular hypertrophy
    (E) overriding of the aorta over the septal defect

114. All of the following gaseous anesthetics may cause liver toxicity EXCEPT

    (A) methoxyflurane
    (B) halothane
    (C) enflurane
    (D) isoflurane
    (E) chloroform

115. All of the following factors have been clearly associated with poor adherence to medical regimens EXCEPT

    (A) field dependence
    (B) very old age
    (C) male sex
    (D) socially marginal status
    (E) severe physical illness

116. The lateral umbilical folds are formed by the elevations of peritoneum covering which of the following structures?

    (A) umbilical arteries
    (B) umbilical vein
    (C) inferior epigastric arteries
    (D) urachus
    (E) deep circumflex iliac arteries

117. Left coronary blood flow is greatest

    (A) near the end of systole
    (B) in early systole
    (C) at the peak aortic systolic pressure
    (D) near the end of diastole
    (E) in early diastole

118. Introns are correctly described as

    (A) noncoding intervening sequences splitting genes for a single protein
    (B) noncoding intervening sequences separating genes for different proteins
    (C) all noncoding sequences of DNA
    (D) untranslated regions of mature mRNA that separate different protein messages
    (E) untranslated regions of mature mRNA that intervene in the message for a single protein

119. Rh_0-specific immune globulin (RhoGAM) therapeutic preparations are correctly described as composed of

    (A) anti-inflammatory agents
    (B) blocking antibodies
    (C) antilymphocyte antibodies
    (D) antiallergen antibodies
    (E) enhancing antibodies

120. Cells that exhibit neoplastic transformations may show all of the following changes EXCEPT

    (A) increased sensitivity to contact inhibition of growth
    (B) decreased sensitivity to density-dependent inhibition
    (C) loss of anchoring ability for growth
    (D) infinite potential for replication and survival
    (E) the ability to produce malignant transformations in synergistic hosts

121. All of the following may cause hypokalemia EXCEPT

    (A) carbenicillin
    (B) furosemide
    (C) triamterene
    (D) amphotericin B
    (E) glycyrrhizic acid

122. A patient complains of pain in the chest and nausea. A thorough medical workup does not reveal any organic pathologic condition. It is learned that the patient's mother, who died recently, had exactly these symptoms. This patient's symptoms may be caused by

    (A) generalized anxiety disorder
    (B) pathologic grief reaction
    (C) posttraumatic stress disorder
    (D) major depression
    (E) none of the above

123. The pampiniform plexus of veins is associated with which of the following structures?

    (A) liver
    (B) heart
    (C) lungs
    (D) testes
    (E) uterus

124. In the normal heart, the major source of energy for oxidative metabolism is

    (A) glucose
    (B) lactate
    (C) fatty acids
    (D) pyruvate
    (E) amino acids

125. Addition of a competitive inhibitor to an enzymatic reaction will result in which of the following changes to a Lineweaver–Burk plot of that reaction?

    (A) increase in the slope
    (B) increase in the slope and decrease in the Y intercept
    (C) decrease in the slope
    (D) decrease in the slope and increase in the Y intercept
    (E) decrease in both the slope and the Y intercept

126. Antibody against autologous IgG would be synthesized in

    (A) central lymphoid organs
    (B) peripheral lymphoid organs
    (C) thymic tissue
    (D) macrophages
    (E) phagosomes

127. In order to heal properly, wounds require all of the following EXCEPT

    (A) fibroblast secretion of tropocollagen
    (B) cross-linkage of collagen

    (C) fibroblast synthesis of elastic fibers
    (D) the presence of collagenase
    (E) the hydroxylation of collagen

128. The most serious result of acute acetaminophen intoxication is

    (A) hypoglycemic coma
    (B) methemoglobinemia
    (C) respiratory depression
    (D) renal tubular necrosis
    (E) hepatic necrosis

129. The single best approach that physicians may use in dealing with a chronically angry patient is to

    (A) express their own emotions freely
    (B) let the patient use catharsis
    (C) be neutral and objective
    (D) consult a psychiatrist
    (E) use sarcasm to defuse the anger

130. The dartos muscle is located in which of the following structures?

    (A) spermatic cord
    (B) anterior abdominal wall
    (C) diaphragm
    (D) scrotal wall
    (E) small intestine

131. All of the following statements regarding systemic hemodynamics are true EXCEPT that the

    (A) greatest cross-sectional area is within the capillaries rather than small veins
    (B) greatest percentage of blood volume is in the small veins and the least is in the arterioles
    (C) greatest drop in pressure occurs in the arterioles rather than the large arteries
    (D) compliance of the venous circulation is less than the arterial circulation
    (E) velocity of blood flow is lowest in the capillaries

132. Which of the following has its highest concentration in erythrocyte plasma membranes?

    (A) cholesterol
    (B) plasmalogens
    (C) gangliosides
    (D) a lipid containing glycerol, two fatty acids, and serine phosphate
    (E) phosphatidyl ethanolamine

133. The sketch below represents the organism that may cause

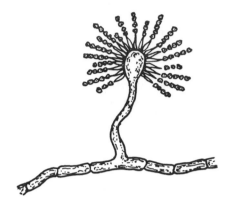

(A) phycomycosis
(B) tinea barbae
(C) tinea corporis
(D) tinea pedis
(E) aspergillosis

134. The most important component in the formation of the hemostatic plug is

(A) red blood cells
(B) fibrin
(C) lymphocytes
(D) platelets
(E) collagen

135. The phenothiazine antipsychotic that is LEAST likely to have extrapyramidal side effects is

(A) chlorpromazine
(B) trifluoperazine
(C) thioridazine
(D) haloperidol
(E) prochlorperazine

136. All of the following are often associated with decreased sexual activity EXCEPT

(A) mania
(B) depression
(C) chronic schizophrenia
(D) diabetes mellitus
(E) multiple sclerosis

137. The tail of the epididymis is continuous with which of the following structures?

(A) testes
(B) prostate
(C) ductus deferens
(D) bladder
(E) seminal vesicle

138. In a healthy individual with normal cardiovascular function, cardiac output is controlled ultimately by

(A) the heart
(B) the sympathetic nervous system
(C) the central nervous system
(D) the peripheral circulation
(E) none of the above

139. Under normal conditions, the brain relies primarily on glucose as an energy source. Of the total calories consumed by the body, this accounts for

(A) 5 percent
(B) 20 percent
(C) 50 percent
(D) 60 percent
(E) 75 percent

140. A patient is suffering from eruptions and multiple draining sinuses with copious suppuration. The lesions are located in the cervicofacial region. Microscopic examination of material taken from the lesions reveals small sulfur granules. This patient is most likely suffering from

(A) amebiasis
(B) mucormycosis
(C) histoplasmosis
(D) candidiasis
(E) actinomycosis

141. The lesion shown below is characteristic of

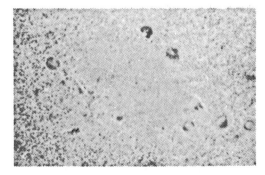

(A) an abscess
(B) a granuloma
(C) a keloid
(D) an infarct
(E) a thrombus

142. Which of the following oral hypoglycemic agents has the longest duration of action?

    (A) tolazamide

    (B) tolbutamide

    (C) acetohexamide

    (D) chlorpropamide

    (E) isopropamide

143. If a diagnostic test is positive in 98 of 100 patients with a particular disease and is negative in 90 of 100 controls without the disease, which of the following statements is true?

    (A) Specificity is 98 percent and sensitivity is 90 percent.

    (B) Specificity is 90 percent and sensitivity is 98 percent.

    (C) Positive predictive accuracy is 98 percent.

    (D) Negative predictive accuracy is 98 percent.

    (E) None of the above

DIRECTIONS (Questions 144 through 232): Each set of matching questions in this section consists of a list of up to ten lettered options followed by several numbered items. For each item, select the ONE lettered option that is most closely associated with it. Each lettered heading may be selected once, more than once, or not at all.

Questions 144 through 147

For each hormone listed below, select the metabolic derangement that would most likely result from its deficiency.

    (A) osteoporosis

    (B) ketoacidosis

    (C) sodium wasting

    (D) somnolence

    (E) hypoglycemia

144. Aldosterone

145. Cortisol

146. Insulin

147. Thyroid hormone

Questions 148 through 150

The Lineweaver-Burk plot below is based on an enzyme-catalyzed reaction in the absence of an inhibitor, the presence of a competitive inhibitor, and the presence of a noncompetitive inhibitor. For each description below, indicate the lettered point on the graph with which it is associated.

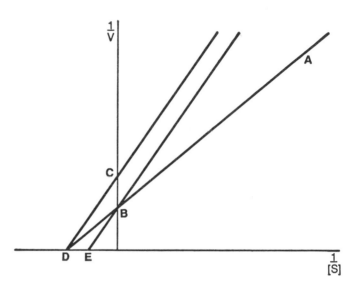

148. K_m of the uninhibited enzyme

149. V_{max} of the competitively inhibited enzyme

150. The point that contains all the necessary information to determine the substrate concentration at which half the active sites will be occupied in the presence of the noncompetitive inhibitor.

Questions 151 through 153

    (A) benign hyperplasia

    (B) sinus histiocytosis

    (C) metastatic carcinoma

    (D) non-Hodgkin's disease

    (E) metastatic melanoma

    (F) Hodgkin's disease

    (G) sarcoidosis

    (H) angiosarcoma

    (I) lipid granuloma

    (J) tuberculosis

151. A 4 cm lymph node is removed from an otherwise healthy 32-year-old dentist. Microscopically, the nodal architecture is effaced by a polymorphous infiltrate of neutrophils, plasma cells, eosinophils, and Reed–Sternberg cells.

152. Numerous enlarged inguinal lymph nodes are removed from a 45-year-old female. Microscopically, the nodal architecture is effaced by anaplastic non-cohesive cells with prominent nucleoli and cytoplasmic melanin. Two years earlier the woman had a "black" lesion removed from the ipsilateral foot.

153. An enlarged axillary lymph node is removed from a 61-year-old female. Microscopically, the nodal architecture is effaced by anaplastic gland-forming cells. Special studies on the tissue confirm the presence of estrogen and progesterone receptor proteins.

Questions 154 through 157

For each antihypertensive agent, select the side effect with which it is most commonly associated.

    (A) bradycardia
    (B) tachycardia
    (C) first-dose syncope
    (D) depression
    (E) sedation

154. Hydralazine

155. Propranolol

156. Prazosin

157. Methyldopa

Questions 158 through 161

For each age listed below, select the developmental stage, described by Erikson, with which it is most likely to be associated.

    (A) basic trust vs mistrust
    (B) initiative vs guilt
    (C) industry vs inferiority
    (D) identity vs role diffusion
    (E) autonomy vs shame, doubt
    (F) intimacy vs isolation
    (G) integrity vs despair
    (H) generativity vs stagnation

158. first year

159. fourth year

160. tenth year

161. fifteenth year

Questions 162 through 165

    (A) systemic lupus erythematosis
    (B) primary biliary cirrhosis
    (C) amyloidosis
    (D) pemphigus
    (E) pernicious anemia

162. Autoantibodies against parietal cells or intrinsic factor

163. Autoantibodies against surface antigens in keratinocytes

164. Autoantibodies against mitochondria

165. Autoantibodies against nuclear antigens

Questions 166 through 168

For each phase of the cardiac cycle listed below, choose the portion of the electrocardiogram with which it is most closely associated.

    (A) P wave
    (B) QRS complex
    (C) ST segment
    (D) T wave
    (E) QT interval

166. Ventricular repolarization

167. Atrial contraction

168. Plateau phase of cardiac action potential

Questions 169 through 171

    (A) a substitution mutation changes only one specific amino acid of the protein coded
    (B) a codon codes for one specific amino acid
    (C) deletions or insertions cause frame-shifts starting at the codon for the amino acid affected
    (D) the sum of purines in double-stranded DNA is equal to the sum of pyrimidines
    (E) most of the 64 possible base triplets have been shown to code for amino acids

169. Proof that the genetic code is degenerate

170. Proof that the genetic code is nonoverlapping

171. Proof that the sequence of bases in DNA is read sequentially from a fixed starting point

Questions 172 through 174

For each reaction described below, choose the enzyme that catalyzes it.

    (A) glucokinase
    (B) glucose 6-phosphate dehydrogenase
    (C) glycogen phosphorylase
    (D) glucose 6-phosphatase
    (E) glycogen synthase

172. Inorganic phosphate is a substrate.

173. UDP-glucose is a substrate.

174. ATP is a substrate.

Questions 175 through 178

For each of the findings described below, choose the disease with which it is usually associated.

    (A) Marfan's syndrome
    (B) Pompe's disease
    (C) Tay-Sachs disease
    (D) Niemann-Pick disease
    (E) Lesch-Nyhan syndrome

175. Connective tissue disorder with skeletal, ocular, and cardiovascular abnormalities

176. Accumulation of GM_2 ganglioside in the nervous system

177. Spingomyelin buildup in reticuloendothelial cells

178. Cardiac and neurologic glycogen storage disease

Questions 179 through 184

For each of the following agents, select the pharmacologic effect with which it is associated.

    (A) blockade of muscarinic receptors
    (B) selective blockade of β_1-adrenergic receptors
    (C) inhibition of breakdown of cholinergic neuro-transmitters
    (D) stimulation of α_1-adrenergic receptors
    (E) blockade of postganglionic nicotinic receptors

179. D-Tubocurarine

180. Physostigmine

181. Phenylephrine

182. Atropine

183. Metroprolol

184. Norepinephrine

Questions 185 through 189

For each age listed below, select the vocalization or language likely to be heard at that age.

    (A) cooing and vowel sounds
    (B) consonant sounds
    (C) conjunctions
    (D) pronouns
    (E) babbling

185. 3 months

186. 5 months

187. 6 months

188. 24 months

189. 36 months

Questions 190 through 194

For each diuretic agent, select the group in which it is classified.

    (A) carbonic anhydrase inhibitors
    (B) loop diuretics
    (C) thiazide diuretics
    (D) potassium-sparing diuretics
    (E) osmotic diuretics

190. Mannitol

191. Ethacrynic acid

192. Spironolactone

193. Triamterene

194. Furosemide

Questions 195 through 197

    (A) facial nerve
    (B) vagus
    (C) both
    (D) neither

195. Carries taste fibers

196. Is predominantly afferent

197. Innervates the stapedius muscle

Questions 198 and 199

The following illustration represents a continuous record of the relative cell volume of a red blood cell as it is changed from being immersed in a large volume of normal plasma to being in a large volume of a test solution and then returned to the plasma. Changes in cell volume are passive (not due to cell volume regulation).

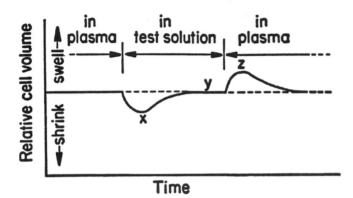

198. The change in cell volume that has peaked at point x on the above diagram resulted from

    (A) net exit of water from cell
    (B) net extracellular water entry into cell
    (C) net solute entry into cell
    (D) no net water movement
    (E) increased rate of solute entry into cell

199. The cell volume change that has peaked at point z is a result of

    (A) net exit of water from cell
    (B) no net water movement
    (C) net entry of water into cell caused by prior net entry of solute
    (D) net solute exit that occurred during prior exposure to test solution
    (E) neither net solute nor water movement

Question 200 through 202

For each characteristic of the citric acid cycle, choose the correct number.

    (A) two
    (B) three
    (C) twelve
    (D) fifteen
    (E) twenty-four

200. NADH molecules produced in one turn of the cycle

201. CO_2 molecules released in one turn of the cycle

202. Moles of nucleoside triphosphate that can be generated as a result of one turn of the cycle

Questions 203 and 204

    (A) clonidine
    (B) propranolol
    (C) labetalol
    (D) hydralazine
    (E) captopril

203. Blocks both α- and β-adrenergic receptors

204. Effects are related primarily to the renin–angiotensin system.

Questions 205 and 206

    (A) trauma to the head
    (B) usually seen with anemia
    (C) ruptured aneurysm in circle of Willis
    (D) right heart failure
    (E) left heart failure

205. Subarachnoid hemorrhage

206. Subdural hemorrhage

Questions 207 through 216

    (A) first pharyngeal arch
    (B) head somites
    (C) third pharyngeal arch
    (D) second pharyngeal arch
    (E) first pharyngeal pouch
    (F) second pharyngeal pouch
    (G) fourth and sixth pharyngeal arches
    (H) third pharyngeal pouch
    (I) fourth pharyngeal pouch

207. Which of the above structures gives rise to the stapes?

208. Which of the above structures gives rise to the stylopharyngeal muscle?

209. The superior parathyroid gland is formed from which of the above structures?

210. The malleus and incus are formed from which of the above structures?

211. The thyroid, arytenoid, corniculate, and cuneiform cartilages of the larynx are formed from which of the above structures?

212. The auditory tube is formed from which of the above structures?

213. The muscles of facial expression are formed from which of the above structures?

214. The muscles of mastication are formed from which of the above structures?

215. The thymus gland is formed from which of the above structures?

216. The anterior two-thirds of the tongue is formed from which of the above structures?

Questions 217 through 223

    (A) operant conditioning
    (B) classical conditioning
    (C) cognitive map
    (D) stimulus generalization
    (E) shaping
    (F) reciprocal inhibition
    (G) Premack's principle
    (H) extinction

217. A child likes to play pinball, and neglects eating food. The parents are told to allow the child to play pinball only after eating.

218. A child who was bitten by a snake is afraid of a rope.

219. A child who developed a phobia of ropes after being bitten by a snake is exposed to a rope repeatedly. He is no longer phobic of the rope.

220. A bell is rung just before presenting food to a dog. Eventually, the dog salivates at the sound of the bell alone.

221. A patient who is phobic of spiders is put in a relaxed state by suggestion and soothing music. While in this relaxed state, a photograph of a spider is presented to the patient.

222. In order to induce an animal to press a lever, food is given when the animal approaches the lever. Then, food is given when it touches the lever. Then, food is given only when the animal actually presses the lever.

223. When a person thinks about biting into a sour apple, salivation occurs.

Questions 224 through 226

The graph below represents a patient who has a febrile episode. Temperatures measured are rectal and in degrees C. Match each numbered statement with the appropriate letter choice from the graph (letters A through G). For this set of questions, letter choices may be used once, more than once, or not at all.

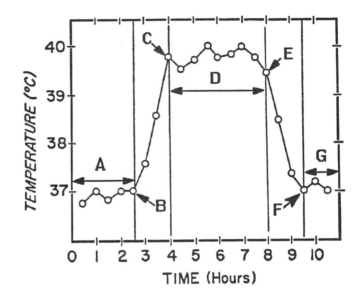

224. Period during which patient claims to be fairly comfortable (although the patient's set point is above normal)

225. Point at which patient begins to behave as if in a hot environment (sweats and complains of "burning up")

226. Point at which patient begins to behave as if in a cold environment (complains of chills and has shivering)

Questions 227 and 228

    (A) benign reactive follicular hyperplasia
    (B) malignant nodular lymphoma
    (C) Hodgkin's disease
    (D) metastatic carcinoma
    (E) metastatic melanoma

227. Nodal architecture preserved by numerous enlarged, varying-sized germinal follicles populated by a mixture of benign lymphoid cells

228. Nodal architecture effaced by numerous similar-sized nodules containing atypical lymphoid cells

Questions 229 through 232

    (A) *Yersinia pestis*

    (B) *Treponema pallidum*

    (C) *Rickettsia typhi*

    (D) *Bordetella pertussis*

    (E) *Rickettsia rickettsii*

229. Etiologic agent of Rocky Mountain Spotted Fever

230. Etiologic agent of syphilis

231. Etiologic agent of plague

232. Etiologic agent of whooping cough

DIRECTIONS (Questions 233 through 311): Each of the numbered items or incomplete statements in this section is followed by answers or by completions of the statement. Select the ONE lettered answer or completion that is BEST in each case.

233. A 2-year-old girl comes to your office with a three-day history of fever to 102°F, runny nose, conjunctivitis, cough, and diffuse erythematous macular rash over her face, chest, and back. The rash appears confluent when you examine her mouth. You would expect to find

    (A) Forscheimer's spots

    (B) bad breath

    (C) Koplik's spots

    (D) a large number of vesicles on her tongue

    (E) strawberry tongue

234. The protein coat (capsid) of true viruses is known to

    (A) serve as an antigen in serologic tests

    (B) function to maintain infectivity of nucleic acid in the extracellular state

    (C) serve as an antigen in vaccines

    (D) aid in the penetration of the virion into susceptible cells

    (E) all of the above

235. Amino acids whose side chains contribute to the charge of a protein at pH 7 include

    (A) cysteine

    (B) glycine

    (C) tyrosine

    (D) lysine

236. A 6-year-old farm boy develops restlessness, hallucinations, and convulsions, and dies 2 days later. At autopsy, the only significant finding is eosinophilic inclusions in neurons. These findings are consistent with

    (A) rabies

    (B) polio

    (C) herpes simplex encephalitis

    (D) western equine encephalitis

    (E) eastern encephalitis

237. The reagent cyanogen bromide cleaves

    (A) peptide bonds on the α-carboxyl side of arginine residues

    (B) peptide bonds on the α-carboxyl side of lysine residues

    (C) disulfide bridges

    (D) peptide bonds between the α-carboxyl of methionine and the α-amino group of the adjacent amino acid

238. Antibody-mediated antiviral immunity may operate through which of the following mechanisms?

    (A) complement-independent neutralization

    (B) complement-dependent neutralization

    (C) opsonization

    (D) lysis of infected host cells

    (E) all of the above

239. Which of the following population groups is most likely to develop carcinoma of the colon?

    (A) North American whites with low fiber diets

    (B) Black Africans with high fiber diets

    (C) Japanese with high fiber diets

    (D) infants and neonates

    (E) adolescents

240. The risk factors for suicide include

    (A) young age

    (B) female sex

    (C) Catholic religion

    (D) living alone

    (E) absence of a medical disorder

241. The enzyme, succinyl-CoA-acetoacetate transferase (3-ketoacid CoA transferase), is found in all the following tissues EXCEPT

    (A) skeletal muscle

    (B) kidney

    (C) brain

    (D) lung

    (E) liver

242. A virus causes diseases by

   (A) rendering vital target cells nonfunctional

   (B) disrupting the mucosa to allow bacteria to enter and produce a superimposed infection and disease

   (C) stimulating the host to produce immune substances that are deleterious to the host

   (D) altering the growth properties of the cell

   (E) all of the above

243. In the photomicrograph of a cytologic preparation shown below, malignant cells may be characterized by all of the following features EXCEPT

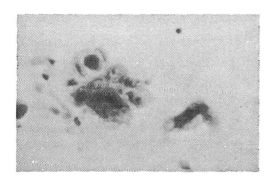

   (A) decreased mitotic rate

   (B) elevated nuclear to cytoplasmic ratio

   (C) hyperchromic nuclei

   (D) cellular pleomorphism

   (E) enlarged nucleoli

244. Depression may be associated with

   (A) cancer of the pancreas

   (B) antihypertensive drugs

   (C) hypothyroidism

   (D) Cushing's syndrome

   (E) all of the above

245. All of the following apply to the normal uterus EXCEPT that

   (A) it is anteflexed

   (B) it is anteverted

   (C) it has an inner mucous coat called the endometrium

   (D) it has a middle muscular coat called the perimetrium

   (E) the body of the uterus is enclosed between the layers of the broad ligament

In the illustration below, an animal receives a continuous infusion of gastrin. The production of gastric acid and pancreatic bicarbonate secretion is monitored before and after administration of peptide x (at arrow).

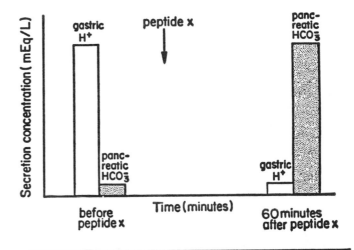

246. At the arrow, a peptide is administered. Which of the following is most likely to produce the changes observed?

   (A) motilin

   (B) angiotensin II

   (C) cholecystokinin (CCK)

   (D) somatostatin

   (E) secretin

247. Compounds derived from the amino acid, tyrosine, include all of the following EXCEPT

   (A) histamine

   (B) melanin

   (C) dopamine

   (D) p-hydroxyphenylpyruvate

   (E) epinephrine

248. Influenza viruses are correctly described as

   (A) being of three antigenic types (A, B, and C)

   (B) having a segmented genome

   (C) typed according to the ribonucleoprotein in the virion

   (D) having RNA as their genetic information

   (E) all of the above

249. Thrombosis and embolism may be associated with all of the following EXCEPT

(A) stasis of blood
(B) damage to vessel surface
(C) infarction
(D) may contain platelets, fibrin, and blood cells
(E) form best with hypocoagulable states

250. The following statements concerning acute grief reaction are true EXCEPT that

(A) depressive symptoms are common
(B) waves of somatic distress are common
(C) hallucinations and illusions may occur
(D) all symptoms must subside within four to eight weeks
(E) antidepressant therapy may be indicated

251. For descriptive purposes, the perineum is divided into two unequal triangles by an imaginary transverse line joining the anterior ends of which of the following structures?

(A) inferior pubic rami
(B) ischial rami
(C) ischial tuberosities
(D) sacrotuberous ligaments
(E) anterior superior iliac spines

The illustration below represents filtration through the glomerular membrane and shows the locations of the Starling forces.

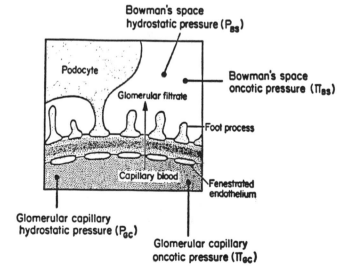

252. In which of the following is there a positive ultra-filtration pressure ($+P_{uf}$) for formation of glomerular filtrate? Numbers = mm Hg.

	P_{GC}	P_{BS}	Π_{GC}	Π_{BS}
(A)	40	20	30	10
(B)	40	15	25	0
(C)	40	10	20	0
(D)	50	20	30	0
(E)	55	25	40	5

253. All of the following enzymes are found in the liver, but not muscle, EXCEPT

(A) glucose 6-phosphatase
(B) hexokinase
(C) pyruvate carboxylase
(D) fructose 1,6-biphosphatase
(E) glucokinase

254. Receptors for C3b are present in the membranes of all of the following EXCEPT

(A) macrophages
(B) B lymphocytes
(C) neutrophils
(D) T lymphocytes
(E) monocytes

255. Which one of the following types of change seen in cell injury is not associated with the nucleus?

(A) pyknosis
(B) karyolysis
(C) karyorrhexis
(D) apoptosis
(E) cloudy swelling

256. Depressive syndrome is characterized by all of the following EXCEPT

(A) suicidal thoughts
(B) auditory hallucinations
(C) apathy
(D) anhedonia
(E) anorexia

257. All of the following muscles converge at the perineal body EXCEPT the

(A) transverse perineal
(B) ischiocavernosum
(C) bulbospongiosus
(D) levator ani
(E) external anal sphincter

258. Mixed micelles ("biliary micelles") within the intestinal lumen contain all of the following EXCEPT

(A) apolipoproteins
(B) bile salts
(C) cholesterol
(D) lecithin
(E) lipid-soluble vitamins

259. The conversion of fibrinogen to fibrin is catalyzed by

(A) prothrombin
(B) thrombin
(C) antithrombin III
(D) plasmin
(E) heparin

260. A remnant of the cranial end of the mesonephric duct is known as which of the following?

(A) a hydrocele of the testis
(B) a hematocele of the testis
(C) the appendix of the testis
(D) the appendix of the epididymis
(E) the processus vaginalis

261. All of the following structures are located in the inferior boundary of the omental foramen EXCEPT the

(A) first part of the duodenum
(B) portal vein
(C) hepatic artery
(D) bile duct
(E) inferior vena cava

262. In obsessive-compulsive disorder, all the following statements are true EXCEPT that

(A) the patient may be disabled
(B) fixation in the anal sadistic phase causes the syndrome
(C) the superego may be rigid
(D) serotonergic antidepressant drugs may be helpful
(E) psychosurgery may be helpful

263. All of the following structures are associated with the auditory pathway EXCEPT the

(A) lateral lemnisus
(B) mamillary bodies
(C) inferior colliculus
(D) medial geniculate body
(E) cochlear nuclei

264. In a young, healthy individual performing a forced expiration from total lung capacity down to residual volume, airflow over the last half of the vital capacity measurement is limited by

(A) the maximal force that can be generated by the expiratory muscles
(B) dynamic collapse of large intrathoracic airways (3rd–4th generation)
(C) the intra-pleural pressure
(D) collapse of extrathoracic airways
(E) airway collapse at the level of terminal bronchioles

265. Which of the following characteristics is indicative of regions of the eukaryotic genome that are actively transcribed?

(A) reduced sensitivity to DNase I digestion
(B) presence of the nonhistone proteins HMG1 and HMG2
(C) reduced levels of 5-methylcytosine
(D) elevated levels of the core histones
(E) reduced levels of the core histones

266. All of the following statements concerning bacterial spores are true EXCEPT that they

(A) are stable to heating at 80°C for several minutes
(B) require alanine, adenine, or other effector molecules for germination
(C) may form when nutritional conditions become unfavorable for bacterial growth
(D) are an important constituent of all gram negative organisms
(E) contain high levels of calcium dipicolinate

267. Serum sickness can be associated with all of the following EXCEPT

(A) circulating immune complexes
(B) complement activation
(C) fever, arthralgias, or vasculitis
(D) delayed hypersensitivity
(E) glomerulonephritis

268. Which class of cholinesterase inhibitors tend to form relatively irreversible covalent bonds with the enzyme?

(A) edrophonium
(B) carbamates
(C) chlorinated hydrocarbons
(D) organophosphates
(E) none of the above

269. Psychological defense mechanisms may be described as all of the following EXCEPT

    (A) maladaptive modes of adjustment leading to psychopathology
    (B) accentuated during hospitalization
    (C) unconsciously mobilized
    (D) reduce anxiety
    (E) may be associated with hormonal states

270. The pyramidal decussation occurs in which of the following structures?

    (A) the diencephalon
    (B) the internal capsule
    (C) the pons
    (D) the midbrain
    (E) the medulla

271. With different levels of dynamic exercise under steady-state conditions,

    (A) cardiac output is almost linearly related to oxygen uptake
    (B) stroke volume is linearly related to oxygen uptake up to maximal oxygen consumption ($\dot{V}_{O_2 max}$)
    (C) arterial diastolic blood pressure decreases substantially
    (D) blood pressure in the pulmonary artery approaches that of the systemic arteries
    (E) blood perfusion of the skin decreases

272. Which of the following arteries provides the blood supply to the jejunum and ileum?

    (A) celiac trunk
    (B) superior mesentery
    (C) inferior mesentery
    (D) superior pancreatoduodenal
    (E) left gastric

273. All of the following statements concerning the aortic hiatus are correct EXCEPT that

    (A) the thoracic duct passes through it
    (B) the azygos vein usually passes through it
    (C) this aperture is posterior to the diaphragm
    (D) it passes posterior to the median arcuate ligament
    (E) it transmits the anterior and posterior vagal trunks

274. Which item is LEAST likely to delay wound healing?

    (A) diabetes mellitus
    (B) excessive scar formation at wound site
    (C) infection of wound

    (D) closely opposed clean wound edges
    (E) foreign material in wound

275. Neuromuscular blocking agents bind to which type of receptor?

    (A) nicotinic
    (B) muscarinic
    (C) beta-adrenergic
    (D) alpha-adrenergic
    (E) none of the above

276. Factors that influence how a patient perceives a symptom include all of the following EXCEPT

    (A) the frequency of the symptom in a given population
    (B) the familiarity of the symptom
    (C) the predictability of the outcome of the illness
    (D) the degree of threat associated with the illness
    (E) all of the above are correct statements

277. All of the following cranial nerves innervate voluntary muscles derived from embryonic somites EXCEPT the

    (A) oculomotor
    (B) hypoglossal
    (C) facial
    (D) abducens
    (E) trochlear

278. An excised, degassed lung is either filled with saline or with air. Which of the following is correct?

    (A) The saline-filled lung is less compliant.
    (B) In the saline-filled lung, the recoil pressure, at any given volume, is lower than in the air-filled lung.
    (C) The maximal volume attainable in the saline-filled lung is significantly greater than that in the air-filled lung.
    (D) The difference in recoil pressure between the two conditions, at any given volume, is entirely due to the intrinsic elasticity of the lung parenchyma.
    (E) The compliance of the lung increases when it is inflated with air *after* removal of saline (lavage).

279. Hydrolysis of a phospholipid by which of the following produces phosphatidic acid?

    (A) phospholipase A$_1$
    (B) phospholipase A$_2$
    (C) phospholipase C

(D) phospholipase D

(E) lipoprotein lipase

Questions 280 and 281

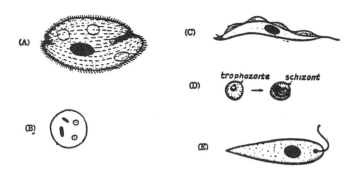

280. Malarial parasite

281. Causes Kala-azar

282. When presynaptic α_2-adrenergic receptors are stimulated, there is

(A) increased vasoconstriction

(B) increased norepinephrine release

(C) decreased norepinephrine release

(D) inhibition of norepinephrine re-uptake

(E) increased heart rate

283. Which of the following factors will increase the likelihood of a person's seeking medical help?

(A) unpleasant experience with physicians

(B) being Hispanic

(C) high level of stress

(D) low socioeconomic class

(E) all of the above

284. The cranial portion of the parasympathetic system is associated with all of the following cranial nerves EXCEPT the

(A) oculomotor

(B) trigeminal

(C) facial

(D) glossopharyngeal

(E) vagus

285. A tetraplegic patient has a complete spinal transection between cervical and thoracic levels. Which of the following statements apply to this patient?

(A) The maximal inspiratory pressures are more compromised than the expiratory ones.

(B) The inspiratory reserve volume is greatly reduced (less than 10 percent of normal).

(C) Functional residual capacity equals residual volume.

(D) Vital capacity is only slightly compromised.

(E) The ventilatory response to limb exercise is characterized by an increase in tidal volume contributed by the expiratory reserve volume.

286. The carbon atoms of fatty acids synthesized in humans can be derived from all of the following EXCEPT

(A) citrate

(B) glucose

(C) cholesterol

(D) leucine

(E) phenylalanine

287. When both lactose and glucose are present in the environment, very little lac mRNA is transcribed because

(A) the sigma subunit of RNA polymerase binds the holoenzyme

(B) cAMP levels are low

(C) the repressor binds the operator efficiently

(D) the catabolite activator protein bends DNA

(E) allolactose is the inducer of the lac operon

288. Acute rejection of a renal transplant is characterized by

(A) an infiltrate composed of mononuclear cells

(B) necrotizing arteritis with a neutrophilic infiltrate

(C) a granulomatous polymorphous infiltrate

(D) fibrosis and scarring

(E) slow cortical atrophy over several months

289. H_1-histamine antagonists frequently affect the autonomic nervous system by acting as

(A) cholinesterase inhibitors

(B) muscarinic antagonists

(C) muscarinic agonists

(D) α_1-agonists

(E) blockers of acetylcholine release

290. The basic elements of informed consent include all of the following EXCEPT

(A) a reasonable explanation of the procedures

(B) advising patients that they are free to withdraw consent at any time

(C) a description of potential risks and benefits

(D) a discussion of potential alternatives

(E) advising patients that they are entitled to a lawyer

291. Which of the following structures is primarily concerned with homeostasis?

    (A) the thalamus
    (B) the cerebellum
    (C) the basal ganglia
    (D) the hypothalamus
    (E) the reticular system

292. Which of the following generally occurs with exercise training of a previously sedentary individual?

    (A) a decrease in maximal oxygen consumption
    (B) a decrease in resting heart rate
    (C) a decrease in the maximal cardiac output
    (D) a decrease in resting stroke volume
    (E) a generalized increase in sympathetic tone

293. Both bacterial and eukaryotic nuclear DNA are

    (A) associated with histones
    (B) linear molecules
    (C) approximately the same size
    (D) methylated at the C-5 position of cytosine
    (E) replicated in a semiconservative manner

294. Hairy cell leukemia is

    (A) a benign disorder of erythrocytes
    (B) a benign disorder of keratinocytes
    (C) a malignant disorder of B-cell lymphocytes
    (D) a malignant disorder of megakaryocytes
    (E) a malignant disorder of neutrophils

295. The lung lesion depicted below is a

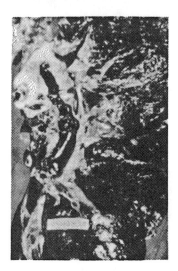

    (A) pulmonary embolus
    (B) bronchogenic carcinoma
    (C) granulomatous inflammatory process

    (D) congenital malformation
    (E) cyst

296. Which diuretic agent has as its primary mechanism of action the inhibition of carbonic anhydrase?

    (A) furosemide
    (B) spironolactone
    (C) hydrochlorothiazide
    (D) mannitol
    (E) acetazolamide

297. The following statements about anxiety are true EXCEPT that

    (A) it usually increases sympathetic tone
    (B) it may improve performance
    (C) it may be a conditioned response
    (D) it may be enhanced by stimulation of locus ceruleus
    (E) all of the above are true statements

298. Which of the following cortical areas is associated with receptive aphasia?

    (A) Broca's arena
    (B) Wernicke's area
    (C) Brodmann area 17, 18, 19
    (D) the precentral gyrus
    (E) the postcentral gyrus

299. Which sequence of events correctly describes the process of the digestion of dietary triglyceride in preparation for absorption?

    (A) emulsification → hydrolysis by acid lipases → incorporation into micelles → hydrolysis by pancreatic lipase
    (B) hydrolysis by acid lipases → emulsification → hydrolysis by pancreatic lipase → incorporation into micelles
    (C) incorporation into micelles → hydrolysis by acid lipases → hydrolysis by pancreatic lipase → emulsification
    (D) hydrolysis by pancreatic lipases → incorporation into micelles → hydrolysis by acid lipases → emulsification
    (E) emulsification → hydrolysis by acid lipases → hydrolysis by pancreatic lipase → incorporation into micelles

300. Blood gas analysis of an arterial blood sample shows

    pH = 7.55 P_{O_2} = 40 mm Hg
    HCO_3^- = 21 mM P_{CO_2} = 25 mm Hg

This blood sample was probably taken from

(A) a patient with severe chronic lung disease

(B) a native of a coastal region who has been vacationing in the Peruvian Andes for two weeks

(C) an experimental subject who has been breathing a gas mixture of 10 percent O_2 and 90 percent N_2 for a few minutes

(D) an emergency room patient severely overdosed with heroin

(E) an emergency room patient acutely overdosed with aspirin

301. Stem cells

(A) have CD_3 molecules on their surface

(B) have CD_4 molecules on their surface

(C) have CD_8 molecules on their surface

(D) have CD_{12} molecules on their surface

(E) lack CD_3, CD_4, and CD_8 molecules on their surface

302. The process of apoptosis is best described as

(A) liquefaction necrosis

(B) swelling of the endoplasmic reticulum

(C) hypertrophy

(D) individual cell necrosis

(E) dysplasia

303. Which drug or treatment is generally contraindicated in the management of congestive heart failure?

(A) furosemide

(B) digoxin

(C) captopril

(D) propranolol

(E) sodium restriction

304. To study the psychiatric morbidity of Spielmeyer-Vogt syndrome, all patients with the syndrome being treated in the city, as identified by medical records, were interviewed by psychiatric clinicians. A demographically controlled control group was also interviewed. This is an example of

(A) prospective cohort study

(B) case control study

(C) cross sectional prevalence survey

(D) lifetime prevalence study

(E) census survey

305. A person who lacks CD_8 lymphocytes will most likely

(A) not show cytotoxicity for virus infected cells

(B) have an enhanced capacity to destroy tumor cells

(C) have an enhanced ability to kill allograft cells

(D) show suppression of immunoglobulin production by B cells

(E) show suppression of delayed hypersensitivity reactions

306. Which of the following statements concerning the figure below, depicting viral multiplication, is true?

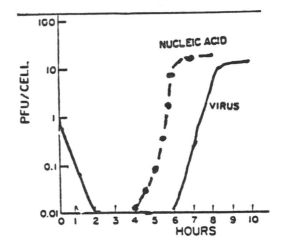

(A) The time interval, 0–6 hr, represents the eclipse period.

(B) The time interval, 0–6 hr, represents the absorption of virus to host cells.

(C) The viral multiplication curve is similar to the bacterial growth curve.

(D) The time interval, 0–3 hr, represents the late period.

(E) The time interval, 0–4 hr, represents the period at which the virions are at the peak of their infectivity.

307. Inducers function in the regulation of gene expression by

(A) preventing transcription of mRNA

(B) binding to the operator region of DNA

(C) mediating removal of the sigma subunit of RNA polymerase

(D) altering the conformation of repressors

(E) hybridizing to the promoter region of DNA

308. All of the following statements apply to the ductus deferens EXCEPT that

   (A) it joins the duct of the seminal vesicle to form the ejaculatory ducts

   (B) it passes through the inguinal canal

   (C) it crosses the urethra

   (D) it is the continuation of the duct of the epididymis

   (E) it crosses over the external iliac vessels to enter the pelvis minor

309. Extensive diffuse pulmonary fibrosis is LEAST likely to occur with prolonged inhalation of

   (A) silica

   (B) *Thermopolyspora polyspora*

   (C) asbestosis

   (D) nitrogen dioxide

   (E) carbon monoxide

310. The effects of nitroglycerin include

   (A) dilation of veins

   (B) decreased oxygen supply to the heart

   (C) decreased sympathetic stimulation of the heart

   (D) calcium channel blockade

   (E) inhibition of the sodium/potassium ATPase pump

311. Studies in humans and animals of childhood experience and adult function indicate all of the following EXCEPT that

   (A) male mice raised in isolation after weaning are more likely to be aggressive in later life

   (B) closure of one eye for a few days during the first six months of life in rhesus monkeys results in permanent impairment in depth perception

   (C) being in day care for 8 hours a day throughout infancy causes deficits in cognition and attachment behavior in adulthood

   (D) rats that are stimulated, handled, and stressed in infancy have faster rates of growth, larger bodies, and greater resistance to being killed by starvation or drowning

   (E) all of the above are true statements

Answers and Explanations

1. **(B)** The average adult brain weighs about 1,400 g, approximately 2 percent of the total body weight. The brain, a gelatinous mass, is invested by a succession of three connective tissue membranes called meninges and is protected by an outer capsule of bone, the skull. *(Noback, p 5)*

2. **(D)** Except for arachidonic, all of the fatty acids listed in the question are nonessential and cannot be precursors for the synthesis of essential fatty acids in humans. Prostaglandins are synthesized from arachidonic acid (*cis*-5,8,11,14-eicosatetraenoic acid) or other 20-carbon fatty acids that have at least three double bonds. Prostaglandins are 20-carbon fatty acids that contain a 5-carbon ring. They are hormonelike in their action, but unlike hormones, they often directly modulate the activities of the cells in which they are synthesized. *(Stryer, pp 991–992)*

3. **(D)** Primary hyperparathyroidism is a group of diseases characterized by overproduction of parathormone in a setting of no previous parathyroid hypersecretion. It occurs in 2.5 per 1,000 people. The overproduction of parathormone causes bone destruction with increased calcium release and elevated calcium levels in the blood. Subsequently, the kidneys are overloaded with calcium, with leakage of both calcium and phosphorus in the urine. Eventually, there is renal stone formation. This disease is also associated with peptic ulcers, pancreatitis, hypertension, CNS disturbances, and multiple endocrine neoplasia types I and II. The bone disease consists of bone destruction and new bone formation and the development of cysts and fibrosis. The renal disease includes stone formation, polyuria, polydipsia, and renal failure. Laboratory analysis of serum shows hypercalcemia with hypophosphatemia and elevated levels of parathormone. Primary hyperparathyroidism may be caused by adenomas, chief cell or water clear cell hyperplasias, or carcinomas. Parathyroid adenomas are the major cause in most patient series of primary hyperparathyroidism. *(Rubin and Farber, pp 1146–1149)*

4. **(C)** The cell bodies of the first-order neurons are located in the dorsal root ganglia of the spinal nerves and the sensory ganglia of the cranial nerves. The thalamus contains third-order sensory neurons. The cortex contains sensory, motor, and association neurons. The cerebellum contains no first-order sensory neurons and the superior cervical sympathetic ganglion contains post-ganglionic sympathetic motor cells. *(Noback, p 53)*

5. **(B)** Vitamin B_{12}, or cobalamin, is unique in that its corrin ring requires a cobalt atom in order to function. Cobalamin enzymes are involved in hydrogen rearrangement reactions, as in the synthesis of deoxyribonucleosides from ribonucleosides or as in the conversion of methylmalonyl coenzyme A (CoA) into succinyl CoA. The methylation of homocysteine by N^5-methyltetrahydrofolate to form methionine also requires the involvement of cobalamin as a methylated intermediate. Deficiencies of vitamin B_{12} or cobalt result in anemic symptoms. Pernicious anemia is a disease in which vitamin B_{12} is not absorbed because of a lack of a protein called intrinsic factor. This protein is normally synthesized by the gut epithelium and is required for vitamin B_{12} absorption. *(Stryer, pp 506–509)*

6. **(C)** Squamous cell carcinoma is the most common type of bronchogenic carcinoma, accounting for 60 percent of all reported cases. It is found in males more often than in females and is the form of lung cancer most closely correlated with a history of smoking. This type of tumor is thought to arise from bronchial mucosa and is thus central in location. Its increasing incidence in women is thought to be secondary to the increasing number of women smoking cigarettes in the past 20 years. *(Rubin and Farber, pp 554–556)*

7. **(B)** The first-order sensory neurons of the olfactory, optic, and bipolar neurons. The bipolar cells in the nasal mucous, retina, and the spiral ganglia are first-order neurons. First-order sensory neurons in the dorsal root ganglia and the semilu-

nar ganglion are pseudounipolar first-order sensory neurons. Neurons in the spinal cord are not bipolar or first-order sensory neurons. *(Noback, p 53)*

8. **(B)** Acetic acid is a weak acid, as indicated by its pK_a, and dissociates into a hydrogen ion and its conjugate base, acetate (i.e., $CH_3 - COOH \rightarrow H^+ + CH_3 - COO^-$). A solution of a weak acid and its salt is referred to as a buffer. The pH of any buffer solution can be determined by use of the Henderson-Hasselbalch equation.

$$pH = pK_a + \log A^-/HA$$

When the acetic acid has been converted into 80 percent acetate, the ratio A^-/HA is 4, and substituting the values provided in the problem into the Henderson-Hasselbalch equation yields:

$$pH = 4.75 + \log 4 = 5.35$$

(Stryer, pp 41–42)

9. **(D)** Mesothelioma is the most common malignant tumor of the pleura. It is a highly invasive lesion and has been linked to asbestos fibers—especially in persons in the shipbuilding and insulation industries. A history of smoking also increases the risk of developing a mesothelioma. Histologically, the tumor may be either sarcomatous (composed of mesenchymal stromal cells), carcinomatous (resembling tubular or papillary structures), or a combination of these two types. These tumors are highly malignant, and most patients die within 1 year of diagnosis. *(Cotran, pp 807–808)*

10. **(C)** Although metabolic acidosis may occur and [H⁺] increase, the initial compensatory response to hemorrhage results in a large increase in total peripheral vascular resistance. The loss of blood volume initially decreases cardiac output, but baroreceptor-mediated sympathetic drive causes vasoconstriction. Thus, vascular resistance increases, heart rate increases, and blood pressure returns toward normal. Slightly later, the kidneys may secrete renin, and the production of angiotensin II via converting enzyme activity ultimately ensues. Fluid also will shift from the interstitial compartments to the vascular space, helping to partly restore cardiac output. Other humoral agents, including epinephrine, vasopressin, and glucocorticoids, may also be released to further compensate for the cardiovascular effects of hemorrhage. *(Guyton, pp 263–265)*

11. **(D)** The SA node is located at the superior end of the crista terminalis at the junction of the anteromedial aspect of the superior vena cava and the right auricle. The sinuatrial node is a collection of specialized cardiac muscle fiber (nodal tissue) in the wall of the right atrium, which initiates the impulses for contraction. It is the natural pacemaker of the heart. *(Moore, p 104)*

12. **(D)** Temporary occlusion of both common carotid arteries will decrease vascular pressure within the carotid sinus area. This important peripheral baroreceptor responds to changes in pressure and is an important reflex in maintaining relatively constant arterial pressure on a short-term basis. A decrease in pressure will depress the number of impulses that travel from the carotid sinus nerve. Since these impulses normally inhibit the central vasoconstrictor area and excite the vagal center, a decrease in impulses will reflexively cause arterial pressure to rise and heart rate and contractility to increase. The entire circulation will be stimulated to constrict, and thus there will be a reduction in venous capacitance. *(Guyton, pp 198–199)*

13. **(C)** The normal yield from the complete oxidation of glycogen is about 4.2 kcal/g. Approximately the same amount of energy is derived from the combustion of proteins. In contrast, oxidation of fatty acids derived from triacylglyceride stores is much greater, about 9.5 kcal/g. Despite the fact that glycogen is an important and easily mobilized energy store, fats are the major energy reservoir. *(Stryer, p 471)*

14. **(E)** The condition of psoriasis is characteristically a scaly hyperkeratotic lesion of the skin, with the characteristic features described as parakeratosis, which is abnormal keratin maturation with nucleated material in the stratum corneum and with resultant thickness of the epidermis with club-shaped papillae extending into the dermal collagen. From time to time in various stages of the disease, collections of neutrophil leukocytes in the form of microabscesses can be seen in the upper layers of the epidermis. These are sometimes referred to as Pautrier's microabscesses. The condition is clearly distinguishable microscopically from other thickening of the epidermis, which may be mistaken clinically for basal cell carcinoma or even melanoma or squamous cell carcinoma. The condition of pemphigus vulgaris is a bullous or vesicular type of lesion that may have produced crusting on the surface and may be clinically similar but is microscopically quite distinct. Psoriasis is thought to be related to an abnormality of cell proliferation and control, resulting from some forms of injury, but its real etiology is still largely unknown. *(Rubin and Farber, pp 1209–1214)*

15. **(B)** The atrioventricular node is composed of specialized cardiac muscle cells that are located in the interatrial septum on the ventricular side of the orifice of the coronary sinus. The SA node ini-

tiates the impulses for contraction, and it is the natural pacemaker of the heart. The SA node may be located by following the nodal artery from the right coronary artery. *(Moore, p 104)*

16. **(D)** Although short-term regulation of arterial BP is primarily affected by the integrated responses of peripheral baroreceptors and the central and sympathetic nervous systems, the primary determinant of regulation of BP in the long run is the relationship of urine output to fluid intake. This system is normally capable of returning BP to normal levels (infinite gain), which is different from the short-term nervous regulation. By adjusting extracellular fluid and blood volumes, renal–body fluid mechanisms alter venous return. Individual beds then adjust their resistance because of the interplay of local and neuronal factors, and thus arterial pressure is slowly readjusted to control levels. The total peripheral vascular resistance is thus altered by those mechanisms rather than being the variable that directly determines BP. *(Guyton, pp 205–209)*

17. **(A)** The primary precursors for gluconeogenesis in liver are lactate and alanine, which are produced in muscle during intense activity. Alanine is formed from pyruvate by transamination in a reaction catalyzed by alanine aminotransferase. Alanine is converted back to pyruvate in liver and employed in the synthesis of glucose. *(Stryer, pp 444–445,496)*

18. **(D)** Constrictive pericarditis is a condition in which the normally thin and delicate pericardium is replaced by dense fibrous tissue with, in some circumstances, calcification within the fibrous tissue, resulting in a rigid, constricting pericardium that causes eventual malfunction of the myocardium and congestive failure. Although there are many reasons why the pericardium may cause an obstructive function to the heart, many of the others result from the acute accumulation of fluid or fluid and fibrin as seen in some cases of acute rheumatic fever or acute staphylococcal infections. In uremia and in lupus erythematosus, there may be hemorrhagic or even fibrinous pericarditis, but it rarely extends long enough to produce the complete constrictive form of the disease with dense fibrosis that is so typically seen in tuberculosis. In fact, tuberculosis is by far the most common cause of this otherwise relatively rare disorder. *(Rubin and Farber, p 536)*

19. **(E)** Identification is the psychologic defense mechanism by which an individual becomes like an admired (or otherwise psychologically important) person. Identification is an important phenomenon in personality development. *(Leigh and Reiser, pp 79–100)*

20. **(E)** The extraperitoneal fat is located between the peritoneum and the transversalis fascia. The internal spermatic fascia, the femoral sheath, deep inguinal ring, and the psoas fascia are all formed from transversalis fascia. As the processus vaginalis evaginates the transversalis fascia at the deep inguinal ring, it carries a thin layer of fascia before it that becomes the internal spermatic fascia. It constitutes the filmy, innermost covering of the spermatic cord. *(Moore, p 147)*

21. **(B)** Atrial fibrillation is a common arrhythmia that accompanies several forms of chronic heart disease. It probably represents some form of reentry phenomenon in which part of the tissue may be excited at an inappropriately early part of the cardiac cycle. Since the atria do not contract, there are no P waves. Activation of conducting tissue in the atrioventricular node becomes variable in time from cycle to cycle, and thus the QRS complex interval becomes less constant. The strength of ventricular contraction is related to the timing of filling, and thus failure of the atria to effectively contract alters ventricular filling. This produces an extremely irregular pulse. Direct current shock is an effective mechanism to return the heart to normal rhythm and reverse atrial fibrillation. However, atrial fibrillation per se is not a life-threatening event, and placing the entire myocardium into refractory period frequently is not the appropriate course of action. A number of drugs are available to prolong the effective refractory period of selective parts of the heart, and these drugs would represent an effective manner in which to revert atrial fibrillation to normal atrial contraction. *(Berne and Levy, p 393)*

22. **(D)** None of the amino acids composing the peptide Val-Ala-Pro-Glu-Gly have any charged side chains except for glutamate, which bears a charged carboxyl group. Thus, we only have to consider the amino and carboxyl groups of the C- and N-terminals along with the glutamic acid carboxyl group. At neutral pH, the carboxyl groups will be dissociated, since their pKs are always at a low pH. Likewise, the positively charged N-terminal amino group will not be dissociated, since its pK is always at a high pH. Thus, at pH 7, the peptide will contain two negative charges and one positive charge for an overall negative charge. Increasing the pH will only increase the negativity of the peptide, since the amino group will become more dissociated and less charged as its pK is approached. The isoelectric point of the peptide will be found at pH lower than 7. *(Lehninger, pp 71–76; Stryer, pp 17,42)*

23. **(B)** Wire-loop lesions in glomeruli in renal biopsy specimens, though not pathognomonic, are generally associated with renal involvement by sys-

temic lupus erythematosus. The formation of the wire loops is caused by subendothelial electron-dense deposits that produce thickened, refractile capillary walls. Small subepithelial deposits, or spikes, may also be present and produce extension of the deposits through the basement membrane. Wire-loop lesions also may be seen in glomerular lesions of patients with cryoglobulinemia. Diabetes mellitus, hypertension, and acute tubular necrosis may be associated with histologic changes in the renal glomeruli or tubules or both. These entities are not typically associated with wire-loop lesions, however. In the hepatorenal syndrome, renal dysfunction appears to be functional rather than associated with anatomic renal changes. (Rubin and Farber, pp 864–867)

24. **(B)** Society's sick-role expectations, as described by Parsons, include exemption from normal social role expectations, the recognition that the individual is not responsible for being sick and that he or she cannot be expected to get well simply by wanting to get well, being sick is an undesirable state, and the individual should try to get well, and that the sick person should seek competent help to get well. The idea that an individual is responsible for the maintenance of his or her health is contrary to the second expectation described above. (Leigh and Reiser, pp 17–24)

25. **(C)** An indirect inguinal hernia leaves the abdominal cavity lateral to the inferior epigastric artery and veins. The herniating mass is medial to the crest of the ilium, anterior superior iliac spine, deep inguinal ring, and the superficial circumflex iliac vessels. (Moore, pp 147–149)

26. **(D)** The prolonged depolarization of the plateau phase of the cardiac action potential is attributable to slowly inactivating voltage-gated calcium channels. (Guyton, pp 99–100)

27. **(D)** Alanine, cysteine, glycine, and serine are all converted to pyruvate during amino acid degradation. Thus, each of these amino acids can give rise to glucose via conversion of pyruvate to oxaloacetate and then phosphoenolpyruvate. In addition, ketone body formation can proceed by conversion of pyruvate to acetyl-CoA. In contrast, leucine can only be converted to potential ketone body precursors. The degradation of leucine leads to the formation of acetyl-CoA and acetoacetate. (Stryer, pp 503–511)

28. **(D)** The classic complement pathway is usually activated by the antigen-antibody union then involving complement components C1q, C4, C2, and C3–C9. The alternate complement pathway proceeds through C3–C9, and it can be activated by aggregated immunoglobulins IgA, IgG_4, IgE, lipopolysaccharides, and endotoxins but not IL-1, β-interferon, lipoproteins, or the complement component C1. IL-1 activates T cells. β-Interferon is an antiviral protein, and the complement component C1 binds to the antigen-antibody complex and initiates the cascade of the classic complement pathway. (Joklik et al, pp 286–295)

29. **(D)** Red infarcts are localized areas of ischemic necrosis resulting from a vascular interruption. These infarcts usually occur secondary to venous occlusion, with necrosis of the tissue due to ischemia accompanied by congestion and hemorrhage. Red infarcts occur in loose tissues that have a double circulation and are easily congested. The lungs are classically affected. As with arterial interruption, there is necrosis. At the same time, large amounts of hemorrhagic blood accumulate in the pulmonary parenchyma, so the infarct remains red. The intestines and brain are other organs that may have red infarcts. The heart, spleen, and kidneys classically have pale infarcts because they are solid tissues. Infarcts may occur with arterial occlusions, but there is no seepage or reflux of blood, since there is no dual blood supply, and the tissue is solid. (Cotran, pp 111–114)

30. **(C)** Acetaminophen is an effective analgesic and antipyretic agent but has only weak anti-inflammatory activity because of weak peripheral prostaglandin inhibitory properties. Indomethacin, aspirin, phenylbutazone, and tolmetin have prominent anti-inflammatory properties and hence may be useful in the treatment of patients with acute gout, rheumatoid arthritis, and other diseases associated with inflammation. (Gilman et al, pp 654–664)

31. **(B)** Temporal pairing of a neutral stimulus with a stimulus that produces an inherent response (food in the case described in the question) characterizes classical conditioning. Operant conditioning involves reward and punishment. (Leigh and Reiser, pp 45–47)

32. **(D)** The inferior limit of the posterior wall of the rectus sheath is marred by a crescentic border called the arcuate line. The aponeurosis of the external abdominal oblique ends medially in the linea alba. Inferiorly, it folds back on itself to form the inguinal ligament. The medial part of the inguinal ligament is reflected horizontally back and is attached to the pecten pubis at the lacunar ligament. The opening in the aponeurosis is called the superficial inguinal ring. (Moore, pp 133,136)

33. **(B)** A PTH-like effect would be expected to stimulate bone resorption, vitamin D conversion, and elevate serum calcium levels. Serum calcitonin would consequently be expected to rise. A PTH-like effect on the kidneys would increase calcium absorption while markedly increasing phosphate excretion. *(Guyton, pp 874–877)*

34. **(C)** Aldosterone is the major mineralocorticoid hormone. It acts by enhancing renal reabsorption of sodium ions and excretion of potassium ions. Cortisol and cortisone are the primary glucocorticoids that promote glycogen synthesis and gluconeogenesis and increase fat and protein degradation. Progesterone is required for implantation of a fertilized ovum in the uterus and maintenance of pregnancy. Pregnenolone is a common precursor in the biosynthesis of all the above hormones. *(Stryer, pp 565–568)*

35. **(C)** Killing of microbes by phagocytes is regulated by both oxygen-dependent and oxygen-independent mechanisms. The oxygen-dependent mechanisms involve the participation of superoxide anion, hydrogen peroxide, singlet oxygen, and hydroxyl radicals, all of which are powerful microbicidal agents. Ferrous ions are not part of the oxygen-dependent microbicidal mechanisms of phagocytes. *(Jawetz et al, pp 113–115)*

36. **(C)** Chemical carcinogenesis is the induction of cancer by chemical agents. Although the mechanisms are still poorly understood, chemical carcinogenesis is dose dependent. As the dose is increased, over time the risk of developing cancer also is increased. This dose relationship is irreversible and additive. A variable latency period, from the time of insult to the time of cancer induction, may range from several months to years. When the cells with malignant induction divide, they transmit the carcinogenic effects to their daughter cells, so malignant clones arise. Chemical promoters, which are often hormonal, interact with the chemical carcinogens to decrease the latency period and increase the number of tumor cells. All cells undergoing active proliferation are more susceptible to carcinogenic induction. Susceptibility to chemical carcinogenesis is largely genetically determined, varying greatly among cells and tissue strains. *(Cotran, pp 271–273)*

37. **(B)** Propylthiouracil inhibits the synthesis of thyroid hormones and thus is effective in treating hyperthyroidism. Although the complete mechanism of action is not fully understood, it is believed that propylthiouracil interferes with the incorporation of iodine into tyrosyl residues of thyroglobulin and inhibits the coupling of the iodotyrosyl residues to form iodothyronines. However, propylthiouracil does not inactivate existing thyroxine and tri-iodothyronine, nor does it interfere with the effectiveness of exogenous thyroid hormones. *(Gilman et al, pp 1373–1377)*

38. **(A)** The limbic system is concerned with basic instinctual and emotive behaviors and memory. Higher functions, such as thinking (cognition), are performed by the cerebral cortex. *(Leigh and Reiser, pp 52–59)*

39. **(A)** The disposition of the peritoneum in the adult appears meaningless and complex if its developmental changes and modifications are not considered. The primordia of the viscera are located outside this peritoneal sac in the extraperitoneal tissue. Later, as the viscera develop, they protrude into the peritoneal sac to varying degrees. The kidneys protrude only slightly and are called retroperitoneal. The transverse colon, stomach, spleen, and sigmoid colon protrude completely, and the peritoneum forms the serosa of the walls of these organs. *(Moore, pp 152–153)*

40. **(C)** The stimulation of afferent nerves to salivary gland acini results in the secretion of a solution that resembles plasma. This is accompanied by a loss of cellular potassium ions, which is brought about by a rise in the intracellular concentration of calcium ions. In experiments in which single ionic channels have been recorded directly, it has been demonstrated that the basolateral plasma membranes of salivary gland acinar cells contain calcium-activated potassium channels. It is believed that these account for the efflux of potassium following stimulation. Na^+-K^+-Cl^- cotransport and the ouabain-sensitive Na^+-K^+ pump may each contribute to the reuptake of potassium ions by these cells. *(Petersen and Maruyama)*

41. **(A)** Although peptide bonds define the primary structure (the sequence of amino acids) and, hence, supply the information necessary to specify the three-dimensional structure of a protein, they play no active role in stabilizing the tertiary structure of proteins. Four major types of weak bonds are important in tertiary structure—hydrogen bonds between R groups of the amino acids composing the protein, hydrogen bonds between the peptide groupings of α-helical and β-pleated sheet regions, ionic bonds between positively and negatively charged R groups, and hydrophobic interactions between nonpolar R groups. Study has revealed that hydrophobic interactions are the most important forces involved in maintaining the tertiary structure of proteins. *(Stryer, pp 28–30)*

42. **(D)** The penicillin binucleate core structure is a cyclized dipeptide formed by condensation of L-cysteine and D-valine. Several different side chains are found at the R portion of the figure

that accompanies the question. These impart important biologic characteristics to the molecule, such as acid stability, resistance to β-lactamase, broadened spectrum, and so forth. *(Joklik et al, pp 154–162)*

43. **(C)** Adrenocortical carcinoma is a rare malignant tumor of the adrenal cortex. It almost never affects children. These tumors are consistently large, bulky, and unilateral, with extension into the soft tissues and retroperitoneum apparent at the time of diagnosis. They often show necrosis and hemorrhage, invade vascular and lymphatic structures, and frequently metastasize. The tumor is considered to be an adenocarcinoma and ranges in structure from well differentiated to anaplastic. About half of the tumors are functional and secrete steroids, especially cortisol. Clinically, affected patients may have symptoms of Cushing's syndrome—hypoglycemia, virilization, feminization, or a combination of these. These tumors are thought to arise from the adrenal cortical cells and are not of neural crest origin. *(Rubin and Farber, pp 1150–1154)*

44. **(B)** Eight to 12 hours after the last dose of heroin, an addicted individual may experience nonpurposive symptoms, such as lacrimation, rhinorrhea, yawning, and sweating. After 12 to 14 hours, the sufferer may fall into a restless sleep. The syndrome progresses, and symptoms such as restlessness, gooseflesh, anorexia, tremor, and dilated pupils appear. At 48 to 72 hours, nonpurposive symptoms reach their peak, and the addicted person experiences increasing irritability, insomnia, anorexia, violent yawning, sneezing, lacrimation, coryza, weakness, depression, nausea, vomiting, intestinal spasm, diarrhea, increased heart rate and blood pressure, chilliness alternating with flushing and excessive sweating, and myalgias and arthralgias. *(Gilman et al, pp 526–531)*

45. **(D)** Benzodiazepines are antianxiety agents. They are habit-forming and have additive sedative action with alcohol. Patients who use these drugs should be cautioned to drive carefully, especially after drinking alcohol. Antipsychotic drugs, such as phenothiazines, impair conditioned avoidance learning in animals. *(Leigh and Reiser, pp 437–455)*

46. **(D)** The lesser omentum includes the hepatogastric and hepatoduodenal ligaments. The falciform attaches the liver to the anterior abdominal wall. The greater omentum includes the gastrocolic, gastrosplenic, and gastrophrenic ligaments. The lesser omentum is a fold of peritoneum that connects the lesser curvature of the stomach and the proximal part of the duodenum to the liver. *(Moore, p 154)*

47. **(D)** Inhibition or loss of the 21 β-hydroxylase or 11 β-hydroxylase enzyme in the pathways for the synthesis of steroids results primarily in a deficiency of glucocorticoids in the adrenal cortex. Because glucocorticoids normally act to inhibit the release of ACTH, the secretion of ACTH from the pituitary is enhanced. Deficiencies in these enzymes do not, however, prevent the synthesis of androgens in the adrenal cortex, and their release from this organ becomes enhanced by the elevated ACTH levels. Such deficiencies also result in adrenal hyperplasia. *(Ganong, pp 308–309)*

48. **(B)** Fibroblasts synthesize procollagen intracellularly. Procollagen is a triple helix containing glycosylated residues and hydroxylated proline. Once procollagen is secreted, it must be hydrolyzed by extracellular peptidases to form tropocollagen. The peptidases cleave the nonhelical peptides of the N-terminal and C-terminal ends. Tropocollagen spontaneously associates into collagen fibers in the extracellular space. *(Stryer, pp 261–270)*

49. **(C)** The importance of the capsule in the virulence of the pneumococcus is apparent from the observations that only encapsulated strains are virulent, and vaccine efficacy is type specific (the organisms are divided into more than 80 types on the basis of antigenic differences in the capsular carbohydrate composition). Cell wall teichoic acids and peptidoglycan are found in rough pneumococci (and most other bacteria as well) and are not intimately involved in the pathogenesis of disease. M protein is the potent antiphagocytic cell wall component of group A streptococci. *(Joklik et al, pp 432–442)*

50. **(A)** There have been many classifications of the histologic appearance of non-Hodgkin's lymphoma. In more recent times, it has become apparent that a particular classification that recognizes certain types of differentiation of the lymph node into nodular, diffuse, and cleaved nuclei or noncleaved of the cells can be related to the grade of aggressiveness of the tumor and, therefore, can be used as both a clinical and a histologic classification. The least aggressive of the lymphomas would be those that still retain the nodular pattern and in which the cells are small, with cleaved nuclei resembling the central germinal center cells from which they arose. Although nodular large, cleaved cell would be the next in degree of aggressiveness and would be probably classified as intermediate, all of the others are diffuse with varying degrees of cellular cleaving and are usually in the intermediate to high grade of aggressiveness. *(Rubin and Farber, pp 1094–1104)*

51. **(C)** Phenothiazines antagonize dopaminergic neurotransmission and chronically can cause a

variety of extrapyramidal symptoms, including parkinsonism, akathisia, and tardive dyskinesia. On withdrawal of drug treatment, parkinsonism usually abates, but akathisia and tardive dyskinesia can sometimes worsen temporarily. *(Gilman et al, pp 398–400)*

52. **(C)** The majority of adults with and without psychiatric disorders who commit aggressive acts are more likely to commit them against familiar persons, usually family members. Some XYY syndrome persons may be more prone to engage in aggression. Other metabolic disorders predisposing to aggression include Sanfilippo syndrome, Spielmeyer-Vogt syndrome, and phenylketonuria. While males are more likely to commit homicide, battery, or rape; domestic violence is engaged in equally by both sexes. The rate of aggression among psychiatric inpatients may be as high as 10–15 percent during the year prior to hospitalization. *(Kaplan and Sadock, pp 271–282)*

53. **(A)** Each spinal nerve contains nerve fibers classified into one of four functional components, namely: (1) General somatic afferent, (2) General visceral afferent, (3) General somatic efferent, and (4) General visceral efferent. Special visceral efferent is branchiomeric musculature. *(Noback, p 107)*

54. **(A)** Androgens stimulate the synthesis of proteins, and this effect accounts for much of the increase in rate of growth that occurs during puberty. Within long bones, androgens also eventually cause the epiphyses to fuse with the shaft of the bone. When this takes place, no further linear bone growth occurs. Other effects of androgens include some increase in the amount of retention of ions, such as calcium and phosphate. *(Ganong, pp 346–348)*

55. **(D)** The rate-limiting step in the synthesis of heme is the condensation of glycine and succinyl-CoA to form δ-aminolevulinate. The mitochondrial enzyme δ-aminolevulinate synthetase catalyzes this reaction. δ-Aminolevulinate dehydrogenase catalyzes the condensation of two molecules of δ-aminolevulinate to porphobilinogen. Four molecules of porphobilinogen condense to form a linear tetrapyrrole, which undergoes a series of reactions to produce protoporphyrin IX. Chelation of iron by this molecule yields heme. *(Lehninger, pp 718–719; Stryer, pp 594–595)*

56. **(C)** The Retroviridae are characterized by the presence of a reverse transcriptase (RNA-dependent DNA polymerase) in the virion. This family contains oncornaviruses that cause leukemias, sarcomas, lymphomas, and mammary carcinomas in animals as well as a few nononcogenic species,

such as the lentivirus that causes visna in sheep. They are RNA viruses that are able to insert their genome into the DNA of the host cell through the action of the transcriptase. In this form they are nonantigenic, as they are hidden in the genetics of the host cell. Once the virus is expressed again and mature particles are produced, the virus will take on the antigenic characteristics of its capsid proteins. *(Joklik et al, pp 878–886)*

57. **(A)** The photograph that accompanies the question demonstrates severe hydronephrosis of the kidney. Hydronephrosis refers to dilatation of the renal pelvis and calices associated with progressive atrophy of the kidney due to obstruction of the flow of urine from the kidney. The obstruction may be located at any site along the urinary outflow tract and may be partial or total, unilateral or bilateral. Since glomerular filtration may continue for some time after the development of the obstruction, the renal pelvis and calices become dilated by the continued urine production. The resultant back-pressure produces atrophy of the renal parenchyma with obliteration of the pyramids. The degree of hydronephrosis depends on the extent and rapidity of the obstructive process. *(Cotran, pp 1071–1073)*

58. **(D)** Resistant bacteria produce penicillinase, which hydrolyzes the β-lactam ring to form penicilloic acid, a molecule with no antibacterial activity. Penicillinase is produced by a number of clinically important bacteria, most notably *Staphylococcus*. In infections with these organisms, therapy often is based on penicillinase-resistant penicillins. *(Gilman et al, pp 1067–1068)*

59. **(A)** An individual usually is not consciously aware of signal anxiety, a type of anxiety that serves as a signal of an impending danger intrapsychically. Panic anxiety, neurotic anxiety, and psychotic anxiety are severe forms of anxiety and are pathologic. *(Leigh and Reiser, pp 41–78)*

60. **(D)** The pain and temperature inputs are conveyed via two types of first-order afferent neurons with their cell bodies in the dorsal root ganglia or the cranial nerve equivalent. Third-order neurons are located in the thalamus. The dorsal gray column contains second-order sensory neurons. The anterior gray column contains motor neurons and the lateral funiculus contains fibers. *(Noback, p 131)*

61. **(C)** Aromatase is the enzyme that controls the conversion of testosterone to estradiol. It also catalyzes the formation of estrone from androstenedione. The major proportion of circulating estradiol in adult men is formed directly by aromatization of these circulating androgens. Lesser

amounts may be secreted by both the Leydig's cells and the Sertoli's cells in the testes and by the adrenal cortex. *(Ganong, pp 374–375)*

62. **(D)** The activation of factor X is the final reaction of both the extrinsic and intrinsic pathways of clotting. Activated factor X proteolytically cleaves prothrombin to thrombin, which in turn cleaves fibrinogen to fibrin. Accelerin stimulates the activation of factor X, and fibrin-stabilizing factor (factor XIII) stabilizes the clot by cross-linking fibrin. All of these factors are part of the common pathway. The defect in hemophilia is a deficiency in factor VIII, or the antihemophilic factor. This factor acts as the last step of the intrinsic pathway. Factor VIII acts in concert with factor IX, a proteolytic enzyme, to activate factor X. *(Stryer, pp 248–251)*

63. **(E)** There are five genera of DNA animal viruses. The HAPPPy mnemonic device (**H**erpes, **A**deno, **P**apova, **P**arvo, and **P**ox) enumerates these. All others are RNA viruses. Variola is a poxvirus, as is molluscum contagiosum; measles is caused by a paramyxovirus. *(Joklik et al, pp 769–781)*

64. **(C)** Down's syndrome is the most common chromosome abnormality, occurring in 1 of 800 live births. It is characterized by a trisomy 21 karyotype with an extra G group chromosome (chromosome 21), making 47 total chromosomes. In the majority of cases, the parents are phenotypically and genetically normal, and Down's syndrome is secondary to a meiotic error in the ovum. The risk of having a Down's syndrome child is proportional to increasing maternal age. The clinical features of Down's syndrome include fat facies, epicanthic folds, oblique palpebral fissures, and severe mental retardation. The majority of affected individuals die early from cardiac or infectious complications. Thirty percent have a ventricular septal defect.

Trisomy 13 is also called Patau's syndrome, and affected children have microcephaly and severe mental retardation, with absence of a portion of the forebrain. These children die soon after birth. Trisomy 18, or Edwards' syndrome, is also a very severe genetic defect, and the average life span is 10 weeks. Affected children have severe mental retardation and cardiac anomalies, including a ventricular septal defect. The chromosome abnormality is an extra chromosome 18 due to a meiotic error. Patients with an XO karyotype have Turner's syndrome and are phenotypically females. Only 3 percent of affected fetuses survive to birth. Fetuses that survive birth have severe edema of the hands, feet, and neck. They have a webbed neck, short stature, and congenital heart disease. At puberty, there is failure to develop normal secondary sex characteristics, so their genitalia remain immature. The ovaries are atrophic and infertile, with primary amenorrhea. Klinefelter's syndrome, or testicular dysgenesis, is characterized by an XXY karyotype. It occurs in 1 of 600 live births. Affected individuals usually are diagnosed after puberty and have eunuchoid habitus, long legs, and small atrophic testes and penis. Secondary male characteristics fail to develop. These men are infertile and often have a low IQ. *(Cotran, pp 129–132)*

65. **(D)** In patients with endogenous asthma and nasal polyps, a single dose of aspirin may cause bronchoconstriction and vasomotor collapse. Analgesic nephropthy, hepatotoxicity, and infertility are rare side effects, which occur most often during protracted or high-dose therapy. Hemolytic anemia may occur as an uncommon side effect in patients with glucose 6-phosphate dehydrogenase deficiency. *(Gilman et al, pp 644–652)*

66. **(D)** Rationalization is a defense mechanism in which the person gives a post hoc plausible explanation for an unacceptable action. *(Leigh and Reiser, pp 79–100)*

67. **(E)** Pain and temperature pathways comprise the lateral spinothalamic, spinotectal, and spinoreticular. The fasciculi cuneatus and gracilis carry discriminative general senses, light touch, and subconscious proprioception. The corticospinal is motor and the dorsal spinocerebellar is proprioception. *(Noback, pp 131,143–144,153,161)*

68. **(B)** Acidophilic cells of the anterior pituitary are those cells that stain with acidic dyes. The major peptide hormones found in cells of this type are growth hormones and prolactin. Tumors of acidophilic cells may lead to excessive secretion of growth hormone, which, in children, produces gigantism and, in adults, results in acromegaly. Acromegaly is associated with changes in facial features and enlargement of the hands and feet. Dwarfism may be the result of deficiencies in growth hormone or of growth factors. Cushing's syndrome is caused by excess secretion of glucocorticoids and may result from tumors of ACTH-containing cells in the pituitary. In contrast to the growth hormone-containing cells, the cells that synthesize ACTH may be chromophobic or basophilic. Adrenogenital syndrome results from excessive secretion of androgens. *(Ganong, pp 204–205)*

69. **(A)** The proteolytic blood enzyme thrombin has a specificity for arginine–glycine bonds similar to trypsin. Thrombin is synthesized as prothrombin, which contains γ-carboxyglutamate residues deriving from vitamin K-dependent, posttranslational modification of glutamate. In order to be ac-

tivated, prothrombin is proteolytically cleaved by factor X_a after being anchored to platelet membranes in a calcium-γ-carboxyglutamate-dependent reaction. The γ-carboxyglutamate end of the prothrombin molecule is removed, leaving an active thrombin. Fibrinogen is converted to fibrin by the proteolytic cleavage of four arginine–glycine bonds. The A and B fibrinopeptides released spontaneously associate to form a clot of insoluble fibrin fibers. *(Stryer, pp 250–251)*

70. **(C)** Koplik's spots on the buccal mucosa are characteristic of infection with morbilli (measles) virus. Microscopic examination of these lesions would reveal giant cells containing viral nucleocapsids. Macroscopically, these lesions will appear as small, erythematous macules with white centers. Rubeola (red measles) is an acute febrile disease characterized by fever, maculopapular rash, and respiratory symptoms. A cell culture-produced attenuated vaccine is available. There is only one antigenic variety of measles virus, so the vaccine is monovalent. It should not be given until after 12 months of age to allow maternal antibody, which could interfere with the infection established by the vaccine strain, to dissipate from the infant's circulation. *(Joklik et al, pp 1011–1014)*

71. **(E)** Atherosclerosis is a complex condition that is primarily and initially an intimal disease. It has now been long established and associated with an elevated serum cholesterol, but the lipoproteins are considered to be of equal importance in that a high level of LDL in association with elevated cholesterol is a very poor prognostic sign in the potential of an individual to develop severe atheroma and its complications. High levels of HDL appear to balance out the negative effect of cholesterol and are, therefore, considered good prognostic signs. *(Rubin and Farber, pp 459–461)*

72. **(A)** The rate of cortisol secretion in normal persons is approximately 20 mg/day and is subject to fluctuations occurring throughout the day. Endogenous glucocorticoid concentrations in plasma follow a diurnal cycle, with peak concentrations occurring during early morning hours, a gradual decline in mid- to late afternoon, and the lowest concentrations occurring at night. This diurnal variation is not observed in patients with Cushing's disease. *(Wyngaarden and Smith, p 89)*

73. **(B)** Persons who unsuccessfully attempt suicide tend to be young and female, unlike persons who complete suicide. Suicidal attempt often occurs at times of interpersonal difficulties and is not infrequent among Catholics. *(Leigh and Reiser, pp 101–144)*

74. **(B)** The first-order sensory neurons for pain and temperature of the face are located in the trigeminal ganglion. The second-order neurons for pain and temperature are located in the nucleus of the spinal tract of the trigeminal nerve. The main sensory nucleus contains second-order neurons for discriminative general senses of the face. The mesencephalic root is concerned with proprioception. *(Noback, pp 135,148,152)*

75. **(D)** The major site of melatonin synthesis is within parenchymal cells of the pineal gland. It is formed by *N*-acetylation of 5-hydroxytryptamine followed by methylation. The rate of its synthesis is phase locked to the light–dark cycle, being high in the dark and very markedly diminished in the light portions of the cycle. Its synthesis and release are primarily regulated by sympathetic nerves whose activity appears to be entrained to the light–dark cycle via the suprachiasmatic nuclei. Sympathetic input regulates the *N*-acetyltransferase reaction within the pineal cells by controlling intracellular cyclic AMP levels. *(Ganong, pp 394–395)*

76. **(D)** Conversion of pyruvate to acetyl-CoA results in the production of 1 mol of NADH. Oxidation of the resultant acetyl-CoA to CO_2 and water via the citric acid cycle yields 3 mol of NADH, 1 mol of $FADH_2$ and 1 mol of guanosine triphosphate (GTP). Oxidation of each mol of NADH during electron transport yields 3 mol of ATP, whereas oxidation of $FADH_2$ results in the formation of 2 mol of ATP. Therefore, beginning with pyruvate, the yield is 12 mol of ATP from 4 mol of NADH, 2 mol of ATP from 1 mol of $FADH_2$, and 1 mol of ATP equivalent (GTP) from substrate level phosphorylation, giving a total of 15 mol of ATP. *(Stryer, pp 373–374,377–379)*

77. **(B)** The DiGeorge syndrome is a form of glandular aplasia due to defective embryonic development of the third and fourth pharyngeal pouches, which give rise to the thymus, parathyroid, and thyroid glands. This anomaly results in a depletion of thymic-dependent areas in lymphoid tissues. In Bruton's hypogammaglobulinemia, B-dependent areas are depleted. Hence, antibody formation is severely restricted. In severe combined immunodeficiency disease, both B cell and T cell functions are absent, and the affected individual is completely without any immune capability. Job's disease, or lazy leukocyte syndrome, is characterized by a defect in the chemotactic response of neutrophils. *(Joklik et al, pp 329–332)*

78. **(C)** Celsus and Virchow defined clinical signs of acute inflammation that included redness, heat, swelling, pain, and loss of function. The heat and redness are related to dilatation of the vascula-

ture. The swelling is a result of exudation of fluid, proteins, and cells into the interstitial tissue. Pain is thought to be secondary to prostaglandin secretions. Virchow describes loss of function as a result of the combined effects of the other factors of the inflammatory response. Numbness, which implies neurologic involvement, is not characteristic of the local acute inflammatory response. *(Cotran, pp 39–41)*

79. **(C)** Phenylbutazone impairs platelet aggregation and displaces anticoagulant drugs from their binding with blood proteins. Barbiturates, glutethimide, and rifampin all induce microsomal enzyme systems in the liver that increase drug metabolism and thus reduce the response. Cholestyramine, a plasma cholesterol-lowering agent, binds anticoagulants in the intestine, reducing their absorption. *(Craig and Stitzel, p 377)*

80. **(E)** Pain receptors are considered to be free nerve endings. Meissner's and Vater-Pacini corpuscles are thought to be involved with touch and proprioception. Rods are retinal light-sensitive cells. *(Leigh and Reiser, pp 211–243)*

81. **(B)** The fibers terminating in the nucleus gracilis originate from below T_6, including the lower extremities, and those in the nucleus cuneatus originate from above T_6, including the upper extremities. The longest neuronal fibers in the body are those of the fasciculus gracilis. They extend without interruption from receptors in the foot through the spinal nerves, dorsal roots (location of their cell bodies), and fasciculus gracilis to the nucleus gracilis. *(Noback, p 146)*

82. **(C)** Aldosterone is synthesized and secreted by cells of the adrenal cortex. A primary role for mineralocorticoids, such as aldosterone, is to stimulate the renal reabsorption of sodium ions. After adrenalectomy, the excretion of sodium ions in the urine is significantly increased and plasma sodium ion concentrations fall. At the same time, plasma potassium concentrations increase. If mineralocorticoids are not administered, blood pressure and the volume of the plasma decrease and death ensues. Although the loss of glucocorticoids, such as cortisol and corticosterone, may also become lethal in certain circumstances, such as fasting, their loss in adrenalectomy is not as critical as is the loss of aldosterone. Neither the loss of the androgen dehydroepiandrosterone, secreted by the adrenal cortex, nor the loss of catecholamines, such as epinephrine, secreted by the adrenal medulla, produce similar life-threatening changes in body functions. *(Ganong, p 320)*

83. **(E)** The atoms composing the CO_2 and ammonia (NH_4^+) that form the carbamoyl group of carbamoyl phosphate are ultimately incorporated into urea. Likewise, the atoms forming the amino group of aspartate constitute the remainder of the urea molecule. Thus, of the molecules listed in the question, only argininosuccinate contains all of the atoms destined to become urea. *(Stryer, pp 500–502)*

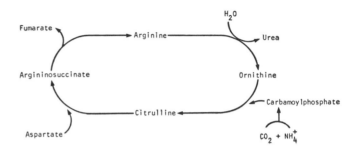

84. **(C)** For sterilization of surgical instruments sensitive to heat, the method of choice is ethylene oxide. The autoclave uses high temperatures for sterilization. Both phenol and ethyl alcohol are used for disinfection, but neither can be relied on to kill spores. Ethylene oxide is effective against all types of bacteria, including the tubercle bacilli and spores. It is a gas and can be used for the sterilization of fragile and heat-labile materials and other items packaged in cloth or paper containers. Sterilization is complete in 4 to 12 hours, which must be followed by 12 to 24 hours of aeration to allow dissipation of the dissolved gas. Ionizing radiation would not penetrate many surgical instruments evenly and hence would not sterilize effectively. *(Joklik et al, pp 195–196)*

85. **(B)** Sarcoid is a multisystem disease of unknown cause. It affects all organ systems, and young women are most often the victims. The characteristic lesions are noncaseating epithelioid granulomas that contain multinucleated giant cells. Schaumann's bodies or crystalline inclusion bodies may be identified. The lung and thoracic lymph nodes are the most commonly involved sites, and pulmonary involvement may be quite serious, causing severe restrictive lung disease. Besides tissue biopsy as a method of diagnosing sarcoid, the Kveim test is the most commonly used clinical diagnostic procedure: Antigenic tissue suspensions from patients with sarcoid are injected into the skin, and positive reactions show papules 4 to 6 weeks later. Biopsy specimens of the papules show noncaseating granulomas. The findings are rarely unequivocally positive, and the reliability of this test is being questioned. Pa-

tients with sarcoid usually have a progressive downhill course over years, and steroid therapy can only ameliorate their disease. *(Cotran, pp 427–429)*

86. **(E)** Propranolol is useful in treating angina by decreasing myocardial oxygen consumption during rest and exercise. Propranolol decreases cardiac demand for oxygen because of its negative chronotropic effect (especially during exercise), its negative inotropic effect, and its minor depression of arterial pressure. *(Gilman et al, p 780)*

87. **(D)** Lithium salts are particularly effective in treating acute mania. They also may be effective in preventing recurrences of unipolar depression, but not to the extent of their use in treatment of mania. Lithium is not particularly effective in panic disorders, anxiety disorder, or schizophrenia. *(Leigh and Reiser, pp 439–455)*

88. **(E)** A loss of pain occurs in lesions involving the lateral spinothalamic tract, which is located in the lateral funiculus. A lesion in the posterior funiculus involving the fasciculi cuneatus and gracilis may result in loss of vibratory sense, the inability to recognize a common object by feel and palpation, a loss of two-point discrimination, and a loss of position sense. *(Noback, pp 131,156)*

89. **(E)** Activity in the sympathetic afferent nerves to the pancreas results in the enhanced secretion of glucagon from the α cells within the pancreatic islets. The stimulation of sympathetic afferents also inhibits insulin secretion from the β cells. The increase in glucagon secretion is a β-adrenergic response that uses a cyclic AMP second messenger mechanism. Thus, agents that elevate cyclic AMP promote glucagon secretion. An inhibitory α-adrenergic receptor also is present, but the β-adrenergic response usually is dominant on sympathetic stimulation. The secretion of glucagon is enhanced also by elevated amino acid concentrations in plasma and is inhibited by glucose and insulin. *(Ganong, p 237)*

90. **(B)** In mammals, unlike plants, there is no mechanism for synthesizing net glucose from acetyl-CoA or substances whose metabolism will lead only to the production of acetyl-CoA. The ketone body β-hydroxybutyrate can only be metabolized to acetoacetyl-CoA and, ultimately, to acetyl-CoA. In contrast, glycerol can enter the gluconeogenic or glycolytic pathways at the level of dihydroxyacetone phosphate. Propionate, the end product of β oxidation of odd-chain fatty acids, and the amino acid glutamate can be converted to the citric acid cycle intermediates succinyl-CoA and α-ketoglutarate, respectively. These intermediates, as well as the citric acid cycle intermediate oxaloacetate, can all be converted to phosphoenolpyruvate for use in gluconeogenesis. *(Stryer, pp 438–442)*

91. **(A)** In a positive viral hemagglutination test, the virus is the hemagglutinating particle. Antibody specific to the viral hemagglutinin will block this activity and inhibit hemagglutination. The assay is similar to a neutralization test, with the erythrocyte taking the place of a susceptible nucleated host cell. Many different viruses possess hemagglutinating activity. Hence, this assay can be used to identify serum antibodies that are reactive with numerous different viral agents. The limiting ingredient is the availability of the viruses. *(Joklik et al, p 946)*

92. **(D)** Malignant melanoma is a neoplasm of melanocytes that usually occurs in patients 40 to 60 years old. It most often arises in the skin but may originate in other mucosal surfaces. These tumors may arise either de novo, from preexisting benign nevi, or in rare cases in familial groups. Lentigo maligna, one subtype, tends to arise in sun-exposed areas of the skin. Clinically, these tumors are raised lesions with irregular notched borders and may be red, white, or black or have black and brown foci. Malignant melanoma arises from melanocyte cells in the epidermis. These malignant cells form clusters or nodules and spread laterally within the epidermis or vertically into the dermis. Tumor in the papillary dermis only occurs as a result of direct tumor spread or recurrence. Tumor cells are frequently pigmented with melanin granules and have large eosinophilic nucleoli. Malignant melanomas frequently metastasize, either by lymphatic vessels to regional lymph nodes or hematogenously to the skin, lungs, and liver. Nodular melanoma has the worst prognosis and is the most likely form to metastasize. *(Rubin and Farber, pp 1243–1254)*

93. **(A)** Epinephrine is the drug of choice for treating severe anaphylactic shock, since it has both α and β effects. The α β effect constricts the smaller arterioles and precapillary sphincters, thereby markedly reducing cutaneous blood flow. Veins and larger arteries also respond to epinephrine. The β effects of epinephrine cause relaxation of the bronchial smooth muscle and induce a powerful bronchodilatation, which is most evident when the bronchial muscle is contracted, as in anaphylactic shock. Neither norepinephrine nor dopamine would be the drug of choice, since neither has action on the β_2 receptors and, therefore, would not cause the bronchodilatation needed for treating anaphylactic shock. Isoproterenol has a powerful action on all β receptors but almost no action on the α receptors, so vasodilatation instead of vasoconstriction would be produced.

Phenylephrine would be a poor drug of choice for anaphylactic shock, since it has little effect on the β receptors and causes no bronchodilatation. *(Gilman et al, pp 192–198)*

94. **(C)** Suicide and suicidal attempt occur more frequently among people who seem to think of suicide or consider it as an option. Most people who commit suicide have seen a physician or given warnings of their intent. Suicide may occur when a patient's mood seems to be lifting. At this time, these persons may either gain more energy or experience a sense of resolution as the option of suicide has been decided. *(Leigh and Reiser, pp 101–144)*

95. **(C)** The lower motor neurons of the spinal cord are often called anterior horn cells because the cell bodies are located in the anterior horn of the spinal cord. The posterior funiculus contains fibers of the lemniscal system. The corticospinal contains axons of upper motor neurons. The dorsal root ganglion contains first-order sensory neurons. The ventral root contains axons of lower motor neurons. *(Noback, pp 110–117, 160–161)*

96. **(C)** The thyroid gland synthesizes and secretes thyroxine (3,5,3′,5′,-tetraiodothyronine, T_4) and 3,5,3′-triiodothyronine (T_3) as well as lesser amounts of reverse triiodothyronine (3,3′,5′-triiodothyronine, RT_3) and monoiodotyrosine. Of these, T_3 is most active in stimulating oxygen consumption in the body, being three to five times as potent as T_4, although it is secreted in smaller amounts. RT_3 and monoiodotyrosine are not active. Thyroglobulin is a glycoprotein of the thyroid gland that plays a major role in the synthesis of the thyroid hormones and that may be released into the circulation. It is not, however, believed to play a role in the actions of the thyroid hormones. *(Ganong, pp 268–269)*

97. **(C)** Of the enzymes listed in the question, only glucokinase and glucose 6-phosphatase are found in the liver and not in most other tissues. A deficiency in glucokinase would lead to increased blood sugar levels, not hypoglycemia. This would occur because of the liver's decreased ability to phosphorylate free glucose for use. In contrast, a defect in glucose 6-phosphatase would cause the symptoms observed in von Gierke's disease. This endoplasmic reticulum enzyme catalyzes the dephosphorylation of glucose 6-phosphate, allowing glucose to be released into the blood when levels are low. A lesion at this point would result in massive storage of glycogen in liver. *(Stryer, pp 465–466)*

98. **(D)** Complement-fixation procedures are performed in two stages. The test system consists of antigen and antibody (one of which is unknown) plus complement. The indicator system consists of sheep erythrocytes and hemolysin (an antisheep-RBC serum), which will sensitize the cells to the lytic action of complement. If complement is fixed in the test system, it is effectively bound (or consumed) in the antigen-antibody complexes there and is not free to participate in the lysis of the sensitized erythrocytes present in the indicator system. *(Jawetz et al, pp 121–122)*

99. **(B)** The photomicrograph shows the characteristic appearance of hyperplastic ducts surrounded by what appears to be fibrous tissue and also smooth muscle. The pattern is a uniform one, in which the ducts are evenly distributed in this background of muscle and fibrous tissue. This is characteristic of so-called fibroadenoma of the breast, which tends to occur in younger females and is usually discrete and of a rubbery consistency. It is, however, very important that this be distinguished from the other forms of lumps in the breast, such as the various forms of carcinoma. Intraductal carcinoma and Paget's disease usually are both clinically and pathologically easily distinguishable from this lesion. The fibroadenoma is an entirely benign condition. *(Kissane, p 1730)*

100. **(B)** The major action of atropine is to competitively antagonize the muscarinic action of acetylcholine at postganglionic parasympathetic neuroeffecter junctions. Atropine and scopolamine are, therefore, known as antimuscarinic agents. Because of the relatively small effect at the nicotinic receptor sites at autonomic ganglia, atropine produces a partial block only at relatively high doses. An example of an agent that prevents the release of acetylcholine is botulin toxin, whereas hemicholinium exerts its anticholinergic action by interference with high affinity choline uptake. *(Gilman et al, pp 152–153)*

101. **(B)** In REM sleep, there is autonomic activation and a suppression of skeletal muscle activity. Thus, sleepwalking does not occur during REM but rather in the slow wave phase of sleep (stages 4 and 3). *(Leigh and Reiser, pp 271–302)*

102. **(B)** The linea semilunaris is a curved line that extends from the ninth costal cartilage to the pubic tubercle. This semilunar line indicates the lateral border of the rectus abdominis muscle. The lines are obvious in persons with good abdominal muscular development. In such persons, three or more transverse grooves are also visible in the skin overlying the tendinous intersections of the rectus abdominis muscles. *(Moore, p 128)*

103. **(B)** Wernicke's area, which is located at the posterior end of the superior temporal gyrus, is be-

lieved to play an important role in the understanding of language, either written or spoken. Patients with lesions in this area have a form of fluid aphasia in which the ability to vocalize is not impaired but the subject matter of speech is not intelligible. Moreover, the ability to understand either speech or writing is impaired. This is in contrast to lesions of Broca's area, in which understanding is preserved but the ability to vocalize speech is impaired. Deficits in the processing of visual information, dyslexia, or disorders of short-term memory may each result from cerebral lesions but are not specifically associated with Wernicke's area. *(Ganong, pp 228–229)*

104. (A) The double-reciprocal Lineweaver-Burk plot that accompanies the question illustrates a competitively inhibited enzyme. In competitive inhibition, the intercept on the *y* axis, which is equal to $1/V_{max}$, does not change. This points out that at significantly high substrate concentration, the inhibition can be overcome. In noncompetitive inhibition, the V_{max}, and hence the *y*-axis intercept, does change. Noncompetitive inhibition cannot be overcome by increasing the substrate concentration. Allosteric enzymes do not obey Michaelis-Menten kinetics and cannot be plotted as straight lines on double-reciprocal curves. Likewise, irreversibly inhibited enzymes cannot be treated by Michaelis-Menten kinetics. *(Stryer, pp 189–191,193–195)*

105. (C) The graft-versus-host reaction occurs when immunocompetent lymphoid cells are transferred to a histoincompatible recipient who is unable to reject them. The donor cells then mount an immune response against the foreign histocompatibility antigens of the recipient and attempt to reject them. This usually occurs in bone marrow transplantation performed as a therapeutic modality in patients with certain leukemias or other blood diseases, such as aplastic anemia. *(Joklik et al, pp 125–126)*

106. (C) Staging of a cancer requires clinical and pathologic judgment regarding the extent of spread of the lesion. It does not depend on the tumor's microscopic appearance. T is used to grade the size and extent of the primary tumor. N indicates the presence of lymph node metastases, and M indicates distal metastases. T0 indicates a carcinoma in situ or tumor confined to the mucosa. T1 is a superficial invasive tumor without extension into the underlying muscle wall or deeper connective tissue. T2 indicates muscle wall extension, and T3 shows full-thickness involvement of the organ by tumor. A T4 lesion has local extension and spread and is larger. An N0 tumor shows no lymph node involvement, whereas N1 has positive lymph node metastases. M0 tumors show no distant metastases, and M1 indicates distant tumor. The tumor described in the question invades the muscle wall but does not extend through the wall or into adjacent organs or tissue, so it is classified as T2. The lymph nodes are involved, thus N1, but there are no other metastases, so it is M0. Thus it is regarded as a T2,N1,M0 tumor. *(Rubin and Farber, pp 156–157)*

107. (C) The uptake and elimination of gaseous anesthetics are influenced by pulmonary ventilation, blood flow to tissues, and the solubility of the agent in tissue as well as in blood. Increased pulmonary ventilation increases the exchange of the agent across alveolar membranes, thus increasing the transfer of gas to blood when the alveolar gas tension is high relative to the blood. Conversely, if air ventilated to the lungs has a lower alveolar tension relative to blood, the rate of removal of gas from blood will increase. The solubility of an agent in blood and tissue is important. Agents that are highly soluble raise the blood or tissue tension of an agent slowly. High blood flow to tissues accelerates the delivery or removal of an agent from that tissue. The extent of liver metabolism does not influence the uptake and elimination of inhalational anesthetics. However, metabolism may be a determinant of toxicity. *(Gilman et al, pp 271–277)*

108. (D) The three basic models of the doctor–patient relationship are activity–passivity, guidance–cooperation, and mutual participation models. Activity–passivity model is the traditional model, in which the patient is a passive recipient of treatment. Guidance–cooperation model implies patient cooperation with the treatment regimen. Mutual participation implies a model of doctor–patient relationship in which the physician aids the patient in self-help. *(Simons, pp 19–32)*

109. (A) The main arteries of the anterior abdominal wall are the inferior epigastric and deep circumflex iliac arteries, which are branches of the external iliac artery, and the superior epigastric artery, which is a terminal branch of the internal thoracic artery. The superficial epigastric, circumflex iliac, and external pudendal are branches of the femoral artery. *(Moore, pp 132,142)*

110. (B) Skeletal muscle constitutes the major mass of the body, and thus alterations in its resistance will greatly affect systemic BP (i.e., product of cardiac output times resistance). For instance, when carotid sinus pressure is elevated, a reflex is elicited that inhibits activity in the vasoconstrictor regions of the brain and causes vasodilatation in the skeletal muscle bed and others. A separate sympathetic colinergic pathway has been described as arising from areas in the cortex and hypothalamus and producing vasodilatation in skeletal muscle. This reflex may induce vasodilatation in anticipation of exercise. In addition to these extrinsic neuronal regulatory mechanisms, local metabolic factors contribute to the regulation of muscle blood flow. This is especially true in stimulated or exercising muscle. For instance, metabolically active muscle can be shown to autoregulate, that is, increase its resistance as perfusion pressure rises to maintain constant blood flow and, conversely, decrease resistance when pressure decreases. Skeletal muscle is very heterogeneous. Within the same muscle group, blood flow is high to red muscle and relatively low to white muscle. Precapillary sphincter contraction and relaxation further confound local flow patterns via intermittent activity and perhaps by shunting of blood to non-nutrient pathways. *(Berne and Levy, pp 520–521)*

111. **(E)** Mutations are caused by changes in the base sequence of DNA. Substitution of one base pair for another is the most common type of mutation. A transition substitution refers to the replacement of one purine by another purine or one pyrimidine by another. Transversions refer to replacement of either a purine or a pyrimidine with either a pyrimidine or a purine, respectively. Frame-shift mutations (insertions or deletions) are less common than substitutions. The formation of thymine dimers is not the most common cause of mutations. In fact, most cells have repair mechanisms for dealing with DNA so affected. *(Stryer, pp 635–638)*

112. **(B)** Isografts are tissue exchanges between genetically identical individuals (inbred animals or identical twins). Allografts (also called homografts) are exchanges between genetically nonidentical individuals of the same species. Xenografts (heterografts) cross species boundaries. *(Joklik et al, p 125)*

113. **(C)** The classic description of Fallot's tetralogy, a congenital heart disease, includes pulmonary stenosis, ventricular septal defect, and overriding of the aorta over the septal defect and, as a result of these abnormalities, right ventricular hypertrophy.

Coarctation of the aorta is a totally separate congenital anomaly and may occur in both infants and adults depending on its relationship to the ducts and on whether or not the ductus arteriosus closes. It is not a characteristic part of the tetralogy of Fallot, although theoretically the two could occur in the same individual. *(Kissane, p 743)*

114. **(D)** Liver toxicity is an uncommon but significant adverse reaction associated with the use of halogenated anesthetics. The mechanism of injury with halothane, methoxyflurane, and enflurane appears to involve hypersensitivity or hepatotoxic metabolites or both. The potential for hepatotoxicity appears to correlate with the degree of liver metabolism. Halothane, methoxyflurane, and enflurane undergo liver biotransformation. All of these agents have been reported to cause liver damage. Isoflurane undergoes little biotransformation in vivo. This agent does not appear to be hepatotoxic. *(Lewis et al)*

115. **(C)** There is controversy concerning the factors influencing adherence to medical regimens. Among the demographic factors, female sex has clearly been associated with poor adherence. Field dependence has been associated with poor adherence among individuals suffering from alcoholism. Severe physical illness, contrary to what one would suspect, also has been associated with poor adherence. *(Simons, pp 38–47)*

116. **(C)** The lateral umbilical folds, formed by elevations of peritoneum covering the inferior epigastric arteries, run superomedially on each side. The medial umbilical folds are formed by elevations of peritoneum covering the medial umbilical ligaments, the obliterated parts of the fetal umbilical arteries. The median umbilical fold is formed by an elevation of peritoneum covering the median umbilical ligament, the fibrous remnant of the urachus. *(Moore, p 142)*

117. **(E)** When cardiac muscle contracts, it squeezes blood vessels that course through it, and this extravascular compression has a significant effect on coronary blood flow. In early systole, there is an actual reversal of blood flow, and although coronary blood flow increases during systole, it is not until the ventricle relaxes that maximal left coronary artery blood flows are obtained. Since aortic pressure is maximal during systole, it is obvious that choice **C** in the question is incorrect. Peak flows are obtained in early diastole, when the ventricle is relaxed and aortic pressure has not declined to its diastolic level. *(Berne and Levy, pp 511–512)*

118. **(A)** Although in bacteria a continuous sequence of triplet codons encode for each protein, genes may be discontinuous in eukaryotic cells. Noncoding intervening sequences of DNA that split genes in eukaryotes are called introns. Mature mRNA translated from such DNA does not contain the intron message. However, newly synthesized mRNA may contain intron message. These intervening sequences in the primary transcripts are specifically excised and ligated so that the mature mRNA contains no intron message. The coding sequences of split genes are called exons. *(Stryer, pp 110–113)*

119. **(B)** Erythroblastosis fetalis can occur when an Rh_0-positive child is being carried by an Rh_0-negative mother. If the mother makes antibodies against the $Rh_0(D)$ antigen, these may cross the placenta and destroy fetal erythrocytes. The induction of this immune response can be blocked if an antibody specific for the Rh_0 antigen is injected into the mother at the time of her first exposure to the fetal RBCs, which usually occurs at parturition. Rh_0 immune globulin (RhoGAM) is a human γ-globulin preparation rich in antibodies specific for the Rh_0 antigen. It is used to prevent the sensitization of the mother, which will then protect a subsequent antigenically incompatible fetus from this disease. *(Joklik et al, p 123)*

120. **(A)** Neoplastic transformation is a phenotypic change in cells that characterizes the malignant state and is passed on to progeny. These transformed cells show anaplasia and transplantability. They also show decreased sensitivity to contact inhibition and to density-dependent inhibition for growth. Thus, these tumor cells are more mobile and do not cease to grow when in contact with other cells or when more than a monolayer of confluent cells is present. Instead, they continue to replicate and pile up. Unlike normal cells, these tumor cells also can grow and divide on fluid media and have lost the need for anchorage to grow. Malignant transformed cells have an infinite ability to replicate and survive under appropriate conditions. These transformed cells are capable of tumorigenesis, so they are able to produce a neoplasm when placed within a synergistic host. *(Cotran, pp 243–249)*

121. **(C)** Hypokalemia is a frequent complication of therapy with loop diuretics (e.g., furosemide) as well as thiazide-type agents. These agents cause an increase in the amount of sodium delivered to distal sites of the nephron, where sodium is exchanged for potassium. Diuretics, such as triamterene and spironolactone, are potassium-sparing in that they produce a weak diuresis and cause potassium retention. Amphotericin B causes hypokalemia by producing renal tubular acidosis (type IV). Large doses of certain penicillins (e.g., carbenicillin) may produce hypokalemia by acting in the nephron as nonreabsorbable anions, which are paired with potassium for urinary excretion. Glycyrrhizic acid, a flavoring agent in certain foods and medications, may cause hypokalemia through its aldosterone-like effects. *(Lindeman and Papper)*

122. **(B)** Pathologic grief reactions include distorted reactions in which there may be acquisition of symptoms belonging to a deceased loved one. Posttraumatic stress disorder involves unusual and catastrophic disasters, not simple bereavement. *(Leigh and Reiser, pp 110–112)*

123. **(D)** The veins leaving the posterior surface of the testis anastomose to form a pampiniform plexus. This large, vine-like venous plexus, forming a large part of the spermatic cord, surrounds the ductus deferens and arteries in the spermatic cord. It is located within the internal spermatic fascia and ends in the testicular vein. The pampiniform plexus of veins sometimes becomes varicose (dilated and tortuous), producing a condition known as varicocele. *(Moore, p 145)*

124. **(C)** Although the heart is versatile in its use of substrates, more than 60 percent of myocardial oxygen consumption is derived from free fatty acids. Glucose and lactate are the major carbohydrate sources but make up only 30 to 35 percent of the sources for myocardial energy. In the normal heart, pyruvate uptake is very low, and oxidation of amino acids provides little to myocardial energy expenditure. In general, the heart uses the substrate in greatest supply. For example, ketone bodies may be used in diabetic acidosis. However, under normal conditions, free fatty acids are the major substrate. *(Berne and Levy, p 517)*

125. **(A)** A Lineweaver-Burk analysis of enzyme kinetics in the presence and absence of an inhibitor allows the characterization of the type of inhibition. The analysis is based on a transformation of the Michaelis–Menten equation, which produces a straight line when the reciprocal of the velocity is plotted against the reciprocal of substrate concentration (i.e., $1/v$ vs $1/[S]$). The intercept on the Y axis is equal to $1/V_{max}$, and the slope is equal to K_m/V_{max}. Addition of a competitive inhibitor to an enzymatic reaction results in a higher value for K_m but no change in V_{max}. This means that in a Lineweaver-Burk analysis, the slope will increase, but the Y intercept will remain unchanged. *(Stryer, pp 189–191,193–195)*

126. **(B)** Antibodies are synthesized in peripheral lymphoid tissues, such as the spleen and lymph nodes. The central lymphoid tissues are the thymus (responsible for T cell development) and the bursa of Fabricius (in birds) or certain gut-associated lymphoid tissues (in mammals), which are thought to be responsible for B cell development. Macrophages are important accessory cells in the induction of an immune response and are a prerequisite for most humoral immune responses. They process the antigen in some way and present it to T and B cells, which collaborate in the production of antibody molecules. In all probability, the antigen does not go through the normal phagocytic process (i.e., engulfment into a phagosome, lysosomal fusion with the phagosome to form a phagolysosome, the development of this inclusion to a digestive vacuole, and so forth) but rather is mildly degraded or modified and is reinserted into the membrane of the phagocytic cell. *(Joklik et al, pp 205–206)*

127. **(D)** The rapidity with which wounds heal is primarily related to fibroblast proliferation and secretion of collagen. Collagen is the major component contributing to the tensile strength of the wound. It is produced by fibroblasts as tropocollagen. Collagen is composed of a triple helix of three α chains, which are hydroxylated and have lysine oxidations. These modifications allow cross-linkages between the chains, and these cross-links are the most important factor contributing to the stability and strength of collagen and scar tissue. Fibroblasts also synthesize elastic fibers, which aid in the repair of wounds. Collagenase is an enzyme that cleaves collagen and digests it, retarding healing. It is rarely found in uncomplicated, healing wounds. *(Cotran, pp 77–82)*

128. **(E)** Dose-dependent, potentially fatal hepatic necrosis is the most serious consequence of acute acetaminophen poisoning. Renal failure and hypoglycemia also may occur. Methemoglobinemia and respiratory depression are manifestations of phenacetin poisoning. Although acetaminophen is a metabolite of phenacetin, symptoms of their toxicities are very different. *(Gilman et al, p 658)*

129. **(C)** In dealing with a chronically angry patient, physicians should be as neutral and objective as possible. It may be helpful for the physician to recognize that these patients arouse anger, but an angry reaction will only increase the patient's angry behavior. Sarcasm used by a physician in this situation tends to increase the patient's anger. *(Simons, pp 101–120)*

130. **(D)** The superficial fascia of the wall of the scrotum is devoid of fat, but it contains a thin sheet of smooth muscle called the dartos muscle. Because its fibers are attached to the skin, contraction of them causes the scrotum to wrinkle when cold, which helps to regulate the loss of heat through its skin. *(Moore, p 149)*

131. **(D)** Although the capillaries are the smallest vessels, by virtue of their large number and parallel existence, their effective cross-sectional area is very large. Since velocity is inversely related to cross-sectional area, the velocity in the capillaries is very low. This large surface area and low velocity promote exchange of substances between blood and tissue. Resistance to blood flow primarily occurs in arterioles with smooth muscle, and thus this is the site of the largest pressure drop. Blood

volume is greatest in small veins by nature of their high compliance. *(Berne and Levy, pp 361–363)*

132. **(A)** The lipid composition of erythrocytes, as well as most mammalian plasma membranes, is approximately half cholesterol and half phospholipid. Of the phospholipids, most is either phosphatidyl choline or spingomyelin, with phosphatidyl ethanolamine also contributing a lesser, but considerable, amount. Gangliosides and phosphatidyl serine also are present but constitute smaller percentages of the lipid. Plasmalogens are phospholipids containing a long-chain unsaturated alcohol in ester linkage at the 1' position. They are especially abundant in the membranes of nerve and muscle cells. *(Stryer, pp 284–287)*

133. **(E)** The organism represented in the sketch that accompanies the question is septate (note the divisions, or cross-walls) in the hypha. This observation rules out any of the phycomycetes, since these organisms are coenocytic. The position of the conidiospores in strings arising from the columnella is characteristic of the genus *Aspergillus*. The dermatophytes that are the causative agents of the tinea infections usually have single conidiospores and are characterized by their macroconidial forms. *(Jawetz et al, p 312)*

134. **(D)** The simplest form of a blood clot at a site of injury is a hemostatic plug. It is composed of an aggregation of platelets with a web of fibrin, which prevents leakage of blood into the extravascular spaces. Platelets are the most important component in the formation of this plug. When the blood vessel is injured, cells and plasma start to leak out, but platelets are immediately attracted to the site of injury. They accumulate, pile up, and stop the leakage. They also release tissue thromboplastin, which activates the intrinsic blood coagulation pathway, causing the fibrin mesh to form. The fibrin tightens the plug and traps other cells, strengthening the platelet plug and forming a more permanent plug. RBCs and lymphocytes are seen in hemostatic plugs as they are trapped from the circulating blood by the aggregation of platelets and fibrin. They act as filler material in the plug and have no other defined role in the formation of hemostatic plugs. Collagen is important in the initiation of hemostasis, as when blood vessels are damaged. The collagen fibrils in the subendothelial wall of the vessel are exposed to the circulation and are the substance that the platelets initially stick to when they form a hemostatic plug. *(Cotran, pp 97–99)*

135. **(C)** Extrapyramidal reactions are most likely to occur with piperazine-type phenothiazines, including trifluoperazine and prochlorperazine, as well as the butyrophenone haloperidol. Thioridazine, a piperidine-type phenothiazine, is least likely to cause extrapyramidal reactions. Prochlorperazine is mainly used as an antiemetic. *(Gilman et al, pp 398–400)*

136. **(A)** Common causes of sexual dysfunction include many types of neuropathy and chronic illnesses. Diabetic neuropathy is probably the most common organic cause of sexual dysfunction. Depression and anxiety are common functional causes of sexual dysfunction. Chronic schizophrenia is often associated with decreased sexual functions. Mania, however, is often associated with increased sexuality. *(Simons, pp 316–401)*

137. **(C)** The tail of the epididymis is continuous with the ductus deferens, the duct that transports sperm from the epididymis to the ejaculatory duct for expulsion into the prostatic urethra. The superior expanded part of the epididymis, called the head, is composed of lobules of the epididymis, which are the coiled ends of the efferent ductules of the testis. These ductules transmit the sperm from the testis to the epididymis. The body of the epididymis consists of the highly convoluted duct of the epididymis. The sperm are stored in the epididymis, where they undergo the final stages of maturation. *(Moore, p 149)*

138. **(D)** The normal heart is capable of pumping all of the blood that is returned to it over a wide range of volumes. By virtue of the Frank-Starling law of the heart, in normal persons the heart is capable of pumping 13 to 15 L/min without excessive backing up of pressure. Accordingly, it is the summation of all peripheral blood flows that return to the heart that ultimately regulates cardiac output. Thus, local metabolic factors and their integrated responses with neurohumoral regulation of specific beds determine venous return, which is identical to cardiac output in the closed circulatory system. Changes in cardiac function or activity in the central or peripheral nervous system contribute to this regulation indirectly. *(Guyton, pp 221–222)*

139. **(B)** Under normal metabolic conditions, the brain oxidizes about 140 g of glucose each day. This amounts to approximately 80 percent of the total glucose consumed each day and about 20 percent of the total O_2 consumed by the body. During starvation, the rate of glucose use by the brain is decreased and that of ketone bodies is increased, such that in late starvation, about 40 g of glucose (from gluconeogenesis) and 100 g of ketone bodies are daily consumed by the brain. *(Lehninger, p 838; Stryer, pp 551–553)*

140. **(E)** Cervicofacial actinomycosis (lumpy jaw) is an endogenous infection that is usually preceded by a tooth extraction or some other traumatic injury to the mouth. The lesion commonly drains to the cheek or submandibular area. The presence of sulfur granules is of great diagnostic importance. These are actually small (approximately 1 mm in diameter) colonies of the organism in a calcium phosphate matrix. They consist of a central filamentous mass of branching bacilli surrounded by radially oriented, club-shaped structures. *(Joklik et al, pp 530–531)*

141. **(B)** The lesion shown in the question is a granuloma, which is a small, circumscribed collection of inflammatory cells. These cells primarily consist of modified macrophages called epithelioid cells. There is an outer rim of lymphocytes. There are also multinucleated giant cells of the Langhans type. Other cells, such as plasma cells, eosinophils, and neutrophils, may be seen in granulomas, but the epithelioid cells are the single diagnostic feature. The center of a granuloma may be necrotic, like that pictured in the question, or it may be a solid mass of epithelioid cells. Granulomas are a form of response to chronic irritants associated with either infectious or noninfectious causes. An abscess is seen in acute inflammatory processes and is a circumscribed collection of pus secondary to liquefactive tissue necrosis. It is accompanied by a neutrophilic response. A keloid is an abnormal formation of collagenous connective tissue in a scar, forming a dense, bulging tumor. It is accompanied by minimal cell response. An infarct is an area of ischemic necrosis of tissue secondary to circulatory obstruction, producing an area with coagulation necrosis and neutrophilic cell response. A thrombus is a clot in a blood vessel formed intravascularly, causing vascular obstruction. They are composed of fibrin, platelets, RBCs, and WBCs. *(Cotran, pp 65–68)*

142. **(D)** In general, the duration of action of the oral hypoglycemic agents correlates with their half-lives. Several compounds (acetohexamide, tolazamide) have active metabolites that may contribute to hypoglycemic activity. Tolbutamide, the shortest-acting agent, has a duration of action of 6 to 12 hours (half-life of 7 hours). Tolazamide produces hypoglycemic activity for 12 to 16 hours or more (half-life of 7 hours). Acetohexamide, although its half-life is 6 hours, has a duration of 12 to 18 hours or more because its metabolite is more active than the parent compound. Chlorpropamide has the longest half-life (35 hours) and longest duration of action (24 to 72 hours). Isopropamide is not an oral hypoglycemic but is an antimuscarinic compound. *(Katzung, pp 595–597)*

143. (B) Sensitivity is defined as the extent to which patients with a particular disease or characteristic are accurately classified as having the disease, according to the diagnostic test. In this question, 98 percent of patients with the disease are accurately classified on the basis of the test result, so the sensitivity of the test is 98 percent. Specificity is defined as the extent to which patients who do not have the disease are correctly classified. In this question, 90 percent of the patients without disease had negative results and would have been correctly classified, so that specificity of the test is 90 percent. Positive and negative predictive accuracy refers to the accuracy of positive and negative results when the test is applied to a particular population, and these values will depend on the prevalence of the disease in the population. *(MacMahon and Pugh, pp 261–263)*

144–147. (144-C, 145-E, 146-B, 147-D) Aldosterone is required for appropriate renal retention of salt and water. Its absence is accompanied by a salt-wasting diuresis. Cortisol is necessary for maintaining serum glucose levels between meals, and hypoglycemia results from its absence. In the absence of insulin, fatty acids are metabolized to ketones in the liver, resulting ultimately in ketoacidosis. The absence of thyroid hormone results in a number of symptoms, including extreme somnolence. *(Guyton, pp 213,839–840,846–847,852,858–859)*

148–150. (148-D, 149-B, 150-D) The kinetic parameters K_m and V_{max} can be determined by plotting reaction rate as a function of varying substrate concentrations in the form of a Lineweaver-Burk plot. V_{max} is determined from the y-intercept and K_m is calculated from the x-intercept. In addition, such plots allow the characterization of competitive and noncompetitive inhibitors. The K_m of an enzyme is increased in the presence of a competitive inhibitor, but the V_{max} remains unchanged, whereas, in the presence of a noncompetitive inhibitor, K_m remains unaltered, but V_{max} is decreased. Therefore, the lines for the uninhibited and competitively inhibited reactions will intersect on the y axis, and the lines for the uninhibited and noncompetitively inhibited enzyme will intersect on the x axis. K_m may be defined as the substrate concentration at which one half of the enzyme's active site will be occupied. Thus, the answers to questions 148 and 150 are both **D.** *(Stryer, pp 190–191,193–197)*

151–153. (151-F, 152-E, 153-C) Hodgkin's disease is a malignancy of lymphoreticular tissue. Adenopathy is a common clinical finding. The diagnostic Reed–Sternberg cell is large and binucleated with prominent multiple eosinophilic nucleoli. The surrounding cellular population is composed variably of lymphocytes, histiocytes, plasma cells, eosinophils, neutrophils, and fibrocytes. Metastatic melanoma is usually seen in lymph nodes draining a primary cutaneous melanoma. The melanoma cells are noncohesive spindle or epithelioid cells with prominent nucleoli, and usually display cytoplasmic melanin. Metastatic carcinoma may be seen in surgically removed lymph nodes. The presence of estrogen and progesterone receptors, the adenocarcinomatous architecture, and the axillary location all would suggest that the metastatic tumor is mammary in origin. *(Rubin and Farber, pp 1108–1115)*

154–157. (154-B, 155-A, 156-C, 157-E) The antihypertensive action of hydralazine is primarily arteriolar venodilatation, which results in reflex tachycardia. This tachycardia may precipitate or aggravate myocardial ischemia. Propranolol is a nonselective β-adrenergic blocking agent. Blockade of cardiac β_1 receptors results in slowing of the heart rate. Prazosin dilates arterioles and venules. This may cause inadequate blood return to the right side of the heart as well as hypotension, which can result in syncopal episodes, particularly after the first dose. This phenomenon can be minimized by administering a small dose initially, preferably at bedtime. Methyldopa routinely causes sedation. This usually dissipates with continued use but uncommonly may persist enough to interfere with daily living activities, particularly mental work. *(Gilman et al, pp 788–801)*

158. (A) In Eriksonian developmental cycle, basic trust and a sense of security are developed during the first two years of life. That roughly parallels the Freudian oral stage. A failure to accomplish the developmental task results in mistrust and insecurity. *(Leigh and Reiser, pp 357–367)*

159. (B) The phase of initiative vs guilt parallels the Freudian oedipal stage of development. During this stage, the child is more energetic and loving, and there is a quality of planning and "attacking" a task. Also during this stage, the child develops a sense of moral responsibility and unconflicted initiative. Failure to master the tasks of this stage may result in guilt and complete repression of initiative. *(Leigh and Reiser, pp 357–367)*

160. (C) The phase of industry vs inferiority parallels Freud's latency period. During this phase, the child receives recognition by learning and producing things. Problems during this period may result in a sense of inferiority and inadequacy. *(Leigh and Reiser, pp 357–367)*

161. (D) Erikson considers adolescence to be a crucial period in developing a sense of identity, an inner sameness and direction. Career choices are made or seriously considered during this stage. Unsuccessful outcome of this stage is "role diffusion," a sense of being undefined and without direction. *(Leigh and Reiser, pp 357–367)*

162–165. **(162-E, 163-D, 164-B, 165-A)** Pernicious anemia is due to a lack of vitamin B_{12}. Autoimmune destruction of gastric parietal cells or immune inactivation of intrinsic factor leads to inadequate absorption of the vitamin. Megaloblastic anemia, leukopenia, thrombocytopenia, and demyelination of the posterolateral spinal cord columns are seen in the fully developed disease. Pemphigus is a bullous skin disorder caused by autoantibodies to surface antigens on keratinocytes. Primary biliary cirrhosis is an autoimmune disorder characterized by chronic destructive cholangitis in the early stages, and micronodular cirrhosis in the late stages of the disease. Anti-mitochondrial antibodies are seen in more than 90 percent of affected individuals. Systemic lupus erythematosis is an autoimmune disease with high titers of anti-nuclear antibodies. Facial rash, renal insufficiency, serositis, and pneumonitis are features of the disorder. *(Rubin and Farber, pp 760–764,1038,1211–1214,1223–1226)*

166–168. **(166-D, 167-A, 168-C)** The depolarization observed in the P wave signals the onset of atrial contraction, whereas the QRS complex is associated with the initiation of ventricular contraction. The sustained depolarization of the plateau phase is represented by the ST interval (which is not normally associated with any voltage deflection). Finally, the T wave is associated with the onset of ventricular repolarization. *(Guyton, p 118)*

169–171. **(169-E, 170-A, 171-C)** The genetic code defines the relationship between the sequence of bases in DNA and the corresponding sequence of amino acids in proteins. Three bases form a codon that codes for an amino acid. Since it has been demonstrated that most of the 64 possible arrangements of bases into codons do code for specific amino acids and since there are only about 20 amino acids, the code is degenerate. If a single base pair is substituted, only one amino acid is changed (provided that a degenerate codon for the same amino acid is not substituted). This demonstrates that the code is not overlapping. Finally, deletions or additions of a single base pair cause a shift of the reading frame subsequent to the point of change. Consequently, all amino acids in the coded protein subsequent to that point will be altered. This demonstrates a sequential reading of bases from a fixed starting point. *(Stryer, pp 99–101)*

172–174. **(172-C, 173-E, 174-A)** Glycogen phosphorylase catalyzes the sequential removal of glucose residues from glycogen yielding glucose 1-phosphate. The reaction is

$$\text{Glycogen}_{(n)} + P_i \rightarrow \text{glucose 1-phosphate} + \text{glycogen}_{(n-1)}$$

The synthesis of glycogen is mediated by glycogen synthase, which catalyzes the addition of glucose residues to a growing glycogen chain. The glucose must be in the activated form of UDP-glucose.

$$\text{Glycogen}_{(n)} + \text{UDP-glucose} \rightarrow \text{glycogen}_{(n+1)} + \text{UDP}$$

Glucokinase catalyzes the formation of glucose 6-phosphate from glucose and ATP. Glucose 6-phosphate dehydrogenase catalyzes the first step of the pentose phosphate pathway. The reaction is

$$\text{Glucose 6-phosphate} + \text{NADP}^+ \rightarrow \text{6-phosphoglu-cono-}\delta\text{-lactone} + \text{NADPH} + \text{H}^+$$

Glucose 6-phosphatase catalyzes the hydrolysis of glucose 6-phosphate to glucose and inorganic phosphate. This enzyme occurs in the liver and allows for the release of free glucose from the liver. *(Stryer, pp 361,428,454–456)*

175–178. **(175-A, 176-C, 177-D, 178-B)** Marfan's syndrome is a rare, usually autosomal dominant disease characterized by abnormally formed connective tissue. Affected patients are very tall and have long extremities and tapering fingers and toes with hyperextensive joints. They have bilateral dislocation of the ocular lens, cystic medial necrosis of the aorta, and floppy mitral valve leaflets. The underlying connective tissue defect is still unknown. Patients usually survive to 40 years of age.

Tay-Sachs disease is an autosomal recessive disease resulting from absence of hexosaminidase A. This GM_2 ganglioside accumulates in neurons of the central and autonomic nervous systems, retina, heart, liver, and spleen. The buildup of the ganglioside in the neurons causes their destruction, with gliosis and lipid deposits in the brain. Affected persons are normal at birth. By age 6 months, there is progressive motor and mental deterioration, and death occurs by age 3 years.

Niemann-Pick disease is an autosomal recessive disease characterized by a deficiency in sphingomyelinase, causing a buildup of sphingomyelin and cholesterol in reticuloendothelial cells and parenchymal cells in tissues. These abnormal cells are lipid laden, foamy, and large. Affected individuals suffer neurologic deterioration and organomegaly and usually die by the age of 3 years.

Pompe's disease is glycogen storage disease type II, which is autosomal recessive. It is caused by absence of the enzyme α-glucosidase in lysosomes, which causes defective glycogenolysis resulting in abnormal buildup of glycogen. The heart and nervous system show the most severe involvement, and patients die of congestive heart failure by 2 years of age.

Lesch-Nyhan syndrome is an X-linked disorder caused by a defect of the enzyme hypoxanthine guanine phosphoribosyltransferase, which is involved in purine metabolism. Affected persons suffer from hyperuricemia, gout, pyelonephritis, and renal stones. Neurologic deficits are the most prominent abnormality and include severe mental retardation, spastic cerebral palsy, and self-mutilating behavior. *(Cotran, pp 136–157)*

179–184. **(179-E, 180-C, 181-D, 182-A, 183-B, 184-D)** Neurohumoral transmission may be classified into two basic types—cholinergic and adrenergic transmission. Cholinergic transmission involves the stimulation of either nicotinic or muscarinic receptors by acetylcholine. Postsynaptic nicotinic receptors may be blocked by D-tubocurarine. Blockade of these receptors at motor end-plates results in muscle paralysis. Muscarinic receptors of postganglionic parasympathetic fibers also are stimulated by acetylcholine. However, these receptors are blocked by atropine and not by D-tubocurarine. The activity of cholinergic neurotransmitters (e.g., acetylcholine) is rapidly terminated by acetylcholinesterase. This enzyme may be inhibited reversibly by anticholinesterases, such as physostigmine.

Adrenergic neurotransmission occurs through stimulation of α or β receptors. Norepinephrine (noradrenalin) is a potent stimulant of postsynaptic α and β receptors. Phenylephrine selectively stimulates only postsynaptic α_1 receptors, β receptors may be classified as either β_1 (e.g., heart) or β_2 (e.g., bronchial muscle) receptors, β_1 receptors may be selectively blocked by metoprolol. *(Gilman et al, pp 96–113)*

185–189. **(185-A, 186-B, 187-E, 188-D, 189-C)** As crying diminishes during infant development, cooing and vowel sounds (e.g., "oo") increase. Words appear at about 1 year, between a range of 8 and 18 months of age. Vocabulary increases to as many as 50 words by 18 months and 200 words by age 2 years. The sequence of appearance of different classes of words is as follows: nouns, verbs, adjectives, and adverbs. Pronouns appear by age 2 years, and conjunctions after the age of 2½ years. *(Lennenberg, pp 128–130)*

190–194. **(190-E, 191-B, 192-D, 193-D, 194-B)** Mannitol is an inert hexose sugar that is filtered, but not reabsorbed, by the nephron. Thus, it increases the osmotic force of the tubule fluid, leading to enhanced diuresis. The high-ceiling loop diuretics, furosemide and ethacrynic acid, block sodium re-

absorption in the thick ascending limb of the loop of Henle. Both spironolactone and triamterene inhibit sodium/potassium exchange in the distal and collecting tubules, thus limiting the loss of potassium in the urine. *(Smith and Reynard, pp 573–583)*

195. **(D)** The obturator nerve innervates the adductor muscles of the thigh. It descends through the psoas major muscle, leaving its medial border at the brim of the pelvis. The obturator nerve leaves the pelvis through the obturator foramen. It pierces the psoas fascia, crosses the sacroiliac joint, passes laterally to the internal iliac vessels and ureter, and enters the pelvis minor. *(Moore, p 231)*

196. **(C)** The greater splanchnic nerve is formed by 4 to 5 roots from the sympathetic trunk between the sixth and tenth ganglia. It usually pierces the corresponding crus of the diaphragm and ends in the celiac ganglion. It is composed of preganglionic sympathetic fibers. *(Moore, p 232)*

197. **(A)** The pudendal nerve arises from the sacral plexus by separate branches of the ventral rami of S_2, S_3, and S_4. It leaves the pelvis between the piriformis and coccygeus muscles to enter the perineum through the lesser sciatic foramen. It innervates the muscles of the perineum. It is also sensory to the external genitalia. *(Moore, p 256)*

198. **(A)** When the red cell was removed from normal isotonic plasma and placed in the test solution, two things happened: (1) the cell shrank, and (2) then it gradually returned to normal size. This would happen if the test solution had two components: (1) a concentration of impermeant solutes giving the same osmolality as plasma, *plus* (2) an additional amount of permeant solute capable of gradually penetrating the red cell membrane (at a slower rate than water). Examples of such permeant solutes are urea and glycerol. When the cell was placed in the test solution, it initially shrank (as if the test solution were hypertonic due to its higher osmolality). However, as the permeant solute became equilibrated (with the same concentration inside the cell as outside), the cell volume returned to normal. That is, although the test solution initially acted as if it were hypertonic due to its total solute concentration, this effect was only transient because of the penetration of the permeant particles.

199. **(C)** When the cell, with its accumulated gain of permeant solute (from prior exposure to test solution), was placed back into plasma, it had by then a total solute osmolality higher than plasma, so there was a period of net entry of water into the cell, causing it to swell (reaching a peak at point z). However, as the accumulated solute diffused out of the cell, the cell eventually lost all of this permeant solute and therefore, ultimately, returned to normal volume. *(Berne and Levy, 1993, pp 12–13)*

200–202. **(200-B, 201-A, 202-C)** A single turn of the citric acid cycle begins with the condensation of acetyl CoA and oxaloacetate to yield citrate. NADH is produced at three steps in the cycle: oxidative decarboxylation of isocitrate to α-ketoglutarate, oxidative decarboxylation of α-ketoglutarate to succinyl CoA, and oxidation of malate to oxaloacetate. During each turn of the cycle, two molecules of CO_2 are released—during the decarboxylation reactions referred to above. In sum, one turn of the cycle yields 3 molecules of NADH, one molecule of $FADH_2$, and one molecule of GTP. In conjunction with electron transport and oxidative phosphorylation, each NADH molecule can yield 3 moles of ATP and each $FADH_2$ can yield two moles of ATP. Thus, one turn of the cycle can yield 15 moles of nucleoside triphosphate. *(Stryer, pp 374–378,420)*

203–204. **(203-C, 204-E)** The treatment of hypertension utilizes drugs with a range of mechanisms of action. Clonidine activates α_2-receptors located in the CNS; propranolol is thought to inhibit β-adrenoceptors not only in the heart but possibly in the brain and kidney as well. Labetalol is unique in that it inhibits both α_1- and β-adrenoceptors. It is, therefore, effective in treating both hypertensive emergencies as well as chronic hypertension. Captopril is an effective antihypertensive agent because of its ability to inhibit the conversion of angiotensin I to angiotensin II (one of the most potent vasoconstrictors). The result is a decrease in vascular tone. Other mechanisms, however, may also be involved in the reduction of blood pressure. *(Gilman et al, pp 798–799,806–807)*

205–206. **(205-C, 206-A)** Trauma to the head can cause both intracerebral hemorrhage and subdural hemorrhage. Subdural hemorrhage is seen more frequently with more trivial head injuries, whereas intracerebral hemorrhage usually requires a severe blow to the head, often associated with a fracture of the skull. It is usually associated, therefore, with searing stress through the cerebral substance, forming rupture of the vessels. A subdural hemorrhage may be slow and accumulative following a trivial injury and easily missed. Severe hypertension may cause rupture of small vessels in the brain, with the classic intracerebral hemorrhage resulting in stroke. Subdural hemorrhage is not associated with hypertension and results usually from trauma. *(Rubin and Farber, pp 1436–1439)*

207. **(E)** The azygos vein empties into the superior vena cava. The inferior petrosal sinus, lingual, facial, superior, and middle thyroid veins drain into the internal jugular veins. *(Woodburne, pp 196,401)*

208. **(B)** The functions of the vagus nerve include special visceral efferent, general visceral efferent, general visceral afferent, special visceral afferent, and general somatic afferent, but not general somatic efferent. *(Woodburne, pp 196–197)*

209. **(A)** The vagus nerve provides motor innervation to the voluntary muscles of the larynx, pharynx, and palate (except the tensor veli palatini), and of the upper two-thirds of the esophagus. *(Woodburne, p 196)*

210. **(A)** The vagus nerve provides parasympathetic preganglionic fibers to the involuntary muscles and glands of the heart, esophagus, stomach, trachea, bronchi, intestines, and other abdominal viscera. *(Woodburne, p 196)*

211. **(B)** The glossopharyngeal nerve provides taste fibers to the posterior one-third of the tongue. *(Woodburne, p 230)*

212. **(B)** The glossopharyngeal nerve provides parasympathetic innervation for the parotid gland after synapse in the otic ganglion. *(Woodburne, p 230)*

213. **(D)** The trigeminal nerve (mandibular division) provides motor supply of the mylohyoid, anterior belly of the digastric, the tensor veli palatini, tensor tympani, lateral and medial pterygoid, masseter, and temporalis. *(Woodburne, p 255)*

214. **(B)** The cell bodies of the inferior ganglion of the vagus are concerned with the visceral afferent components of the vagus. *(Woodburne, p 197)*

215. **(A)** The cell bodies of the superior ganglion of the vagus are concerned primarily with the general somatic afferent (cutaneous) component of the nerve. *(Woodburne, p 197)*

216. **(D)** The middle cervical ganglion commonly lies at the level of the cricoid cartilage in the bend of the inferior thyroid artery or superior to the arch of the artery. *(Woodburne, pp 203–204)*

217. **(G)** Premack's principle holds that a behavior engaged in at a higher frequency can be used to reinforce a lower-frequency behavior. In treating a schizophrenic patient who liked to sit down, doing nothing, a plan was devised in which the patient could sit down for five minutes only after a certain amount of rehabilitation work. *(Kaplan and Sadock, pp 262–271)*

218. **(D)** A stimulus (snake) is generalized to something else that resembles the original stimulus (rope). This type of conditioning may contribute to certain types of phobias and other anxiety conditions. *(Kaplan and Sadock, pp 262–271)*

219. **(H)** Extinction occurs when the conditioned stimulus is presented repeatedly without the unconditioned stimulus. Eventually, the conditioned response gradually weakens and then disappears. *(Kaplan and Sadock, pp 262–271)*

220. **(B)** This is the classical experiment by Pavlov, in which the unconditioned stimulus, food, is paired with the neutral stimulus, bell, until the unconditioned response to food, salivation, becomes conditioned to the sound of the bell. The sound of the bell, then, becomes the conditioned stimulus. *(Kaplan and Sadock, pp 262–271)*

221. **(F)** Reciprocal inhibition means that one state of the person inhibits the elicitation of a contradictory state at the same time. When one is relaxed, one cannot be anxious at the same time. This is one of the techniques to treat phobic symptoms. *(Kaplan and Sadock, pp 262–271)*

222. **(E)** Behavior may be shaped by rewarding intermediate steps until the desired behavior is achieved. Through shaping, complex behaviors can be operantly conditioned. *(Kaplan and Sadock, pp 262–271)*

223. **(B)** Names and images may function as conditioned stimuli. Thus, thinking about biting into a sour apple may evoke the conditioned response of salivation. This type of classical conditioning may occur naturally. *(Kaplan and Sadock, pp 262–271)*

224. **(D)** Endogenous and exogenous pyrogens, resulting from the presence of infecting pathogenic microorganisms, raise the hypothalamic set point and thereby cause a rise in body temperature (fever). Once the patient's temperature has risen to match the newer, higher set point, the patient is comfortable and his new, higher temperature is well-regulated around the new set point.

225. **(E)** If the factors originally responsible for the fever are gone (successfully eliminated by the body's immune system), the hypothalamic set point returns to normal. For a while, the body's core temperature is above the now normal set point. This has the same effect as if the individual were too hot. The patient begins sweating and complains of "burning up" because of his hot skin (due to vasodilation).

226. **(B)** When the set point is first raised, due to pyrogens, the body temperature is temporarily below the new, higher set point, just as if the body were too cool. The hypothalamus causes the usual responses to produce additional heat (shivering) and to conserve the heat present (skin vasoconstriction, lack of sweating). The patient subjectively feels chilled and seeks to raise his body temperature until he is more comfortable (piles on blankets, sits by the fire, gets a heating pad, etc.). *(Guyton, pp 806–807)*

227–228. **(227-A, 228-B)** In the microscopic evaluation of lymph nodes, RFH can, at times, be difficult to differentiate from NL. Several histologic architectural features can be helpful in the decision-making process. In RFH, the nodal architecture is preserved, the follicles are more prominent in the cortex than in the medulla, there is marked variation in the size and shape of the follicles, which are sharply demarcated, and there is only moderate, if any, infiltration of the capsule and pericapsular fat by inflammatory cells. NL, on the other hand, produces effacement of the normal nodal architecture, has follicles or nodules distributed more or less evenly throughout the cortex and medulla of the lymph node, shows slight to moderate variation in the size and shape of the follicles, which are not well demarcated, and demonstrates prominent infiltration of the capsule and pericapsular fat by the neoplastic process. *(Rubin and Farber, pp 1057,1063,1091–1103)*

229–232. **(229-E, 230-B, 231-A, 232-D)** Rocky Mountain Spotted Fever is caused by *R. rickettsii*. Rash, fever, headache, and myalgia are systemic components of the disease. The organism is particularly well demonstrated in endothelial cells sampled by skin biopsy. Syphilis is a systemic infectious disorder with protean clinical findings. The etiologic agent is *T. pallidum*. Bubonic plague is caused by *Yersinia pestis*. Wild rodents and some domesticated animals serve as reservoirs. Fleas transmit the disease to humans. An enlarged, painful lymph node (bubo) arises in the area drained by the flea bite. Massive terminal ecchymoses give rise to the appellation "black death." Whooping cough (pertussis) is caused by *B. pertussis*. Upper respiratory symptoms characterize the disease. Forced inspiratory stridor may produce a "whooping" sound for which the disease is named. *(Rubin and Farber, pp 350–365)*

233. **(C)** The clinical symptoms found in the 2-year-old girl are typical for measles (rubeola) which is the major cause of death in developing countries. Measles is characterized by several days of fever, runny nose, conjunctivitis, cough, macular diffuse, and confluent rash, which starts on the head and then spreads to the rest of the body. Koplik's spots and lymphopenia are encountered in measles. Koplik's spots are red elevations on the buccal mucous membrane. In the center of each may be seen, in strong light, a minute bluish-white speck; they appear in measles prior to skin eruption and are a diagnostic feature of measles. *(Jawetz et al, pp 527–529)*

234. **(E)** The capsid proteins of viruses are external components of the virion and as such are in a position to interact with the immunologic apparatus of the host. Thus, they are the inducers of antibody synthesis both in an infection and in the vaccines that are employed to prevent viral diseases. They also function to protect the viral nucleic acids from nucleases present in the plasma and in phagocytic vacuoles. One of the viral capsid proteins is responsible for adsorption of the virus to susceptible cells, and it, or perhaps other capsid components, may also function in penetration of the virus into the cell. *(Joklik et al, pp 115,631)*

235. **(D)** Cysteine, tyrosine, and glutamine are amino acids with uncharged, polar side chains. Cysteine contains a thiol group, tyrosine possesses a phenolic hydroxyl group, and glutamine contains an amide side chain. Glycine has no side chain. Lysine possesses a side chain ending in an amino group. At pH 7, this amino group is positively charged. *(Stryer, pp 16–21)*

236. **(B)** The symptoms shown by the patient described in the question could have been caused by any of the agents listed. The pathologic process observed in the CNS is similar in all of these. The detection of inclusion bodies is a valuable aid in diagnosis. The rabies inclusion body (Negri body) occurs in the cytoplasm of the infected nerve cell, whereas the inclusion body of herpes simplex (Lipsh&udtz body) has an intranuclear location. Polioviruses do not produce inclusion bodies of diagnostic significance; neither do the togaviruses. *(Hoeprich, pp 864,1093)*

237. **(D)** Cyanogen bromide is one of several chemical reagents that cleaves proteins at specific points. Cyanogen bromide cleaves only on the carboxyl side of methionine residues. Trypsin hydrolyzes peptide bonds on the carboxyl side of lysine and arginine residues. Disulfide bonds can be broken by a variety of reducing agents, e.g., β-mercaptoethanol. *(Stryer, pp 55–56)*

238. **(E)** Viruses can be neutralized by antibody alone if the antibody is directed against a viral component important in adsorption, penetration, or uncoating. Antibody-coated viruses in the circulation or in the tissues are phagocytized and destroyed. This opsonization by antibody is due to the fact that phagocytic cells have a membrane receptor for the Fc portion of certain immunoglobulin molecules, and this antibody–receptor complex serves

to hold the viral particle close to the phagocytic cell until it can be engulfed. Complement can augment this neutralization, and it also can inactivate virions directly by covering their surfaces and, in some instances, lysing the virus even in the absence of specific antiviral antibody. If infected host cells are lysed, the site of viral replication is destroyed, and the infection can be brought under control. *(Davis et al, pp 1023–1024)*

239. **(A)** Carcinoma of the colon and rectum is one of the major cancers in the western world and is frequently seen in North American whites, usually over the age of 50. It is a disease that is relatively rare in black Africans and in Japanese living in Japan, although there is some indication that Japanese living in the USA and changing their diets also may have an increased incidence of this disease. There is some evidence that the incidence may be increasing with urbanization in Africa.

The key to the disease appears to be related to the level of fiber in the diets, which is high in Africa and Japan and low in modern western diets, to a large extent. *(Hutt and Burkitt, pp 27–30)*

240. **(D)** Increased suicide risk is associated with older age, male sex, presence of pain, Protestant religion as opposed to Catholic religion, and living alone. Living alone may contribute to the risk of suicide through loneliness, depression, and reduction in the rescue potential. *(Leigh and Reiser, pp 101–144)*

241. **(E)** The enzyme, 3-ketoacid CoA transferase, is required to transfer CoA from succinyl-CoA to acetoacetate to form acetoacetyl-CoA, which is then cleaved by thiolysis to two molecules of acetyl-CoA. Acetoacetate is a ketone body. It is produced in the liver but cannot be used by this tissue since the liver lacks the CoA transferase. Virtually all peripheral tissues that contain mitochondria possess the transferase and can, therefore, utilize ketone bodies as an energy source. *(Stryer, pp 478–480)*

242. **(E)** Viruses can damage the host and produce disease by all of the mechanisms listed in the question. Cells can be rendered nonfunctional by direct cytopathic effects, depression of synthesis of cellular macromolecules, and alterations of lysosomes or cell membranes. Viral transformation of normal cells to hyperplastic or malignant cells is also a mechanism of disease production. *(Joklik et al, pp 773–778)*

243. **(A)** Malignant cells may show a variety of anaplastic changes. They show irregularities in size and shape of the cell, with extreme variation and overall increase in cell size. The nucleus has an increased amount of DNA and is hyperchromatic. The nuclei are larger than expected for the cell size, with an elevated nucleus/cytoplasm ratio approaching 1 : 1 instead of the normal 1 : 4. The nuclei may show coarsely clumped, irregularly dispersed chromatin, and one or more prominent nucleoli. Some tumors may create tumor giant cells that are multinucleated conglomerations of malignant cells. *(Cotran, pp 243–249)*

244. **(E)** Depression may be symptomatic of a number of organic diseases. Most common medical diseases associated with depression are endocrinopathies, including hypothyroidism, Cushing's syndrome, hyperparathyroidism, etc. Occult malignancies are also associated with depression, especially cancer of the pancreas. Many drugs may cause depressive symptoms, including such antihypertensive drugs as propranolol and reserpine. *(Leigh and Reiser, pp 101–144)*

245. **(D)** The wall of the uterus consists of three layers. The outer, serous coat is called the perimetrium. The middle, muscular coat is called the myometrium. The inner, mucous coat is called the endometrium. The uterus is usually bent anteriorly (anteflexed) between the cervix and the body, and the entire uterus is normally bent or inclined anteriorly (anteverted). The body of the uterus is enclosed between the layers of the broad ligament. *(Moore, pp 284–285)*

246. **(E)** Gastrin infusion stimulates gastric acid secretion. Thus initially, before peptide x was given, there was high gastric acid concentration. Secretin, sometimes called "nature's antacid," must have been peptide x because it is known to inhibit gastric acid secretion and to stimulate pancreatic bicarbonate production. Peptide x could not have been motilin, which has mainly to do with motility. Nor could it have been angiotensin II, which has several functions (e.g., stimulation of aldosterone secretion), none of which include inhibition of gastric acid secretion or stimulation of pancreatic bicarbonate secretion. Nor could it have been CCK, which mainly stimulates pancreatic enzyme secretion and gall bladder contraction. Somatostatin has many inhibitory effects and does not stimulate pancreatic bicarbonate production. *(Johnson, pp 7–10)*

247. **(A)** The cathecolamines, dopamine, norepinephrine, and epinephrine, are all derived sequentially from levodopa. The latter is synthesized from tyrosine by a hydroxylation reaction catalyzed by tyrosine hydroxylase. Levodopa is also the precursor for synthesis of the pigment melanin. p-Hydroxylphenylpyruvate is a breakdown product of tyrosine, which is ultimately converted to acetoacetate and fumarate. Histamine is a vasodilator that is formed from histidine by decarboxylation. *(Stryer, pp 511–512,591–592,1025–1026)*

248. **(E)** All of the statements in the question correctly describe influenza virus. Three serotypes of influenza viruses are known to occur in nature. These are divided into types A, B, and C on the basis of differences in their ribonucleoprotein antigens. Within the types, there are antigenic differences based on changes in the nature of the hemagglutinin and neuraminidase spikes that protrude from the envelope. It is changes in these subtypes that cause the emergence of epidemics and pandemics of influenza, and these changes are also the reason that vaccine prophylaxis of the disease is so difficult. Each pandemic is caused by a new antigenic subtype. Hence, there has not been sufficient time to produce the large quantities of vaccine that would be needed to protect the world's population. Thus, the vaccine is usually reserved for medical personnel and the aged (who are particularly at risk of fatal influenzal disease). It is thought that the segmented genome of the virus may play a role in the antigenic changes that the organism undergoes. *(Joklik et al, pp 642,662,821–823)*

249. **(E)** Emboli are detached intravascular fragments of material that are carried by the blood to distant sites. These emboli are then lodged in vessels that are too small, causing partial or total obstruction. These masses may be solid, liquid, or gaseous and may include air, nitrogen, fragments of bone, marrow, atherosclerotic plaque, tumor, or foreign bodies. Ninety-nine percent of all emboli are of thrombotic origin. Pulmonary emboli are the most common form of emboli. The majority arise in thrombosed veins of the legs. When released, they cause pulmonary obstruction with hypoxia and right-sided heart failure. Pulmonary emboli rarely cause infarction. Systemic emboli arise in the arterial system, usually in the left ventricle or left atrium, and travel to blood vessels of smaller caliber. These emboli cause infarction with hemorrhage secondary to occlusion of the vessel. Other examples of emboli include gas bubbles from deepsea decompression, fat from bone fractures, or amniotic fluid in obstetric complications. *(Rubin and Farber, pp 265–268)*

250. **(D)** While uncomplicated grief reactions usually subside within four to eight weeks, a significant proportion continue to have symptoms up to one to two years after the death of a spouse. In one study, 17 percent of bereaved persons were depressed at the end of 13 months. *(Leigh and Reiser, pp 101–144)*

251. **(C)** For descriptive purposes, the perineum is divided into two unequal triangles by an imaginary transverse line joining the anterior ends of the ischial tuberosities. The midpoint of this line is the central point of the perineum, which overlies the perineal body (central tendon of the perineum). The anal triangle, containing the anus, is posterior to this line and the urogenital triangle, containing the root of the scrotum and penis (or the external genitalia in the female), is anterior to this line. *(Moore, p 295)*

252. **(C)** Filtration pressure (P_{uf}) is calculated from the following equation involving the four Starling forces:

$$P_{uf} = (P_{GC} - P_{BS}) - (\Pi_{GC} - \Pi_{BS})$$

Normally, the filtrate in Bowman's space has such negligible amounts of protein that Π_{BS} is considered to be zero and is often left out of the Starling equation for glomerular filtration. Choices A, B, and D all give zero P_{uf} (i.e., glomerular filtration equilibrium). Choice E gives a negative filtration pressure of –5 mm Hg (favors absorption instead of filtration). *(Vander, pp 25–27)*

253. **(B)** All cells, except liver, phosphorylate glucose to glucose 6-phosphate with a hexokinase. By contrast, glucokinase catalyzes this reaction in liver. Liver glucokinase has a significantly higher K_m for glucose than does hexokinase. As a result, peripheral tissues, but not liver, will take up glucose from blood when blood sugar levels are low. Glucose 6-phosphate, derived from gluconeogenesis or glycogenolysis, is dephosphorylated in liver by glucose 6-phosphatase so that it can cross the liver plasma membrane as free glucose. Pyruvate carboxylase and fructose 1,6-biphosphatase are involved in gluconeogenesis. This process occurs only in liver and kidney. *(Stryer, pp 361,438–440, 454–455,637–639)*

254. **(D)** Phagocytic cells, such as macrophages and neutrophils, have receptors for C3b. B lymphocytes also react with C3b. However, T lymphocytes appear to lack a membrane receptor for this molecule. It is the presence of the C3b receptor on phagocytic cells that is responsible for the opsonization of bacteria and other foreign materials by antibody and complement. The antibody reacts with an antigen on the bacterial surface, and the complement cascade is activated. During this activation, C3b is deposited onto the surface of the organism, and it interacts with the receptor in the phagocyte membrane to bring the two cells together, thus facilitating the phagocytic process. *(Joklik et al, pp 206–207,229,268,280–282,287,351,373)*

255. **(E)** The changes in the nucleus seen in various forms of cell injury include pyknosis, which is a condensation and destruction of the nuclear protein, karyolysis, which is a lysis or disruption of the nuclear material, and karyorrhexis, which has a similar disruptive and irreversible effect. Swelling of the rough endoplasmic reticulum usually occurs in earlier forms of cell injury and is not related to nuclear changes and in some respects, therefore, is reversible. This is typically seen in so-called cloudy swelling and similar cytoplasmic changes recognizable in cell injury. *(Rubin and Farber, pp 14–20)*

256. **(B)** While mood congruent hallucinations may occur during psychotic depression, hallucinations are not the norm in depressive syndrome. Suicidal thoughts, anhedonia, apathy, and anorexia are quite common in depression. *(Leigh and Reiser, pp 101–144)*

257. **(B)** The ischiocavernosus arises from the surface of the ischial tuberosity and ischial rami. The perineal body is the landmark of the perineum where several muscles converge (transverse perineal, bulbospongiosus, levator ani, and some fibers of the external anal sphincter. *(Moore, pp 298,313)*

258. **(A)** Bile salts, along with lecithin (phosphatidyl choline), form small, emulsified droplets with the products of fat digestion (mainly 2-monoglycerides). These small droplets, called mixed micelles (or biliary micelles), are about 5 nanometers in diameter and contain approximately 25 molecules. Very hydrophobic molecules, such as long chain fatty acids, cholesterol, and fat-soluble vitamins, partition themselves into the interior of the micelles. Amphiphilic molecules, with both polar (hydrophilic) and nonpolar (hydrophobic) parts, have the hydrophilic parts facing outward at the surface and the hydrophobic parts within the interior (bile salts, lecithin, and 2-monoglycerides).

Apolipoproteins are not part of mixed micelles. They function in blood partly for stabilization and transport of lipids in an aqueous medium (plasma), but mainly for the specific directing of lipid components to the appropriate tissue destinations (with specific tissue receptors for the various apolipoproteins). *(Berne and Levy, pp 711–713, 842–846)*

259. **(B)** Fibrinogen is converted to fibrin monomers by the action of thrombin, which cleaves several peptide bonds in fibrinogen to yield fibrin. The fibrin monomers, thus formed, aggregate with each other to form a clot. Thrombin itself is derived by proteolytic cleavage of its precursor, prothrombin. Antithrombin III is an inhibitor of thrombin activity. It inactivates the enzyme by forming an irreversible complex with it. This inhibition can be enhanced by the presence of heparin and is the basis of the latter's anticoagulant properties. Fibrin clots can be dissolved by the action of plasmin, a serine protease. *(Stryer, pp 248–256)*

260. **(D)** The appendix of the epididymis is the remnant of the cranial end of the mesonephric duct, which is attached to the head of the epididymis. The appendix of the testis is a vesicular remnant of the cranial end of the paramesonephric duct. It is attached to the superior pole of the testis. The presence of excess fluid or blood in the tunica vaginalis is known as hydrocele or hematocele of the testis. *(Moore, pp 151–152)*

261. **(E)** The boundaries of the omental foramen are the following: anteriorly—the portal vein, hepatic artery, and the bile duct; posteriorly—the inferior vena cava and right crus of the diaphragm; superiorly—the caudate lobe of the liver; and inferiorly—the superior part of the duodenum, portal vein, hepatic artery, and bile duct. *(Moore, p 159)*

262. **(B)** In severe obsessive-compulsive disorder, the patient may be disabled due to the compulsions and may be housebound. In severe cases, psychosurgery, including cingulotomy, have been reported helpful, and serotonergic antidepressants, such as clomipramine and fluoxetine, have been helpful. While most OCD patients have rigid superego, and may, indeed, have fixation in the anal sadistic stage, there seems to be a large biological component in the etiology of the disorder. *(Kaplan and Sadock, pp 984–999)*

263. **(B)** The mamillary bodies are part of the limbic system, the original classic papez circuit for emotion. The auditory pathway receives input from the cochlear nerve and nuclei. The auditory pathways ascend as the lateral lemnisus and terminate in the inferior colliculus, which gives rise to the brachium of the inferior colliculus. The brachium terminates in the medial geniculate body. *(Noback, pp 198,356)*

264. **(B)** During a forced expiration, intrapleural pressure is no longer negative, but becomes positive (above atmospheric pressure). The alveolar pressure is even more positive than this. Air moves out with ever-increasing velocity, while total airway cross-sectional area becomes smaller. As the air approaches the initial generations of the respiratory tree, air pressure in the airways diminishes. The decrease in pressure of the moving air is due to two influences: (1) loss of potential energy as pressure as airflow overcomes resistance, and (2) loss of potential energy as pressure when kinetic energy increases due to velocity increase (Bernoulli's principle). Thus, airway pressure falls with distance from the alveoli and eventually reaches a point beyond which airway pressure is less than the supra-atmospheric intrapleural pressure. Since the pressure outside the airways is higher than that within, they are compressed and increase the resistance to flow. Once airflow is maximal, any further attempts to increase expiratory effort result in additional airway collapse. A flow-limiting segment is produced that prevents additional increase in flow despite intensified expiratory efforts. That is, as expiration begins, increased effort at first results in increased flow, but eventually a maximal flow rate is reached beyond which no amount of effort can increase flow (becomes flow-independent). *(Berne and Levy, 1993, pp 572–573)*

265. **(C)** Regions of the eukaryotic genome that are being actively transcribed are referred to as transcriptionally active chromatin. These regions of the chromosome display several characteristics, which include increased sensitivity of the DNA to digestion by DNAse I and reduced levels of 5-methylcytosine. The C-5 position of cytosine in a majority of the CpG dinucleotide sequences in the genomes of mammalian DNA is methylated. Transcriptionally active chromatin has a lower degree of methylation than does bulk chromatin. The levels of core histones or HMG1 and HMG2 nonhistone proteins have not been correlated with gene activity. *(Stryer, pp 842–844)*

266. **(D)** Spores are not important constituents of gram negative organisms. Bacterial spores are formed when certain gram positive bacteria multiply in culture media that lack the necessary nutrients. Spores are stable to heating for several minutes at 80°C. Spores contain 10–15 percent calcium dipicolinic acid, which is thought to play a role in the resistance of spores to heat. Actually, heating bacterial spores at 80°C for 15–30 minutes is used to initiate spore germination. However, spore germination, in addition to heating at 80°C, requires the presence of L-alanine, or adenosine, which apparently activates an autolysin that degrades the spore cortex and allows the spore to accumulate water, release calcium dipicolinate, and germinate. *(Jawetz et al, pp 27–28)*

267. **(D)** Serum sickness is a type III hypersensitivity disease characterized by circulating immune complexes. The immune complexes are deposited in the skin (vasculitis), kidney (glomerulonephritis), and joints (arthritis). Upon deposition, they evoke an inflammatory response (fever) through complement activation. Delayed hypersensitivity (type IV hypersensitivity) is not involved in serum sickness. *(Rubin and Farber, pp 109–113)*

268. **(D)** Organophosphorus compounds "irreversibly" bind to acetylcholinesterase via alkylphosphorylation. Thus, these compounds tend to have greater toxicity than other cholinesterase inhibitors. However, cholinesterase reactivators such as Pralidoxime can displace this class of cholinesterase inhibitor from the enzyme if administered before "aging" of the phosphate bond occurs. *(Gilman et al, pp 132–141)*

269. **(A)** Psychological defense mechanisms are automatic, unconscious processes that reduce anxiety. These tend to be mobilized and accentuated at times of stress, including hospitalization. Successful deployment of defense mechanisms may be associated with decreased stress hormone activation. While certain defense mechanisms may be accentuated in some psychiatric disorders, defense mechanisms are not necessarily maladaptive. *(Leigh and Reiser, pp 51–52,79–100)*

270. **(E)** The pyramidal decussation occurs in the caudal portion of the medulla. The most distinguishing feature is the crossing of 85 to 90 percent of the corticospinal fibers as the pyramidal decussation. It is composed of interdigitating descending fibers that decussate and course in a caudal and posterior direction to the dorsal aspect of the lateral funiculus of the spinal cord. Dorsal roots are absent. *(Noback, pp 200–201)*

271. **(A)** In dynamic (isotonic) aerobic exercise, work load and body oxygen consumption are directly related (indeed it is often easier to calculate the work load from the oxygen consumption than to measure it directly). No matter whether oxygen consumption or work load is used as the independent variable on a graph (usually as the abscissa) against changes in a given cardiovascular function as the dependent variable (usually as the ordinate), the curve shapes are the same. With increased work load (or increased oxygen consumption), there is an almost perfectly-linear increase in heart rate, whereas the curve for stroke volume increases at first, but then levels off (plateau) at about half maximal work load (or half maximal oxygen consumption). Thus, for severe exercise, the increased levels of cardiac output depend almost entirely on increases in heart rate (at essentially a constant stroke volume).

Although mean arterial blood pressure and systolic arterial blood pressure rise with increasing levels of dynamic exercise, the diastolic blood pressure remains virtually constant. With increasing levels of exercise, blood flow to the skin decreases at first, but then as heat production from the exercising muscles begins to increase, the blood flow to skin also increases to aid in temperature regulation. Blood pressures in the pulmonary circulation are much lower than in the systemic circulation. Even if the cardiac output were to increase four-fold during exercise, there would be only about a doubling of the pulmonary arterial blood pressure (e.g., from 12 to 24 mm Hg), which would be nowhere near systemic arterial pressures. *(Berne and Levy, 1993, pp 533–534)*

272. **(B)** The arteries to the jejunum and ileum arise from the superior mesenteric artery, the second of the impaired branches of the abdominal aorta. The celiac artery supplies the spleen, liver, gallbladder, stomach, pancreas, and duodenum. The distal two-thirds of the transverse colon, descending colon, and upper rectum are supplied by branches of the inferior mesenteric artery, the left gastric supplies the lesser curvature of the stomach and pancreas, and the duodenum is supplied by the superior pancreatic duodenal arteries. *(Moore, pp 180,187,189,197,207)*

273. **(E)** The aortic hiatus is posterior to the diaphragm. It passes posteriorly to the median arcuate ligament anterior to T12 vertebra. The aortic hiatus transmits the thoracic duct, and usually the azygos vein. The anterior and posterior vagal trunks pass through the esophageal hiatus. *(Moore, p 227)*

274. **(D)** Wound healing is delayed by large, gaping defects, excessive scar formation, infection in the wound site, foreign material in the wound site, and metabolic processes such as diabetes mellitus, malnutrition, and scurvy. A clean wound site with closely opposed edges would be likely to heal quickly, without complications or delay. *(Rubin and Farber, pp 75–89)*

275. **(A)** Both competitive and depolarizing neuromuscular blockers act as nicotinic end-plate receptors to interrupt transmission. Competitive blockers function as antagonists at the receptor to prevent the binding of acetylcholine, while depolarizing agents bind with the nicotinic receptor and cause prolonged opening of the ion channel, leading to a depolarization blockade of neuromuscular transmission. *(Smith and Reynard, pp 130–135)*

276. **(E)** Mechanic proposed that four dimensions of an illness or symptom are important in influencing how the illness is perceived. They include commonality, familiarity, predictability of outcome, and the threat and loss likely to result from the illness. For example, since the common cold is both familiar and common, a person with a cold is unlikely to seek medical help. However, coughing up blood is uncommon, unfamiliar, unpredictable, and threatening, and thus is more likely to lead to medical help-seeking behavior. *(Leigh and Reiser, pp 3–15)*

277. **(C)** The facial, trigeminal, glossopharyngeal, and vagus nerves innervate branchiomeric muscles.

The oculomotor, trochlear, abducens, and hypoglossal nerves innervate voluntary muscles derived from embryonic somites. The branchiomeric muscles are derived from the branchial arches and are innervated by the nerves associated with those arches. The muscles of the eye and tongue are innervated by nerves associated with embryonic somites. *(Noback, p 224)*

278. (B) The elastic recoil properties of lungs depend primarily on two factors: (1) elasticity of lung tissue, and (2) surface tension forces at the air/liquid interface at the alveolar surfaces. Filling lungs with saline produces a liquid/liquid interface with no surface tension forces, hence their recoil force is less and their compliance greater (more easily expanded for any given distending pressure). The surface forces at the air/liquid interface are so strong that in the absence of normally present detergent-like surfactant, there is considerable collapse of smaller alveoli. When the saline-filled lungs are drained, much surfactant is washed out, and these lungs become less compliant than before addition of saline. Whether saline-filled or air-filled, lung collagen fibers resist expansion of each to the same maximum volume. *(Berne and Levy, 1993, pp 565–566)*

279. (D) The cleavage sites of the phospholipases are shown on the diagram below. Only digestion with phospholipase D yields phosphatidic acid. Hydrolysis by the other phospholipases leaves unesterified glycerol hydroxyl groups. Lipoprotein lipase hydrolyzes triacyglycerols in lipoproteins. *(Stryer, pp 552)*

280. (D) Malaria is caused by various species of the genus *Plasmodium*. Three main species are recognized: *Plasmodium falcipovum, P. vivax,* and *P. malariae.* These organisms are strictly parasitic and have two hosts—humans and the anopheles mosquitos. In humans, they live inside the erythrocytes, as shown in picture D, where they undergo a cyclic development from trophozoites to schizonts to gametocytes to segmenters to merozoites that infect the new erythrocytes, and the cycle is repeated. Picture A represents *Balantidium coli.* This organism produces an infection of the large intestine similar to amoebic dysentery. The organisms are spread through contaminated water and food. Picture B depicts the cyst form of *Endamoeba hystolytica,* which is the cause of amebic dysentery. *E. hystolytica* penetrates the mucosa of the large intestine, inducing ulceration. It may enter the blood stream and cause abscesses in the liver and also, occasionally, in spleen and brain. Contaminated water is the most common mode of the spread of the infection. Picture C shows the typical morphology of a *T. cruzi,* the causative agent of trypanosomiasis or Chagas' disease. *T. cruzi* is transmitted to humans via infected feces of reduviid bugs (kissing bugs). Picture E represents *Leishmania donovani* in culture. *L. donovani* is the etiological agent of leishmaniasis or kala-azar, which is transmitted to humans by sand flies. *(Jawetz et al, pp 336,338, 344,346,348)*

281. (E) *Leishmania donovani* is the cause of a disease known as kala azar, or leishmaniasis. In the circulating blood, or in the culture, the organisms are flagellated, but differ from the trypanosomes shown in picture C. The clinical symptoms are anemia and cutaneous hemorrhage, with a greatly enlarged liver and spleen. The sand fly, *Phlebotomus,* is believed to transmit the infection from one person to another. Picture A shows *Balantidium coli,* the causative agent of an infection of the large intestine similar to amebic dysentery. Picture B represents *Endamoeba hystolitica,* which is involved with the pathogenesis of amebic dysentery. Both *B. coli* and *E. hystolytica* are spread by contaminated water. Picture D depicts the trophozoite and schizont found in human erythrocytes infected with the malaria parasite, *Plasmodium malariae.* This parasite is transmitted to humans by bites of the anophelene mosquitos. *(Jawetz et al, pp 336,338,344,346,348)*

282. (C) α_2-receptors are located primarily on prejunctional membranes, where they modulate the release of norepinephrine. Activation of these receptors inhibits release of the neurotransmitter. *(Smith and Reynard, p 147)*

283. (C) A high level of stress has been associated with help-seeking behavior, with or without new onset of symptoms. Hispanics were less likely to seek medical help than English-speaking populations in one study. The upper socioeconomic class is associated with medical help-seeking behavior rather than the lower socioeconomic class. *(Leigh and Reiser, pp 3–15)*

284. **(B)** The cranial portion of the parasympathetic system is associated with four cranial nerves: the oculomotor, facial, glossopharyngeal, and vagus. These nerves supply parasympathetic innervation to the head and thoracic and most of the abdominal viscera. The lower abdominal and pelvic viscera receives its parasympathetic innervation from sacral spinal cord segments. The body wall and the extremities do not have a parasympathetic innervation. *(Noback, p 324)*

285. **(C)** Injuries affecting upper cervical segments (above C_3) usually quickly cause death from loss of respiratory muscle function. However, a transsection of the spinal cord between C_8 and T_1 only severs neural connections between the brain stem and some of the muscles involved in respiration (e.g., intercostal and abdominal muscles) while sparing connections to the diaphragm [phrenic nerves come off spinal neurons in segments C_3-C_5 ("C-three, four, and five keep the diaphragm alive")]. In this tetraplegic patient there is essentially complete loss of expiratory muscle function, but only modest loss of inspiratory action (the diaphragm is the major muscle of inspiration). Normal quiet expiration is passive. However, forced expiration, as in the latter part of vital capacity measurement, requires active participation by expiratory muscles. In this patient, you might expect a vital capacity that is at best only about 50 percent of normal. By definition, functional residual capacity (FRC) is the volume at which the respiratory system stays when all respiratory muscles are inactive. On the other hand, residual volume (RV) is the volume left after maximal expiratory effort (involves intercostal and abdominal muscles). RV is normally about one liter less than FRC. Since this patient has no expiratory muscle function, there cannot be a RV less than FRC. That is, in this patient, FRC = RV. *(Berne and Levy, pp 553–554)*

286. **(C)** The immediate source of carbon atoms for fatty acid synthesis is acetyl-CoA. Thus, any precursor of acetyl-CoA can be a source of carbon atoms for fatty acid synthesis. Glucose and other carbohydrates that are converted to glycolytic intermediates can contribute carbon atoms to acetyl-CoA. Likewise, ketogenic amino acids, such as leucine and phenylalanine, derived of protein degradation, can provide carbon atoms to acetyl-CoA. Citrate is the major carrier of mitochondrial acetyl-CoA carbons to the cytosol for fatty acid synthesis, since acetyl-CoA itself cannot move across the inner mitochondrial membrane. After diffusion into the cytosol, citrate is cleaved into acetyl-CoA and oxaloacetate by the enzyme citrate lyase. Cholesterol and other steroids cannot be degraded. They are converted to bile salts and excreted. Thus, although acetyl-CoA is a precursor of cholesterol, once incorporated, the carbon atoms of cholesterol are unavailable for biosynthesis of other compounds. *(Stryer, pp 480–481,503,559)*

287. **(B)** When both lactose and glucose are present in the environment, very little lac mRNA is transcribed because cAMP levels are low. Growing in the presence of glucose and lactose (the less preferred carbon and energy source), enteric bacteria cannot induce the synthesis of enzymes that are required for the degradation of lactose until glucose is metabolized completely. Then a large increase in the cyclic adenosine monophosphate (cAMP) is observed, and the bacteria now initiate transcription of the genes involved in the metabolism of lactose; that is, the lac operon. The increased synthesis of cAMP raises the level of cAMP and the regulatory protein catabolite gene activator protein (CAP) complex. Now, the cAMP-CAP complex can bind to the promoter of the lac operon and initiate transcription of lac messenger ribonucleic acid (mRNA). None of the other statements can explain why, when lactose and glucose are present in the environment, very little lac mRNA is transcribed. *(Joklik et al, pp 115–117)*

288. **(B)** There are three major patterns of rejection of a tissue transplant: hyperacute, acute, and chronic rejection. With the kidney as the example, hyperacute rejection occurs within minutes after the transplantation. Acute rejection manifests itself as sudden deterioration of renal function within days or months to years following transplantation. Two histologic types of acute renal rejection are recognized and may overlap in any given patient. Acute cellular rejection demonstrates an interstitial mononuclear cell infiltrate and edema with mild interstitial hemorrhage. Focal tubular necrosis due to mononuclear cell infiltration may occur. In the absence of an arteritis, this type of rejection responds to immunosuppressive therapy. Acute humoral rejection or rejection vasculitis produces a necrotizing arteritis with endothelial necrosis, neutrophilic infiltration, deposition of immunoglobulin, complement, and fibrin, and thrombosis. This leads to severe glomerular and cortical damage that fails to respond to immunosuppressive therapy. Chronic rejection is a progressive dysfunction of the kidney with gradual increase in serum creatinine levels during a 4- to 6-month period. *(Cotran, pp 183–188)*

289. **(B)** Many H_1 antagonists have significant atropine-like effects related to blockade of muscarinic receptors. These effects include sedation, antiparkinson effects, and decreased rhinorrhea. Some antihistamines, such as diphenhydramine, are, in fact, utilized specifically for their anticholinergic properties. *(Katzung, pp 233–234)*

290. **(E)** An informed consent to a surgical procedure, drugs, or research involves the subject or patient knowing what the proposed procedure is, that he/she may withdraw the consent, knowing what the risks and benefits are, and what the potential alternatives are. *(Kaplan and Sadock, pp 1317–1318)*

291. **(D)** The hypothalamus functions primarily in homeostasis. The cerebellum is the great coordinator of muscle action. The thalamus is the final processing station where ascending influences are organized before being transmitted to the cerebral cortex. The basal ganglia integrate motor activity. The reticular system is associated with attentiveness, awareness, and alertness. *(Noback, pp 233,281,351,361,376)*

292. **(B)** Exercise training results in an increase in the maximal cardiac output, which, in turn, permits greater aerobic capacity of muscles and an increase in the maximal oxygen consumption ($\dot{V}_{O_2max}$). The increase in maximal cardiac output depends to a large extent on a larger stroke volume than was possible before training. Even at rest the stroke volume is higher and permits a lower heart rate for a given level of resting cardiac output. One of the influences decreasing the heart rate is a decrease in sympathetic tone to the heart (probably a greater influence is an increase in parasympathetic tone to the heart). This reflects a general lowering of sympathetic activity in the trained individual both at rest and during submaximal exercise. *(Berne and Levy, 1993, p 536; McArdle et al, pp 283,329,330,333,336,409)*

293. **(E)** Both prokaryotic and eukaryotic DNA are replicated in a semiconservative manner. However, there are many differences between the two kinds of DNA. Bacterial DNA is usually circular, whereas eukaryotic nuclear DNA is linear. The latter is arranged in chromosomes composed of molecules usually 100 times as large as bacterial DNA. In addition, chromosomes contain histone-DNA complexes, a structural arrangement not found in bacteria. *(Stryer, pp 79–84)*

294. **(C)** Hairy cell leukemia is malignant proliferation of B-cell lymphocytes. The disease is most commonly seen in middle-aged and elderly males. Splenomegaly and pancytopenia are usually clinical findings. The hairy cell present in peripheral blood smears shows distinctive thin multiple cytoplasmic projections that resemble hairs. These malignant cells also demonstrate tartate resistant acid phosphatase activity. Hemorrhage and recurrent infections characterize the late stages of the disorder. Some prolongation of survival is achieved by interferon therapy. *(Rubin and Farber, pp 1088–1089)*

295. **(A)** The lesion shown in the question is multiple emboli in the lung, occluding arteries. Pulmonary emboli are a frequent complication of bed rest and are seen in debilitated elderly people. They originate in deep leg veins from thrombi that are disloged and sent into the peripheral circulation via the inferior vena cava, where they obstruct the pulmonary arterial circulation. They may cause pulmonary hemorrhage or infarction, depending on the amount of collateral blood supply. If they are large and obstruct major blood vessels, they may cause sudden death by interrupting cardiac output. If the emboli are multiple, over time they may lead to chronic pulmonary damage and fibrosis, with pulmonary hypertension and right-sided heart failure. *(Rubin and Farber, pp 265–268)*

296. **(E)** Acetazolamide is a potent, reversible inhibitor of carbonic anhydrase, the administration of which results in increased urinary excretion of bicarbonate and sodium ions. Other diuretics, such as furosemide and thiazides, can also inhibit this enzyme; however, it is not their primary mechanism of action. Acetazolamide is frequently used in combination with other diuretics to prevent the development of tolerance. *(Gilman et al, p 716)*

297. **(E)** The physiological arousal associated with anxiety includes increased sympathetic tone. Stimulation of locus ceruleus, which supplies a large portion of noradrenergic neurons to the CNS, is associated with anxiety. The relationship between performance and anxiety seems to be an inverted U curve, so that optimum performance requires a certain degree of anxiety. *(Leigh and Reiser, pp 41–78)*

298. **(B)** Wernicke's, or receptive aphasia, results from a lesion of Wernicke's area. Although hearing and vision are normal, individuals with this disability show an essentially total failure to comprehend either the spoken and/or the written language. Their speech is fluent but meaningless. Their conversations sound normal but are actually devoid of content and full of nonexistent words. *(Noback, p 408)*

299. **(B)** Perhaps as much as 30 percent of fat digestion occurs within the stomach, due to the presence of an acid lipase primarily of gastric origin (gastric lipase). Only after food moves into the small intestine does it mix with the bile salts and lecithin, which together act as effective emulsifying detergents. Reduction of fat into small, emulsified droplets greatly increases surface area available for enzymatic activity in the intestine (primarily pancreatic lipase). The products of pancreatic lipase action (fatty acids and 2-monoglycerides) are incorporated into mixed micelles (also called biliary micelles). These mixed micelles are almost three orders of magnitude smaller than emulsified droplets and serve to solubilize otherwise very water-insoluble lipid products. *(Berne and Levy, pp 709–711)*

300. **(C)** The hypoxemia caused by the oxygen-poor gas mixture breathed resulted in hyperventilation (from stimulation of peripheral chemoreceptors) which, in turn, caused hypocapnia and acute respiratory alkalosis. In simple, acute respiratory alkalosis, one should expect about a 2 mEq/L decrease in plasma bicarbonate for each 10 mm Hg decrease in $PaCO_2$ (secondary to buffer reactions). The plasma bicarbonate found (21 mEq/L) is 3 mEq/L less than normal, just what you would expect for a 15 mm Hg drop in $PaCO_2$ from 40 to 25 mm Hg. Severe chronic lung disease would have resulted in a partially-compensated respiratory acidosis with greater than normal $PaCO_2$ and bicarbonate. High altitude can produce a respiratory alkalosis, but after two weeks renal compensation would have brought the blood pH nearer to normal by decreasing plasma bicarbonate much more below normal (would be called a chronic respiratory alkalosis). Heroin overdose would have caused respiratory depression with hypoxemia but with hypercapnia. An acute overdose with salicylates could produce acute respiratory alkalosis, but would not cause hypoxemia. *(Rose, pp 469–473)*

301. **(E)** Immunological responses depend primarily upon T and B cells, which are the products of differentiation of stem cells. Differentiation of stem cells into T and B cells occurs during the passage of stem cells through the thymus. It is the T cells that have the glycoproteins known as CD_3, CD_4, and CD_8 on their surface. Stem cells lack CD_3, CD_4, or CD_8 on their surface. There is no such molecule as CD_{12} on stem cells, or T lymphocytes. *(Levinson and Jawetz, p 277)*

302. **(D)** The process described as apoptosis is one that for many years was largely overlooked but has now become well recognized as a major form of individual cell deletion in which the nuclear material shrinks within the cell cytoplasm and the cytoplasm shrinks around it, forming small dense bodies. Such bodies are often phagocytosed and removed without disruption of the cell as classically seen in other forms of necrosis. It is clear that this type of cell deletion may occur in people in the normal aging process and in certain types of so-called atrophic processes in the body, including such structures as the endometrium. It is, therefore, a normal regulatory and aging process and distinctly different from the other forms of cell death and necrosis. *(Rubin and Farber, p 15)*

303. **(D)** Propranolol can induce significant hypotension and exacerbate heart failure in patients not also administered cardiotonic and/or diuretic drugs. Beta-adrenergic blockade can also produce AV block when given in combination with digitalis glycosides. *(Gilman et al, p 866)*

304. **(B)** Identified cases are studied in this technique and compared to a control group without the disease or syndrome. This technique is useful for very rare disorders, or for exploratory studies of possible risk factors. *(Kaplan and Sadock, pp 308–326)*

305. **(A)** CD_8 lymphocytes are considered cytotoxic for virus infected cells, allograft, or tumor cells. Therefore, a person who lacks CD_8 T lymphocytes will show a deficiency in cytotoxicity for virus infected cells, tumor, or allograft cells. Another property of CD_8 T lymphocytes is the suppression of antibody by B cells and the reduction of delayed hypersensitivity reactions. Thus, a person who lacks CD_8 T lymphocytes cannot be expected to display functions of CD_8 T lymphocytes that he does not possess. *(Levinson and Jawetz, p 279)*

306. **(A)** The time interval 0–6 hours is called the eclipse period. During this period of viral growth cycle, the virus is absorbed to the host cell, enters the host cell, and the viral nucleic acid is separated from its capsid. These events lead to loss of viral infectivity. The bacterial growth curve is a bell-shaped curve composed of the lag phase in which the cell population is constant, the logarithmic phase of growth in which the number of cells increase in a geometric fashion (1–2–4–8–16, etc.), the stationary phase in which the cell population remains constant, and the phase of decline in which the cells die in an exponential fashion. The time period 6–8 hours represents a portion of the rise period, which marks the appearance of mature virus. The late period, according to the figure, begins at the 4th hour and ends at the 6th hour. During this time period viral nucleic acids and capsid proteins (proteins surrounding and protecting the nucleic acid) are synthesized and assembled into mature virus. *(Joklik et al, pp 790–795)*

307. **(D)** Living cells must respond to their changing environment in order to survive. This means that not all genes and not all gene products are active at the same time. Thus, gene expression is closely regulated. The expression of genes that control utilization of lactose, known as the lactose operon, is an example of gene regulation. The lactose operon is responsible for the synthesis of β-galactosidase, which cleaves lactose into glucose and galactose; lactose permease, which transports lactose into the cell; and β-galactose transacetylase, the function of which is unknown. The lactose operon is inducible. That is, synthesis of the above indicated enzymes occurs only when lactose is present. The operon is controlled by the lacI gene product, which acts as the repressor. *(Joklik et al, pp 114–123)*

308. **(C)** The ductus deferens is the continuation of the duct of the epididymis and ends by joining the duct of the seminal vesicle to form the ejaculatory duct. The ductus deferens ascends in the spermatic cord, passes through the inguinal canal, and crosses over the external iliac vessels to enter the pelvis minor. It crosses the ureter near the posterolateral angle of the bladder. *(Moore, p 179)*

309. **(E)** Honeycomb lung, or diffuse interstitial fibrosis, is a general term for pulmonary fibrosis, which is secondary to many environmental and occupational hazards. It is characterized by diffuse obliteration of the alveolar septa with fibrosis and thickening, bronchiolar dilatation, cyst formation, and squamous metaplasia. Alveolar capillary block leads to dyspnea, tachycardia, cyanosis, and right heart failure. The causes are numerous, including environmental factors, such as silica, *T. polyspora* (farmer's lung), talc, synthetic fibers, beryllium, asbestos, coal dust (anthrocosis), nitrogen dioxide (silo-filler's disease), and flax (byssinosis); connective tissue diseases, such as rheumatoid arthritis, systemic lupus erythematosus, scleroderma, and sarcoidosis; drugs, such as bulsulfan and bleomycin; oxygen; and idiopathic etiologies. *(Kissane, pp 969–981,996–1005)*

310. **(A)** The primary effect of nitroglycerin is the vasodilation of large veins, which leads to a decrease in ventricular preload, arterial pressure, and, ultimately, a decrease in oxygen demand. Nitrates, to a lesser degree, also increase oxygen supply to the heart by selectively dilating large coronary blood vessels. Indirectly, nitroglycerin may, through the baroreceptor reflex, increase sympathetic tone. *(Katzung, p 166)*

311. **(C)** Being in day care for 8 hours a day throughout infancy did not result in any appreciable deficits in cognition or behavior. However, there is an abundance of animal literature that shows that specific deprivations in early life have long-term consequences. *(Kaplan and Sadock, pp 283–299)*

BIBLIOGRAPHY

Anatomy

Hollinshead WH. *Textbook of Anatomy*. 4th ed. Philadelphia: Harper & Row; 1985

Moore KL. *Clinically Oriented Anatomy*. 3rd ed. Baltimore, Md: Williams & Williams; 1992

NoBack CR, Strominger NL, Demarest RJ. *The Human Nervous System*. 4th ed. Philadelphia: Lea & Febiger; 1991

Sadler TW. *Langman's Medical Embryology*. 6th ed. Baltimore, Md: Williams & Wilkins; 1990

Woodburne RT, Burckel WE. *Essentials of Human Anatomy*. 8th ed. New York: Oxford University Press; 1988

Physiology

Berne RM, Levy MN, eds. *Physiology*. 3rd ed. St. Louis: Mosby Year Book; 1993

Davenport HW. *A Digest of Digestion*. 2nd ed. Chicago: Year Book Medical Publishers, Inc.; 1978

Ganong WF. *Review of Medical Physiology*. 14th ed. Los Altos, Calif: Lange Medical Publications; 1989

Guyton AC. *Textbook of Medical Physiology*. 8th ed. Philadelphia: WB Saunders Co.; 1991

Johnson LR. *Gastrointestinal Physiology*. 3rd ed. St. Louis: CV Mosby Co.; 1985

McArdle WD, Katch FI, Katch VL. *Exercise Physiology*. 3rd ed. Philadelphia: Lea & Febiger; 1991

Mountcastle VB. *Medical Physiology*. 14th ed. St. Louis: CV Mosby Co.; 1980

Patton HD, Fuchs AF, et al. *Textbook of Physiology*. 21st ed. Philadelphia: WB Saunders Co.; 1989

Petersen OH, Maruyama Y. Calcium-activated potassium channels and their role in secretion. *Nature*. February 1984; 693–696

Rose DB. *Clinical Physiology of Acid-Base and Electrolyte Disorders*. 3rd ed. New York: McGraw-Hill Information Services Co.; 1989

Vander AJ. *Renal Physiology*. 4th ed. New York: McGraw-Hill Inc.; 1991

Biochemistry

Lehninger AL. *Biochemistry*. 2nd ed. New York: Worth Publishers, Inc.; 1977

Stryer L. *Biochemistry*. 3rd ed. San Francisco: WH Freeman and Co.; 1988

Microbiology

Joklik WK, Willett HP, Amos DB, Wilfert CM. *Zinsser Microbiology*. 20th ed. Norwalk, Conn: Appleton & Lange; 1992

Jawetz E, Melnick JL, Adelberg EA, et al. *Review of Medical Microbiology*. 19th ed. Norwalk, Conn: Appleton & Lange; 1991

Levinson WE, Jawetz E. *Medical Microbiology and Immunology*. 2nd ed. Norwalk, Conn: Appleton & Lange; 1992

Pathology

Cotran RS, Kumar V, Robbins SL. *Robbins Pathologic Basis of Disease.* 4th ed. Philadelphia: WB Saunders Co.; 1989

Hutt MSR, Burkitt DP. *The Geography of Non-Infectious Disease.* Oxford: Oxford UP; 1986

Kissane JM. *Anderson's Pathology.* 9th ed. St. Louis: CV Mosby Co.; 1990

Rubin E, Farber JL. *Pathology.* Philadelphia: JB Lippincott Co.; 1988

Pharmacology

Craig CR, Stitzel RE, eds. *Modern Pharmacology.* 3rd ed. Boston: Little, Brown and Co.; 1990

Gilman AG, Goodman RW, Nies AS, Taylor P, eds. *The Pharmacological Basis of Therapeutics.* 8th ed. New York: Pergamon; 1990

Katzung BG, ed. *Basic & Clinical Pharmacology.* 5th ed. Norwalk, Conn.: Appleton & Lange; 1992

Lewis JH, Zimmerman HJ, Ishak KG, Mullick FG. Enflurance hepatotoxicity: A clinicopathologic study of 24 cases. *Ann Intern Med.* June 1983; 984–992

Lindeman RD, Papper S. Therapy of fluid and electrolyte disorders. *Ann Intern Med.* January 1975; 64–70

Smith CM, Reynard AM, eds. *Textbook of Pharmacology.* Philadelphia: Saunders; 1992

Behavioral Sciences

American Psychiatric Association. *Diagnostic and Statistical Manual of Mental Disorders.* 3rd ed. rev. (DSM-III-R). Washington, DC: American Psychiatric Association; 1987

Balis GU, ed. *The Behavioral and Social Sciences and the Practice of Medicine.* Vol. II. *The Psychiatric Foun-*

dations of Medicine. Stoneham, Mass: Butterworth Publishers, Inc.; 1978

Erikson EH. *Identity and the Life Cycle.* Vol. I. *Psychological Issues.* New York: International Universities Press; 1959

Hine FR, Carson RC, Maddox GL, Thompson RJ, Williams RB. *Introduction to Behavioral Science in Medicine.* New York: Springer-Verlag New York, Inc.; 1983

Kaplan HI, Sadock BJ, eds. *Comprehensive Textbook of Psychiatry.* 5th ed. Baltimore: Williams & Wilkins Co.; 1989

Leigh H, Reiser MF. *The Patient. Biological, Psychological, and Social Dimensions of Medical Practice.* 3rd ed. New York: Plenum Publishing Corp.; 1992

Lennenberg EH. *Biological Foundations of Language.* New York: John Wiley & Sons, Inc.; 1967

Lindemann E. Symptomatology and management of acute grief. *Am J Psychiatry.* May 1944; 141–148

MacMahon B, Pugh T. *Epidemiology, Principles and Methods.* Boston: Little, Brown & Co.; 1970

Mechanic D. Social psychologic factors affecting the presentation of bodily complaints. *N Engl J Med.* May 5, 1972; 1132–1139

Rutter M, Tizard J, Whitmore K. *Education, Health, and Behavior.* London: Longman Group, Ltd; 1970

Scheiber SC, Doyle BB. *The Impaired Physician.* New York: Plenum Publishing Co.; 1983

Simons RC, ed. *Understanding Human Behavior in Health and Illness.* 3rd ed. Baltimore: Williams & Wilkins Co.; 1985

Practice Test Subspecialty List

ANATOMY

1. Central nervous system
4. Peripheral nervous system
7. Special sensory
11. Cardiovascular system
15. Cardiovascular system
20. Muscular system
25. Muscular system
32. Muscular system
39. Digestive system
46. Digestive system
53. Peripheral nervous system
60. Peripheral nervous system
67. Central nervous system
74. Central nervous system
81. Central nervous system
88. Central nervous system
95. Central nervous system
102. Muscular system
109. Cardiovascular system
116. Cardiovascular system
123. Cardiovascular system
130. Muscular system
137. Male reproductive system
195. Peripheral nervous system
196. Autonomic nervous system
197. Peripheral nervous system
207. Embryology—Special sensor
208. Muscular system
209. Embryology—Endocrine
210. Embryology—Special sensor
211. Embryology—Respiratory
212. Embryology—Special sensor
213. Embryology—Muscular
214. Embryology—Muscular
215. Embryology—Lymphatic
216. Embryology—Digestive system
245. Female reproductive system
251. Reproductive system
257. Muscular system
260. Embryology
261. Digestive system
263. Special sensory—Ear
270. Central nervous system

272. Cardiovascular system
273. Muscular system
277. Peripheral nervous system
284. Autonomic nervous system
291. Nervous system
298. Nervous system
308. Male reproductive system

PHYSIOLOGY

10. Cardiovascular regulation
12. Cardiovascular regulation
16. Cardiovascular regulation
21. Cardiac electrophysiology
26. Cardiac electrophysiology
33. Endocrinology
40. Gastrointestinal
47. Endocrinology
54. Endocrinology
61. Endocrinology
68. Endocrinology
75. Endocrinology
82. Endocrinology
89. Endocrinology
96. Endocrinology
103. Nervous system
110. Circulation in specific organs
117. Circulation in specific organs
124. Circulation in specific organs
131. Hemodynamics
138. Cardiac cycle
144. Endocrinology
145. Endocrinology
146. Endocrinology
147. Endocrinology
166. Cardiac electrophysiology
167. Cardiac electrophysiology
168. Cardiac electrophysiology
198. Muscle/Membrane
199. Muscle/Membrane
224. Nervous system
225. Nervous system
226. Nervous system
246. Gastrointestinal

252. Renal
258. Gastrointestinal
264. Respiratory
271. Cardiovascular regulation
278. Respiratory
285. Respiratory/Nervous system
292. Cardiovascular regulation
299. Gastrointestinal
300. Respiratory

BIOCHEMISTRY

2. Lipids
5. Vitamins
8. pH
13. Nutrition
17. Amino acids
22. Amino acids
27. Amino acids
34. Protein
41. Protein
48. Protein
55. Blood
62. Blood
69. Blood
76. Small molecule metabolism
83. Small molecule metabolism
90. Carbohydrate metabolism
97. Carbohydrate metabolism
104. Enzymes
111. Molecular biology
118. Molecular biology
125. Enzymes
132. Lipids
139. Integration of metabolism
148. Enzymes
149. Enzymes
150. Enzymes
169. Molecular biology
170. Molecular biology
171. Molecular biology
172. Enzymes
173. Enzymes
174. Enzymes
200. Carbohydrates
201. Carbohydrates
202. Carbohydrates
235. Amino acids
237. Protein
241. Integration of metabolism
247. Small molecule metabolism
253. Carbohydrate metabolism
259. Blood
265. Molecular biology
279. Lipids
286. Lipids
293. Molecular biology

MICROBIOLOGY

28. Immune response
35. Immune response
42. Physiology
49. Pathogenic bacteriology
56. Virology
63. Virology
70. Virology
77. Immune deficiency disease
84. Physiology
91. Antigen-antibody reaction serology
98. Antigen-antibody reaction serology
105. Immunology transplantation
112. Immunology transplantation
119. Immune response
126. Immune response
133. Mycology
140. Pathogenic bacteriology
233. Virology
234. Virology
236. Virology
238. Virology
242. Virology
248. Virology
254. Cellular immunology
266. Physiology
280. Parasitology
281. Parasitology
287. Physiology
301. Cellular immunology
305. Immune response
306. Viral growth
307. Physiology

PATHOLOGY

3. Endocrine system
6. Respiratory system
9. Respiratory system
14. Miscellaneous
18. Cardiovascular system
23. Kidney and urinary system
29. Circulatory system
36. Processes of neoplasia
43. Endocrine system
50. Blood and lymphatic system
57. Kidney and urinary system
64. Genetic syndromes and metabolic diseases
71. Cardiovascular system
78. Inflammation
85. Genetic syndromes and metabolic diseases
92. Miscellaneous
99. Genital system
106. Processes of neoplasia
113. Circulatory system
120. Processes of neoplasia
127. Inflammation

134. Circulatory system
141. Inflammation
151. Processes of neoplasia
152. Processes of neoplasia
153. Processes of neoplasia
162. Immunologic diseases
163. Immunologic diseases
164. Immunologic diseases
165. Immunologic diseases
175. Genetic syndromes and metabolic diseases
176. Genetic syndromes and metabolic diseases
177. Genetic syndromes and metabolic diseases
178. Genetic syndromes and metabolic diseases
205. Central nervous system
206. Central nervous system
227. Blood and lymphatic system
228. Blood and lymphatic system
229. Infectious diseases
230. Infectious diseases
231. Infectious diseases
232. Infectious diseases
239. Digestive system
243. Processes of neoplasia
249. Cardiovascular system
255. Cell growth, injury and repair
267. Immunologic diseases
274. Cell growth, injury and repair
288. Kidney and urinary system
294. Blood and lymphatic system
295. Respiratory system
302. Cell growth, injury, and repair
309. Respiratory system

PHARMACOLOGY

30. Central and peripheral nervous system
37. Endocrine system
44. Poisoning and therapy of intoxication
51. Central and peripheral nervous system
58. Antibiotics
65. General principles
72. Endocrine system
79. Blood and blood-forming organs
86. Cardiovascular and respiratory systems
93. Cardiovascular and respiratory systems
100. Autonomic nervous system
107. CNS drugs/Gas anesthetics
114. CNS drugs/Gas anesthetics
121. Kidneys, fluids, electrolytes
128. Central and peripheral nervous systems analgesics
135. Central and peripheral nervous systems psychotherapeutic agents
142. Hormone-like drugs/Oral hypoglycemics
154. Cardiovascular and respiratory systems/Antihypertensive agents
155. Cardiovascular and respiratory systems/Antihypertensive agents
156. Cardiovascular and respiratory systems/Antihypertensive agents

157. Cardiovascular and respiratory systems/Antihypertensive agents
179. Autonomic nervous system
180. Autonomic nervous system
181. Autonomic nervous system
182. Autonomic nervous system
183. Autonomic nervous system
184. Autonomic nervous system
190. Kidneys, fluids, electrolytes
191. Kidneys, fluids, electrolytes
192. Kidneys, fluids, electrolytes
193. Kidneys, fluids, electrolytes
194. Kidneys, fluids, electrolytes
203. Cardiovascular antihypertensive agents
204. Cardiovascular antihypertensive agents
268. Autonomic nervous system
275. Central and peripheral nervous systems
282. Autonomic nervous system
289. Autonomic nervous system
296. Kidneys, fluids, electrolytes
303. Cardiovascular and respiratory systems
310. Cardiovascular and respiratory systems

BEHAVIORAL SCIENCES

19. Personality/Psychodynamics
24. Medical sociology
31. Learning theory
38. Brain/Behavior
45. Emotions/Anxiety disorder/Psychopharmacology
52. Emotions/Genetics/Social epidemiology
59. Personality/Psychodynamics
66. Personality/Psychodynamics
73. Suicide/Epidemiology
80. Pain/Neurophysiology
87. Psychopharmacology
94. Suicide/Epidemiology
101. Sleep and dreaming
108. Doctor–patient relationship
115. Medical sociology
122. Grief/Depression
129. Patient management/Individual dynamics
136. Human sexuality
143. Epidemiology
158. Life cycle
159. Life cycle, personality, and psychodynamics
160. Life cycle, personality, and psychodynamics
161. Life cycle, personality, and psychodynamics
185. Life cycle/Psychodynamics
186. Life cycle/Psychodynamics
187. Life cycle/Psychodynamics
188. Life cycle/Psychodynamics
189. Life cycle/Psychodynamics
217. Learning theory
218. Learning theory
219. Learning theory
220. Learning theory
221. Learning theory
222. Learning theory

223. Learning theory
240. Suicide/Sociology/Depression
244. Depression
250. Depression/Grief emotions
256. Depression/Emotions
262. Personality/Psychodynamics
269. Personality/Psychodynamics

276. Medical sociology
283. Medical sociology
290. Ethics, norms, values, and beliefs
297. Emotions/Anxiety disorder/Learning theory
304. Epidemiology
311. Life cycle/Psychodynamics

NAME _____

ADDRESS _____
Street

_____
City   State   Zip

S O C	N U M B E R	⓪①②③④⑤⑥⑦⑧⑨
		⓪①②③④⑤⑥⑦⑧⑨
		⓪①②③④⑤⑥⑦⑧⑨
		⓪①②③④⑤⑥⑦⑧⑨
		⓪①②③④⑤⑥⑦⑧⑨
		⓪①②③④⑤⑥⑦⑧⑨
		⓪①②③④⑤⑥⑦⑧⑨
		⓪①②③④⑤⑥⑦⑧⑨
		⓪①②③④⑤⑥⑦⑧⑨

DIRECTIONS

MAKE ERASURES COMPLETE

Mark your social security number from top to bottom in the appropriate boxes on the right. Refer to the section " HOW TO TAKE THE PRACTICE TEST" in the introduction to the book for more information. PLEASE USE NO. 2 PENCIL ONLY.

1 Ⓐ Ⓑ Ⓒ Ⓓ Ⓔ   31 Ⓐ Ⓑ Ⓒ Ⓓ Ⓔ   61 Ⓐ Ⓑ Ⓒ Ⓓ Ⓔ   91 Ⓐ Ⓑ Ⓒ Ⓓ Ⓔ   121 Ⓐ Ⓑ Ⓒ Ⓓ Ⓔ
2 Ⓐ Ⓑ Ⓒ Ⓓ Ⓔ   32 Ⓐ Ⓑ Ⓒ Ⓓ Ⓔ   62 Ⓐ Ⓑ Ⓒ Ⓓ Ⓔ   92 Ⓐ Ⓑ Ⓒ Ⓓ Ⓔ   122 Ⓐ Ⓑ Ⓒ Ⓓ Ⓔ
3 Ⓐ Ⓑ Ⓒ Ⓓ Ⓔ   33 Ⓐ Ⓑ Ⓒ Ⓓ Ⓔ   63 Ⓐ Ⓑ Ⓒ Ⓓ Ⓔ   93 Ⓐ Ⓑ Ⓒ Ⓓ Ⓔ   123 Ⓐ Ⓑ Ⓒ Ⓓ Ⓔ
4 Ⓐ Ⓑ Ⓒ Ⓓ Ⓔ   34 Ⓐ Ⓑ Ⓒ Ⓓ Ⓔ   64 Ⓐ Ⓑ Ⓒ Ⓓ Ⓔ   94 Ⓐ Ⓑ Ⓒ Ⓓ Ⓔ   124 Ⓐ Ⓑ Ⓒ Ⓓ Ⓔ
5 Ⓐ Ⓑ Ⓒ Ⓓ Ⓔ   35 Ⓐ Ⓑ Ⓒ Ⓓ Ⓔ   65 Ⓐ Ⓑ Ⓒ Ⓓ Ⓔ   95 Ⓐ Ⓑ Ⓒ Ⓓ Ⓔ   125 Ⓐ Ⓑ Ⓒ Ⓓ Ⓔ
6 Ⓐ Ⓑ Ⓒ Ⓓ Ⓔ   36 Ⓐ Ⓑ Ⓒ Ⓓ Ⓔ   66 Ⓐ Ⓑ Ⓒ Ⓓ Ⓔ   96 Ⓐ Ⓑ Ⓒ Ⓓ Ⓔ   126 Ⓐ Ⓑ Ⓒ Ⓓ Ⓔ
7 Ⓐ Ⓑ Ⓒ Ⓓ Ⓔ   37 Ⓐ Ⓑ Ⓒ Ⓓ Ⓔ   67 Ⓐ Ⓑ Ⓒ Ⓓ Ⓔ   97 Ⓐ Ⓑ Ⓒ Ⓓ Ⓔ   127 Ⓐ Ⓑ Ⓒ Ⓓ Ⓔ
8 Ⓐ Ⓑ Ⓒ Ⓓ Ⓔ   38 Ⓐ Ⓑ Ⓒ Ⓓ Ⓔ   68 Ⓐ Ⓑ Ⓒ Ⓓ Ⓔ   98 Ⓐ Ⓑ Ⓒ Ⓓ Ⓔ   128 Ⓐ Ⓑ Ⓒ Ⓓ Ⓔ
9 Ⓐ Ⓑ Ⓒ Ⓓ Ⓔ   39 Ⓐ Ⓑ Ⓒ Ⓓ Ⓔ   69 Ⓐ Ⓑ Ⓒ Ⓓ Ⓔ   99 Ⓐ Ⓑ Ⓒ Ⓓ Ⓔ   129 Ⓐ Ⓑ Ⓒ Ⓓ Ⓔ
10 Ⓐ Ⓑ Ⓒ Ⓓ Ⓔ   40 Ⓐ Ⓑ Ⓒ Ⓓ Ⓔ   70 Ⓐ Ⓑ Ⓒ Ⓓ Ⓔ   100 Ⓐ Ⓑ Ⓒ Ⓓ Ⓔ   130 Ⓐ Ⓑ Ⓒ Ⓓ Ⓔ
11 Ⓐ Ⓑ Ⓒ Ⓓ Ⓔ   41 Ⓐ Ⓑ Ⓒ Ⓓ Ⓔ   71 Ⓐ Ⓑ Ⓒ Ⓓ Ⓔ   101 Ⓐ Ⓑ Ⓒ Ⓓ Ⓔ   131 Ⓐ Ⓑ Ⓒ Ⓓ Ⓔ
12 Ⓐ Ⓑ Ⓒ Ⓓ Ⓔ   42 Ⓐ Ⓑ Ⓒ Ⓓ Ⓔ   72 Ⓐ Ⓑ Ⓒ Ⓓ Ⓔ   102 Ⓐ Ⓑ Ⓒ Ⓓ Ⓔ   132 Ⓐ Ⓑ Ⓒ Ⓓ Ⓔ
13 Ⓐ Ⓑ Ⓒ Ⓓ Ⓔ   43 Ⓐ Ⓑ Ⓒ Ⓓ Ⓔ   73 Ⓐ Ⓑ Ⓒ Ⓓ Ⓔ   103 Ⓐ Ⓑ Ⓒ Ⓓ Ⓔ   133 Ⓐ Ⓑ Ⓒ Ⓓ Ⓕ
14 Ⓐ Ⓑ Ⓒ Ⓓ Ⓔ   44 Ⓐ Ⓑ Ⓒ Ⓓ Ⓔ   74 Ⓐ Ⓑ Ⓒ Ⓓ Ⓕ   104 Ⓐ Ⓑ Ⓒ Ⓒ   134 Ⓐ Ⓑ Ⓒ Ⓓ Ⓔ
15 Ⓐ Ⓑ Ⓒ Ⓓ Ⓔ   45 Ⓐ Ⓑ Ⓒ Ⓓ Ⓔ   75 Ⓐ Ⓑ Ⓒ Ⓓ Ⓔ   105 Ⓐ Ⓑ Ⓒ Ⓓ Ⓔ   135 Ⓐ Ⓑ Ⓒ Ⓓ Ⓔ
16 Ⓐ Ⓑ Ⓒ Ⓓ Ⓔ   46 Ⓐ Ⓑ Ⓒ Ⓓ Ⓔ   76 Ⓐ Ⓑ Ⓒ Ⓓ Ⓔ   106 Ⓐ Ⓑ Ⓒ Ⓓ Ⓔ   136 Ⓐ Ⓑ Ⓒ Ⓓ Ⓔ
17 Ⓐ Ⓑ Ⓒ Ⓓ Ⓔ   47 Ⓐ Ⓑ Ⓒ Ⓓ Ⓔ   77 Ⓐ Ⓑ Ⓒ Ⓓ Ⓔ   107 Ⓐ Ⓑ Ⓒ Ⓓ Ⓔ   137 Ⓐ Ⓑ Ⓒ Ⓓ Ⓔ
18 Ⓐ Ⓑ Ⓒ Ⓓ Ⓔ   48 Ⓐ Ⓑ Ⓒ Ⓓ Ⓔ   78 Ⓐ Ⓑ Ⓒ Ⓓ Ⓔ   108 Ⓐ Ⓑ Ⓒ Ⓓ Ⓔ   138 Ⓐ Ⓑ Ⓒ Ⓓ Ⓔ
19 Ⓐ Ⓑ Ⓒ Ⓓ Ⓔ   49 Ⓐ Ⓑ Ⓒ Ⓓ Ⓔ   79 Ⓐ Ⓑ Ⓒ Ⓓ Ⓔ   109 Ⓐ Ⓑ Ⓒ Ⓓ Ⓔ   139 Ⓐ Ⓑ Ⓒ Ⓓ Ⓔ
20 Ⓐ Ⓑ Ⓒ Ⓓ Ⓔ   50 Ⓐ Ⓑ Ⓒ Ⓓ Ⓔ   80 Ⓐ Ⓑ Ⓒ Ⓓ Ⓔ   110 Ⓐ Ⓑ Ⓒ Ⓓ Ⓔ   140 Ⓐ Ⓑ Ⓒ Ⓓ Ⓔ
21 Ⓐ Ⓑ Ⓒ Ⓓ Ⓔ   51 Ⓐ Ⓑ Ⓒ Ⓓ Ⓔ   81 Ⓐ Ⓑ Ⓒ Ⓓ Ⓔ   111 Ⓐ Ⓑ Ⓒ Ⓓ Ⓔ   141 Ⓐ Ⓑ Ⓒ Ⓓ Ⓔ
22 Ⓐ Ⓑ Ⓒ Ⓓ Ⓔ   52 Ⓐ Ⓑ Ⓒ Ⓓ Ⓔ   82 Ⓐ Ⓑ Ⓒ Ⓓ Ⓔ   112 Ⓐ Ⓑ Ⓒ Ⓓ Ⓔ   142 Ⓐ Ⓑ Ⓒ Ⓓ Ⓔ
23 Ⓐ Ⓑ Ⓒ Ⓓ Ⓔ   53 Ⓐ Ⓑ Ⓒ Ⓓ Ⓔ   83 Ⓐ Ⓑ Ⓒ Ⓓ Ⓔ   113 Ⓐ Ⓑ Ⓒ Ⓓ Ⓔ   143 Ⓐ Ⓑ Ⓒ Ⓓ Ⓔ
24 Ⓐ Ⓑ Ⓒ Ⓓ Ⓔ   54 Ⓐ Ⓑ Ⓒ Ⓓ Ⓔ   84 Ⓐ Ⓑ Ⓒ Ⓓ Ⓔ   114 Ⓐ Ⓑ Ⓒ Ⓓ Ⓔ   144 Ⓐ Ⓑ Ⓒ Ⓓ Ⓔ
25 Ⓐ Ⓑ Ⓒ Ⓓ Ⓔ   55 Ⓐ Ⓑ Ⓒ Ⓓ Ⓔ   85 Ⓐ Ⓑ Ⓒ Ⓓ Ⓔ   115 Ⓐ Ⓑ Ⓒ Ⓓ Ⓔ   145 Ⓐ Ⓑ Ⓒ Ⓓ Ⓔ
26 Ⓐ Ⓑ Ⓒ Ⓓ Ⓔ   56 Ⓐ Ⓑ Ⓒ Ⓓ Ⓔ   86 Ⓐ Ⓑ Ⓒ Ⓓ Ⓔ   116 Ⓐ Ⓑ Ⓒ Ⓓ Ⓔ   146 Ⓐ Ⓑ Ⓒ Ⓓ Ⓔ
27 Ⓐ Ⓑ Ⓒ Ⓓ Ⓔ   57 Ⓐ Ⓑ Ⓒ Ⓓ Ⓔ   87 Ⓐ Ⓑ Ⓒ Ⓓ Ⓔ   117 Ⓐ Ⓑ Ⓒ Ⓓ Ⓔ   147 Ⓐ Ⓑ Ⓒ Ⓓ Ⓔ
28 Ⓐ Ⓑ Ⓒ Ⓓ Ⓔ   58 Ⓐ Ⓑ Ⓒ Ⓓ Ⓔ   88 Ⓐ Ⓑ Ⓒ Ⓓ Ⓔ   118 Ⓐ Ⓑ Ⓒ Ⓓ Ⓔ   148 Ⓐ Ⓑ Ⓒ Ⓓ Ⓔ
29 Ⓐ Ⓑ Ⓒ Ⓓ Ⓔ   59 Ⓐ Ⓑ Ⓒ Ⓓ Ⓔ   89 Ⓐ Ⓑ Ⓒ Ⓓ Ⓔ   119 Ⓐ Ⓑ Ⓒ Ⓓ Ⓔ   149 Ⓐ Ⓑ Ⓒ Ⓓ Ⓔ
30 Ⓐ Ⓑ Ⓒ Ⓓ Ⓔ   60 Ⓐ Ⓑ Ⓒ Ⓓ Ⓔ   90 Ⓐ Ⓑ Ⓒ Ⓓ Ⓔ   120 Ⓐ Ⓑ Ⓒ Ⓓ Ⓔ   150 Ⓐ Ⓑ Ⓒ Ⓓ Ⓔ

151 Ⓐ Ⓑ Ⓒ Ⓓ Ⓔ
Ⓕ Ⓖ Ⓗ Ⓘ Ⓙ
152 Ⓐ Ⓑ Ⓒ Ⓓ Ⓔ
Ⓕ Ⓖ Ⓗ Ⓘ Ⓙ
153 Ⓐ Ⓑ Ⓒ Ⓓ Ⓔ
Ⓕ Ⓖ Ⓗ Ⓘ Ⓙ
154 Ⓐ Ⓑ Ⓒ Ⓓ Ⓔ
155 Ⓐ Ⓑ Ⓒ Ⓓ Ⓔ
156 Ⓐ Ⓑ Ⓒ Ⓓ Ⓔ
157 Ⓐ Ⓑ Ⓒ Ⓓ Ⓔ
158 Ⓐ Ⓑ Ⓒ Ⓓ Ⓔ Ⓕ Ⓖ Ⓗ
159 Ⓐ Ⓑ Ⓒ Ⓓ Ⓔ Ⓕ Ⓖ Ⓗ
160 Ⓐ Ⓑ Ⓒ Ⓓ Ⓔ Ⓕ Ⓖ Ⓗ
161 Ⓐ Ⓑ Ⓒ Ⓓ Ⓔ Ⓕ Ⓖ Ⓗ
162 Ⓐ Ⓑ Ⓒ Ⓓ Ⓔ
163 Ⓐ Ⓑ Ⓒ Ⓓ Ⓔ
164 Ⓐ Ⓑ Ⓒ Ⓓ Ⓔ
165 Ⓐ Ⓑ Ⓒ Ⓓ Ⓔ
166 Ⓐ Ⓑ Ⓒ Ⓓ Ⓔ
167 Ⓐ Ⓑ Ⓒ Ⓓ Ⓔ
168 Ⓐ Ⓑ Ⓒ Ⓓ Ⓔ
169 Ⓐ Ⓑ Ⓒ Ⓓ Ⓔ
170 Ⓐ Ⓑ Ⓒ Ⓓ Ⓔ
171 Ⓐ Ⓑ Ⓒ Ⓓ Ⓔ
172 Ⓐ Ⓑ Ⓒ Ⓓ Ⓔ
173 Ⓐ Ⓑ Ⓒ Ⓓ Ⓔ
174 Ⓐ Ⓑ Ⓒ Ⓓ Ⓔ
175 Ⓐ Ⓑ Ⓒ Ⓓ Ⓔ
176 Ⓐ Ⓑ Ⓒ Ⓓ Ⓔ
177 Ⓐ Ⓑ Ⓒ Ⓓ Ⓔ
178 Ⓐ Ⓑ Ⓒ Ⓓ Ⓔ
179 Ⓐ Ⓑ Ⓒ Ⓓ Ⓔ
180 Ⓐ Ⓑ Ⓒ Ⓓ Ⓔ
181 Ⓐ Ⓑ Ⓒ Ⓓ Ⓔ
182 Ⓐ Ⓑ Ⓒ Ⓓ Ⓔ
183 Ⓐ Ⓑ Ⓒ Ⓓ Ⓔ

184 Ⓐ Ⓑ Ⓒ Ⓓ Ⓔ
185 Ⓐ Ⓑ Ⓒ Ⓓ Ⓔ
186 Ⓐ Ⓑ Ⓒ Ⓓ Ⓔ
187 Ⓐ Ⓑ Ⓒ Ⓓ Ⓔ
188 Ⓐ Ⓑ Ⓒ Ⓓ Ⓔ
189 Ⓐ Ⓑ Ⓒ Ⓓ Ⓔ
190 Ⓐ Ⓑ Ⓒ Ⓓ Ⓔ
191 Ⓐ Ⓑ Ⓒ Ⓓ Ⓔ
192 Ⓐ Ⓑ Ⓒ Ⓓ Ⓔ
193 Ⓐ Ⓑ Ⓒ Ⓓ Ⓔ
194 Ⓐ Ⓑ Ⓒ Ⓓ Ⓔ
195 Ⓐ Ⓑ Ⓒ Ⓓ
196 Ⓐ Ⓑ Ⓒ Ⓓ
197 Ⓐ Ⓑ Ⓒ Ⓓ
198 Ⓐ Ⓑ Ⓒ Ⓓ Ⓔ
199 Ⓐ Ⓑ Ⓒ Ⓓ Ⓔ
200 Ⓐ Ⓑ Ⓒ Ⓓ Ⓔ
201 Ⓐ Ⓑ Ⓒ Ⓓ Ⓔ
202 Ⓐ Ⓑ Ⓒ Ⓓ Ⓔ
203 Ⓐ Ⓑ Ⓒ Ⓓ Ⓔ
204 Ⓐ Ⓑ Ⓒ Ⓓ Ⓔ
205 Ⓐ Ⓑ Ⓒ Ⓓ Ⓔ
206 Ⓐ Ⓑ Ⓒ Ⓓ Ⓔ
207 Ⓐ Ⓑ Ⓒ Ⓓ Ⓔ
Ⓕ Ⓖ Ⓗ Ⓘ
208 Ⓐ Ⓑ Ⓒ Ⓓ Ⓔ
Ⓕ Ⓖ Ⓗ Ⓘ
209 Ⓐ Ⓑ Ⓒ Ⓓ Ⓔ
Ⓕ Ⓖ Ⓗ Ⓘ
210 Ⓐ Ⓑ Ⓒ Ⓓ Ⓔ
Ⓕ Ⓖ Ⓗ Ⓘ
211 Ⓐ Ⓑ Ⓒ Ⓓ Ⓔ
Ⓕ Ⓖ Ⓗ Ⓘ
212 Ⓐ Ⓑ Ⓒ Ⓓ Ⓔ
Ⓕ Ⓖ Ⓗ Ⓘ
213 Ⓐ Ⓑ Ⓒ Ⓓ Ⓔ
Ⓕ Ⓖ Ⓗ Ⓘ

214 Ⓐ Ⓑ Ⓒ Ⓓ Ⓔ
Ⓕ Ⓖ Ⓗ Ⓘ
215 Ⓐ Ⓑ Ⓒ Ⓓ Ⓔ
Ⓕ Ⓖ Ⓗ Ⓘ
216 Ⓐ Ⓑ Ⓒ Ⓓ Ⓔ
Ⓕ Ⓖ Ⓗ Ⓘ
217 Ⓐ Ⓑ Ⓒ Ⓓ Ⓔ Ⓕ Ⓖ Ⓗ
218 Ⓐ Ⓑ Ⓒ Ⓓ Ⓔ Ⓕ Ⓖ Ⓗ
219 Ⓐ Ⓑ Ⓒ Ⓓ Ⓔ Ⓕ Ⓖ Ⓗ
220 Ⓐ Ⓑ Ⓒ Ⓓ Ⓔ Ⓕ Ⓖ Ⓗ
221 Ⓐ Ⓑ Ⓒ Ⓓ Ⓔ Ⓕ Ⓖ Ⓗ
222 Ⓐ Ⓑ Ⓒ Ⓓ Ⓔ Ⓕ Ⓖ Ⓗ
223 Ⓐ Ⓑ Ⓒ Ⓓ Ⓔ Ⓕ Ⓖ Ⓗ
224 Ⓐ Ⓑ Ⓒ Ⓓ Ⓔ Ⓕ Ⓖ
225 Ⓐ Ⓑ Ⓒ Ⓓ Ⓔ Ⓕ Ⓖ
226 Ⓐ Ⓑ Ⓒ Ⓓ Ⓔ Ⓕ Ⓖ
227 Ⓐ Ⓑ Ⓒ Ⓓ Ⓔ
228 Ⓐ Ⓑ Ⓒ Ⓓ Ⓔ
229 Ⓐ Ⓑ Ⓒ Ⓓ Ⓔ
230 Ⓐ Ⓑ Ⓒ Ⓓ Ⓔ
231 Ⓐ Ⓑ Ⓒ Ⓓ Ⓔ
232 Ⓐ Ⓑ Ⓒ Ⓓ Ⓔ
233 Ⓐ Ⓑ Ⓒ Ⓓ Ⓔ
234 Ⓐ Ⓑ Ⓒ Ⓓ Ⓔ
235 Ⓐ Ⓑ Ⓒ Ⓓ
236 Ⓐ Ⓑ Ⓒ Ⓓ Ⓔ
237 Ⓐ Ⓑ Ⓒ Ⓓ Ⓔ
238 Ⓐ Ⓑ Ⓒ Ⓓ Ⓔ
239 Ⓐ Ⓑ Ⓒ Ⓓ Ⓔ
240 Ⓐ Ⓑ Ⓒ Ⓓ Ⓔ
241 Ⓐ Ⓑ Ⓒ Ⓓ Ⓔ
242 Ⓐ Ⓑ Ⓒ Ⓓ Ⓔ
243 Ⓐ Ⓑ Ⓒ Ⓓ Ⓔ
244 Ⓐ Ⓑ Ⓒ Ⓓ Ⓔ
245 Ⓐ Ⓑ Ⓒ Ⓓ Ⓔ
246 Ⓐ Ⓑ Ⓒ Ⓓ Ⓔ

247 Ⓐ Ⓑ Ⓒ Ⓓ Ⓔ
248 Ⓐ Ⓑ Ⓒ Ⓓ Ⓔ
249 Ⓐ Ⓑ Ⓒ Ⓓ Ⓔ
250 Ⓐ Ⓑ Ⓒ Ⓓ Ⓔ
251 Ⓐ Ⓑ Ⓒ Ⓓ Ⓔ
252 Ⓐ Ⓑ Ⓒ Ⓓ Ⓔ
253 Ⓐ Ⓑ Ⓒ Ⓓ Ⓔ
254 Ⓐ Ⓑ Ⓒ Ⓓ Ⓔ
255 Ⓐ Ⓑ Ⓒ Ⓓ Ⓔ
256 Ⓐ Ⓑ Ⓒ Ⓓ Ⓔ
257 Ⓐ Ⓑ Ⓒ Ⓓ Ⓔ
258 Ⓐ Ⓑ Ⓒ Ⓓ Ⓔ
259 Ⓐ Ⓑ Ⓒ Ⓓ Ⓔ
260 Ⓐ Ⓑ Ⓒ Ⓓ Ⓔ
261 Ⓐ Ⓑ Ⓒ Ⓓ Ⓔ
262 Ⓐ Ⓑ Ⓒ Ⓓ Ⓔ
263 Ⓐ Ⓑ Ⓒ Ⓓ Ⓔ
264 Ⓐ Ⓑ Ⓒ Ⓓ Ⓔ
265 Ⓐ Ⓑ Ⓒ Ⓓ Ⓔ
266 Ⓐ Ⓑ Ⓒ Ⓓ Ⓔ
267 Ⓐ Ⓑ Ⓒ Ⓓ Ⓔ
268 Ⓐ Ⓑ Ⓒ Ⓓ Ⓔ
269 Ⓐ Ⓑ Ⓒ Ⓓ Ⓔ
270 Ⓐ Ⓑ Ⓒ Ⓓ Ⓔ
271 Ⓐ Ⓑ Ⓒ Ⓓ Ⓔ
272 Ⓐ Ⓑ Ⓒ Ⓓ Ⓔ
273 Ⓐ Ⓑ Ⓒ Ⓓ Ⓔ
274 Ⓐ Ⓑ Ⓒ Ⓓ Ⓔ
274 Ⓐ Ⓑ Ⓒ Ⓓ Ⓔ
276 Ⓐ Ⓑ Ⓒ Ⓓ Ⓔ
278 Ⓐ Ⓑ Ⓒ Ⓓ Ⓔ
279 Ⓐ Ⓑ Ⓒ Ⓓ Ⓔ
280 Ⓐ Ⓑ Ⓒ Ⓓ Ⓔ
281 Ⓐ Ⓑ Ⓒ Ⓓ Ⓔ
282 Ⓐ Ⓑ Ⓒ Ⓓ Ⓔ
283 Ⓐ Ⓑ Ⓒ Ⓓ Ⓔ

284 Ⓐ Ⓑ Ⓒ Ⓓ Ⓔ
285 Ⓐ Ⓑ Ⓒ Ⓓ Ⓔ
286 Ⓐ Ⓑ Ⓒ Ⓓ Ⓔ
287 Ⓐ Ⓑ Ⓒ Ⓓ Ⓔ
288 Ⓐ Ⓑ Ⓒ Ⓓ Ⓔ
289 Ⓐ Ⓑ Ⓒ Ⓓ Ⓔ
290 Ⓐ Ⓑ Ⓒ Ⓓ Ⓔ
291 Ⓐ Ⓑ Ⓒ Ⓓ Ⓔ
292 Ⓐ Ⓑ Ⓒ Ⓓ Ⓔ
293 Ⓐ Ⓑ Ⓒ Ⓓ Ⓔ
294 Ⓐ Ⓑ Ⓒ Ⓓ Ⓔ
295 Ⓐ Ⓑ Ⓒ Ⓓ Ⓔ
296 Ⓐ Ⓑ Ⓒ Ⓓ Ⓔ
297 Ⓐ Ⓑ Ⓒ Ⓓ Ⓔ
298 Ⓐ Ⓑ Ⓒ Ⓓ Ⓔ
299 Ⓐ Ⓑ Ⓒ Ⓓ Ⓔ
300 Ⓐ Ⓑ Ⓒ Ⓓ Ⓔ
301 Ⓐ Ⓑ Ⓒ Ⓓ Ⓔ
302 Ⓐ Ⓑ Ⓒ Ⓓ Ⓔ
303 Ⓐ Ⓑ Ⓒ Ⓓ Ⓔ
304 Ⓐ Ⓑ Ⓒ Ⓓ Ⓔ
305 Ⓐ Ⓑ Ⓒ Ⓓ Ⓔ
306 Ⓐ Ⓑ Ⓒ Ⓓ Ⓔ
307 Ⓐ Ⓑ Ⓒ Ⓓ Ⓔ
308 Ⓐ Ⓑ Ⓒ Ⓓ Ⓔ
309 Ⓐ Ⓑ Ⓒ Ⓓ Ⓔ
310 Ⓐ Ⓑ Ⓒ Ⓓ Ⓔ
311 Ⓐ Ⓑ Ⓒ Ⓓ Ⓔ